# MR Angiography: From Head to Toe

*Editors*

PRASHANT NAGPAL
THOMAS M. GRIST

MAGNETIC RESONANCE IMAGING CLINICS OF NORTH AMERICA

www.mri.theclinics.com

*Consulting Editors*
SURESH K. MUKHERJI
LYNNE S. STEINBACH

August 2023 • Volume 31 • Number 3

**ELSEVIER**

1600 John F. Kennedy Boulevard • Suite 1800 • Philadelphia, Pennsylvania, 19103-2899

http://www.mri.theclinics.com

**MAGNETIC RESONANCE IMAGING CLINICS OF NORTH AMERICA Volume 31, Number 3 August 2023 ISSN 1064-9689, ISBN 13: 978-0-323-93893-8**

Editor: John Vassallo (j.vassallo@elsevier.com)
Developmental Editor: Shivank Joshi



*Magnetic Resonance Imaging Clinics of North America* (ISSN 1064-9689) is published quarterly by Elsevier Inc., 360 Park Avenue South, New York, NY 10010-1710. Months of issue are February, May, August, and November. Business and Editorial Offices: 1600 John F. Kennedy Blvd., Ste. 1800, Philadelphia, PA 19103-2899. Customer Service Office: 3251 Riverport Lane, Maryland Heights, MO 63043. Periodicals postage paid at New York, NY and additional mailing offices. Subscription prices are $408.00 per year (domestic individuals), $783.00 per year (domestic institutions), $100.00 per year (domestic students/residents), $455.00 per year (Canadian individuals), $1021.00 per year (Canadian institutions), $573.00 per year (international individuals), $1021.00 per year (international institutions), $100.00 per year (Canadian students/residents), and $275.00 per year (international students/residents). International air speed delivery is included in all *Clinics* subscription prices. All prices are subject to change without notice. **POSTMASTER:** Send address changes to *Magnetic Resonance Imaging Clinics*, Elsevier Health Sciences Division, Subscription Customer Service, 3251 Riverport Lane, Maryland Heights, MO 63043. Customer Service (orders, claims, online, change of address): Elsevier Health Sciences Division, Subscription **Customer Service, 3251 Riverport Lane, Maryland Heights, MO 63043. Tel:1-800-654-2452 (U.S. and Canada); 314-447-8871 (outside U.S. and Canada). Fax: 314-447-8029. E-mail: journalscustomerservice-usa@elsevier.com (for print support); journalsonlinesupport-usa@elsevier.com (for online support).**

*Reprints*. For copies of 100 or more of articles in this publication, please contact the Commercial Reprints Department, Elsevier Inc., 360 Park Avenue South, New York, NY 10010-1710. Tel.: 212-633-3874; Fax: 212-633-3820; E-mail: reprints@elsevier.com.

*Magnetic Resonance Imaging Clinics of North America* is covered in the *RSNA Index of Imaging Literature, MEDLINE/PubMed (Index Medicus),* and *EMBASE/Excerpta Medica.*

# Contributors


## CONSULTING EDITORS

**SURESH K. MUKHERJI, MD, MBA, FACR**
Marian University, Head and Neck Radiology, ProScan Imaging, Carmel, Indiana, USA

**LYNNE S. STEINBACH, MD, FACR**
Emeritus Professor of Clinical Radiology on Recall, University of California, San Francisco, San Francisco, California, USA

## EDITORS

**PRASHANT NAGPAL, MD, FSCCT**
Section Chief, Cardiovascular Imaging, Cardiovascular and Thoracic Radiology, Associate Professor, Department of Radiology, University of Wisconsin-Madison School of Medicine and Public Health, Madison, Wisconsin, USA

**THOMAS M. GRIST, MD, FACR**
Department Chair, Radiology, John H. Juhl Professor of Radiology and Medical Physics, Department of Radiology, University of Wisconsin-Madison School of Medicine and Public Health, Madison, Wisconsin, USA

## AUTHORS

**JEANNE B. ACKMAN, MD**
Radiologist, Division of Thoracic Imaging and Intervention, Massachusetts General Hospital, Assistant Professor of Radiology, Harvard Medical School, Boston, Massachusetts, USA

**AYAZ AGHAYEV, MD**
Assistant Professor of Radiology, Harvard Medical School, Cardiovascular Imaging Program, Brigham and Women's Hospital, Boston, Massachusetts, USA

**BRADLEY D. ALLEN, MD, MS**
Assistant Professor, Chief of Cardiovascular and Thoracic Imaging, Department of Radiology, Northwestern University, Feinberg School of Medicine, Chicago, Illinois, USA

**LIISA L. BERGMANN, MD, MBA**
Assistant Professor of Radiology, Departments of Radiology and Medicine, University of Kentucky College of Medicine, Lexington, Kentucky, USA

**CANDICE A. BOOKWALTER, MD**
Department of Radiology, Mayo Clinic, Rochester, Minnesota, USA

**JAMES C. CARR, MD**
Professor, Chair, Department of Radiology, Northwestern University, Feinberg School of Medicine, Chicago, Illinois, USA

**ABHISHEK CHATURVEDI, MD, PhD**
Department of Radiology, University of Rochester Medical Center, Rochester, New York, USA

**RORY L. COCHRAN, MD, PhD**
Diagnostic Radiology Resident, Massachusetts General Hospital, Clinical Fellow in Radiology, Harvard Medical School, Boston, Massachusetts, USA

**JEREMY D. COLLINS, MD**
Department of Radiology, Mayo Clinic, Rochester, Minnesota, USA

**PHILIP A. CORRADO, PhD**
Research Scientist, Accuray Incorporated, Chapel Hill, North Carolina, USA

**MONA DABIRI, MD**
Radiology Department, Children's Medical Center, Tehran University of Medical Science, Tehran, Iran

**DAVID DUSHFUNIAN, MD**
Clinical Research Associate, Department of Radiology, Northwestern University, Feinberg School of Medicine, Chicago, Illinois, USA

**LAURA B. EISENMENGER, MD**
Department of Radiology, University of Wisconsin-Madison, Madison, Wisconsin, USA

**CHRISTOPHER J. FRANCOIS, MD**
Department of Radiology, Mayo Clinic, Rochester, Minnesota, USA

**ISHAN GARG, MD**
Department of Internal Medicine, University of New Mexico Health Sciences Center, Albuquerque, New Mexico, USA

**BRIAN B. GHOSHHAJRA, MD, MBA**
Division Chief of Cardiovascular Imaging, Department of Radiology, Massachusetts General Hospital, Associate Professor of Radiology, Harvard Medical School, Boston, Massachusetts, USA

**THOMAS M. GRIST, MD, FACR**
Department Chair, Radiology, John H. Juhl Professor of Radiology and Medical Physics, Department of Radiology, University of Wisconsin-Madison School of Medicine and Public Health, Madison, Wisconsin, USA

**SANDEEP S. HEDGIRE, MD**
Division of Cardiovascular Imaging, Department of Radiology, Massachusetts General Hospital, Assistant Professor of Radiology, Harvard Medical School, Boston, Massachusetts, USA

**KEVIN M. JOHNSON, PhD**
Associate Professor, Departments of Medical Physics and Radiology, University of Wisconsin-Madison, Wisconsin Institutes for Medical Research, Madison, Wisconsin, USA

**JACQUELINE C. JUNN, MD**
Icahn School of Medicine at Mount Sinai, New York, New York, USA

**TIM LEINER, MD, PhD**
Department of Radiology, Mayo Clinic, Rochester, Minnesota, USA

**MICHAEL MARKL, PhD**
Professor, Vice Chair for Research, Department of Radiology, Northwestern University, Feinberg School of Medicine, Chicago, Illinois, USA

**ANTHONY MAROUN, MD**
Clinical Research Associate, Department of Radiology, Northwestern University, Feinberg School of Medicine, Chicago, Illinois, USA

**JOSEPH SCOTT MCNALLY, MD, PhD**
Department of Radiology, University of Utah, Salt Lake City, Utah, USA

**ALEXANDER MOELLER, MD**
Resident Physician, Department of Radiology, University of Wisconsin-Madison School of Medicine and Public Health, Madison, Wisconsin, USA

**MAHMUD MOSSA-BASHA, MD**
Department of Radiology, University of Washington School of Medicine, Seattle, Washington, USA

**SCOTT K. NAGLE, MD, PhD**
Associate Professor, Department of Radiology, University of Wisconsin-Madison School of Medicine and Public Health, Madison, Wisconsin, USA

**PRASHANT NAGPAL, MD, FSCCT**
Section Chief, Cardiovascular Imaging, Cardiovascular and Thoracic Radiology, Associate Professor, Department of Radiology, University of Wisconsin-Madison School of Medicine and Public Health, Madison, Wisconsin, USA

**ANANYA PANDA, MBBS, MD, FRCR**
Department of Radiology, All India Institute of Medical Sciences, Jodhpur, India

**ANTHONY PERET, MD**
Department of Radiology, University of Wisconsin-Madison, Madison, Wisconsin, USA

**SANDRA QUINN, MD, PhD**
Clinical Research Associate, Department of Radiology, Northwestern University, Feinberg School of Medicine, Chicago, Illinois, USA

**PRABHAKAR SHANTHA RAJIAH, MBBS, MD, FRCR**
Department of Radiology, Mayo Clinic, Rochester, Minnesota, USA

**SCOTT REEDER, MD, PhD**
Professor of Radiology, Departments of Radiology, Medicine and Medical Physics, University of Wisconsin-Madison School of Medicine and Public Health, Madison, Wisconsin, USA

**GRANT S. ROBERTS, PhD**
Research Assistant, Department of Medical Physics, University of Wisconsin-Madison, Wisconsin Institutes for Medical Research, Madison, Wisconsin, USA

**ALEJANDRO ROLDÁN-ALZATE, PhD**
Associate Professor, Departments of Mechanical Engineering and Radiology, University of Wisconsin-Madison, Madison, Wisconsin, USA

**GRISELDA ROMERO-SANCHEZ, MD**
Department of Radiology, Instituto Nacional de Ciencias Medicas y Nutricion Salvador Zubiran, Mexico City, Mexico

**MARK L. SCHIEBLER, MD**
Professor, Department of Radiology, University of Wisconsin-Madison School of Medicine and Public Health, Madison, Wisconsin, USA

**JAE W. SONG, MD, MS**
University of Pennsylvania, Philadelphia, Pennsylvania, USA

**ALMA SPAHIC, MS**
University of Wisconsin-Madison, Madison, Wisconsin, USA

**JITKA STAREKOVA, MD**
Clinical Scientist, Department of Radiology, University of Wisconsin-Madison School of Medicine and Public Health, Madison, Wisconsin, USA

**MICHAEL STEIGNER, MD**
Associate Professor of Radiology, Harvard Medical School, Cardiovascular Imaging Program, Brigham and Women's Hospital, Boston, Massachusetts, USA

**ELIZABETH K. WEISS, BS**
MD/PhD Candidate, Department of Radiology, Northwestern University, Feinberg School of Medicine, Chicago, Illinois, USA

**OLIVER WIEBEN, PhD**
Professor, Vice Chair of Research, Departments of Medical Physics and Radiology, University of Wisconsin-Madison, Wisconsin Institutes for Medical Research, Madison, Wisconsin, USA

# Contents



Several non-contrast magnetic resonance angiography (MRA) techniques have been developed, providing an attractive alternative to contrast-enhanced MRA and a radiation-free alternative to computed tomography (CT) CT angiography. This review describes the physical principles, limitations, and clinical applications of bright-blood (BB) non-contrast MRA techniques. The principles of BB MRA techniques can be broadly divided into (a) flow-independent MRA, (b) blood-inflow-based MRA, (c) cardiac phase dependent, flow-based MRA, (d) velocity sensitive MRA, and (e) arterial spin-labeling MRA. The review also includes emerging multi-contrast MRA techniques that provide simultaneous BB and black-blood images for combined luminal and vessel wall evaluation.



Magnetic resonance angiography (MRA) is a powerful tool for assessing upper and lower extremity artery pathologies. In addition to the classic advantages of MRA, such as the absence of radiation and iodinated contrast exposure, it can provide high temporal resolution/dynamic images of the arteries with high soft tissue contrast. Although it has a relatively lower spatial resolution than computed tomography angiography, MRA does not cause blooming artifacts in heavily calcified vessels, which is crucial in small vessel assessment. Although contrast-enhanced MRA is the most preferred technique to assess extremity vascular pathologies, recent advances in non-contrast MRA protocols provide an alternative imaging technique for patients with chronic kidney disease.



Video content accompanies this article at http://www.mri.theclinics.com.

Aortic pathologic conditions represent diverse disorders, including aortic aneurysm, acute aortic syndrome, traumatic aortic injury, and atherosclerosis. Given the non-specific clinical features, noninvasive imaging is critical in screening, diagnosis, management, and posttherapeutic surveillance. Of the commonly used imaging modalities, including ultrasound, computed tomography, and MR imaging, the final choice often depends on a combination of factors: acuity of clinical presentation, suspected underlying diagnosis, and institutional practice. Further research is needed to identify the potential clinical role and define appropriate use criteria for

advanced hemodynamic parameters. This technique provides several advantages over routine two-dimensional flow imaging techniques, allowing it to become part of clinical practice at major academic medical centers. In this review, we present the current state-of-the-art cardiovascular, neurovascular, and abdominal applications.

**MR Imaging for Intracranial Vessel Wall Imaging: Pearls and Pitfalls** 461

Laura B. Eisenmenger, Alma Spahic, Joseph Scott McNally, Kevin M. Johnson, Jae W. Song, and Jacqueline C. Junn

Conventional vascular imaging methods have primarily focused on evaluating the vascular lumen. However, these techniques are not intended to evaluate vessel wall abnormalities where many cerebrovascular pathologies reside. With increased interest for the visualization and study of the vessel wall, high-resolution vessel wall imaging (VWI) has gained traction. Over the past two decades, there has been a rapid increase in number of VWI publications with improvements in imaging techniques and expansion on clinical applications. With increasing utility and interest in VWI, application of proper protocols and understanding imaging characteristics of vasculopathies are important for the interpreting radiologists to understand.

**MR Angiography of Pulmonary Vasculature** 475

Liisa L. Bergmann, Jeanne B. Ackman, Jitka Starekova, Alexander Moeller, Scott Reeder, Scott K. Nagle, and Mark L. Schiebler

Pulmonary magnetic resonance angiography (MRA) is a useful alternative to computed tomographic angiography (CTA) for visualizing the pulmonary vasculature. For pulmonary hypertension and partial anomalous pulmonary venous return, cardiac MR and pulmonary MRA are useful for flow quantification and treatment planning. For the diagnosis of pulmonary embolism (PE), MRA has been shown to have non-inferior outcomes at 6 months when compared with CTA for PE. Over the last 15 years, pulmonary MRA has become a routine and reliable examination for the workup of pulmonary hypertension, and for the primary diagnosis of PE at the University of Wisconsin.

**MR Angiography: Contrast-Enhanced Acquisition Techniques** 493

Prashant Nagpal and Thomas M. Grist

Video content accompanies this article at http://www.mri.theclinics.com.

Contrast-enhanced MR angiography (CE-MRA) is a frequently used MR imaging technique for evaluating cardiovascular structures. In many ways, it is similar to contrast-enhanced computed tomography (CT) angiography, except a gadolinium-based contrast agent (instead of iodinated contrast) is injected. Although the physiological principles of contrast injection overlap, the technical factors behind enhancement and image acquisition are different. CE-MRA provides an excellent alternative to CT for vascular evaluation and follow-up without requiring nephrotoxic contrast and ionizing radiation. This review describes the physical principles, limitations, and technical applications of CE-MRA techniques.

# MAGNETIC RESONANCE IMAGING CLINICS OF NORTH AMERICA

## FORTHCOMING ISSUES

*November 2023*
**Clinical Value of Hybrid PET/MRI**
Minerva Becker and Valentino Garibotto, *Editors*

*February 2024*
**MR Perfusion**
Max Wintermark and Ananth Madhuranthakam, *Editors*

*May 2024*
**Demyelinating and Inflammatory Lesions of the Brain and Spine**
Reza Forghani and Ashok Srinivasan, *Editors*

## RECENT ISSUES

*May 2023*
**Musculoskeletal MRI-Ultrasound Correlation**
Jan Fritz, *Editor*

*February 2023*
**MR Imaging of the Adnexa**
Erica B. Stein, Kim L. Shampain, and Kim Shampain, *Editors*

*November 2022*
**Postoperative Joint MR Imaging**
Luis Beltran, *Editor*

## PROGRAM OBJECTIVE

The goal of *Magnetic Resonance Imaging Clinics of North America* is to keep practicing physicians up to date with current clinical practice by providing timely articles reviewing the state of the art in patient care.

## TARGET AUDIENCE

All practicing physicians and healthcare professionals who provide patient care utilizing findings from Magnetic Resonance Imaging.

## LEARNING OBJECTIVES

Upon completion of this activity, participants will be able to:

1. Review the techniques, clinical applications and advances of magnetic resonance imaging.
2. Discuss the physical principles, limitations, and clinical applications of magnetic resonance imaging.
3. Recognize conventional vascular imaging methods and discuss contrast versus non-contrast usage in certain clinical scenarios.

## ACCREDITATION

The Elsevier Office of Continuing Medical Education (EOCME) is accredited by the Accreditation Council for Continuing Medical Education (ACCME) to provide continuing medical education for physicians.

The EOCME designates this journal-based CME activity enduring material for a maximum of 10 *AMA PRA Category 1 Credit(s)*™.Physicians should claim only the credit commensurate with the extent of their participation in the activity.

All other healthcare professionals requesting continuing education credit for this enduring material will be issued a certificate of participation.

## DISCLOSURE OF CONFLICTS OF INTEREST

The EOCME assesses conflict of interest with its instructors, faculty, planners, and other individuals who are in a position to control the content of CME activities. All relevant conflicts of interest that are identified are thoroughly vetted by EOCME for fair balance, scientific objectivity, and patient care recommendations. EOCME is committed to providing its learners with CME activities that promote improvements or quality in healthcare and not a specific proprietary business or a commercial interest.

**The planning committee, staff, authors, and editors listed below have identified no financial relationships or relationships to products or devices they or their spouse/life partner have with commercial interest related to the content of this CME activity:**

Jeanne B. Ackman, MD; Ayaz Aghayev, MD; Liisa L. Bergmann, MD, MBA; Candice A. Bookwalter, MD; Abhishek Chaturvedi, MD; Rory L. Cochran, MD, PhD; Jeremy D. Collins, MD; Phil A. Corrado, PhD; Mona Dabiri, MD; David Dushfunian, MD; Laura B. Eisenmenger, MD; Christopher J. Francois, MD; Ishan Garg, MD; Brian B. Ghoshhajra, MD, MBA; Thomas M. Grist, MD; Sandeep S. Hedgire, MD; Jacqueline C. Junn, MD; Kothainayaki Kulanthaivelu, BCA, MBA; Tim Leiner, MD, PhD; Anthony Maroun, MD; J. Scott McNally, MD, PhD; Alexander Moeller, MD; Mahmud Mossa-Basha, MD; Scott K. Nagle, MD, PhD; Prashant Nagpal, MD; Ananya Panda, MBBS, MD; Anthony Peret, MD; Sandra Quinn, BSc, MB BCh, BAO, PhD, MRCPI; Prabhakar Shantha Rajiah, MBBS, MD, FRCR; Scott Reeder, MD, PhD; Grant S. Roberts, PhD; Griselda Romero-Sanchez, MD; Mark L. Schiebler, MD; Jae W. Song, MD, MS; Alma Spahic; Jitka Starekova, MD; Michael Steigner, MD; Elizabeth K. Weiss

**The planning committee, staff, authors, and editors listed below have identified financial relationships or relationships to products or devices they or their spouse/life partner have with commercial interest related to the content of this CME activity:**

Bradley D. Allen, MD, MS: Consultant: Circle Cardiovascular Imaging Inc.

James C. Carr, MD: Advisor: Bayer AG, Bracco, Siemens; Researcher: Bayer Ag, Guerbet, Siemens; Speaker: Bayer AG.

Kevin M. Johnson, PhD: Researcher: GE Healthcare.

Michael Markl, PhD: Researcher: Siemens.

Alejandro Roldán-Alzate, PhD: Researcher: GE Healthcare.

Oliver Wieben, PhD: Researcher: GE Healthcare.

## UNAPPROVED/OFF-LABEL USE DISCLOSURE

The EOCME requires CME faculty to disclose to the participants:

1. When products or procedures being discussed are off-label, unlabelled, experimental, and/or investigational (not US Food and Drug Administration [FDA] approved); and
2. Any limitations on the information presented, such as data that are preliminary or that represent ongoing research, interim analyses, and/or unsupported opinions. Faculty may discuss information about pharmaceutical agents that is outside of FDA-approved labelling. This information is intended solely for CME and is not intended to promote off-label use of these medications. If you have any questions, contact the medical affairs department of the manufacturer for the most recent prescribing information.

**TO ENROLL**

To enroll in the *Magnetic Resonance Imaging Clinics of North America* Continuing Medical Education program, call customer service at 1-800-654-2452 or sign up online at http://www.theclinics.com/home/cme. The CME program is available to subscribers for an additional annual fee of USD 270.00.

**METHOD OF PARTICIPATION**

In order to claim credit, participants must complete the following:

1. Complete enrolment as indicated above.
2. Read the activity.
3. Complete the CME Test and Evaluation. Participants must achieve a score of 70% on the test. All CME Tests and Evaluations must be completed online.

**CME INQUIRIES/SPECIAL NEEDS**

For all CME inquiries or special needs, please contact elsevierCME@elsevier.com.

# Foreword

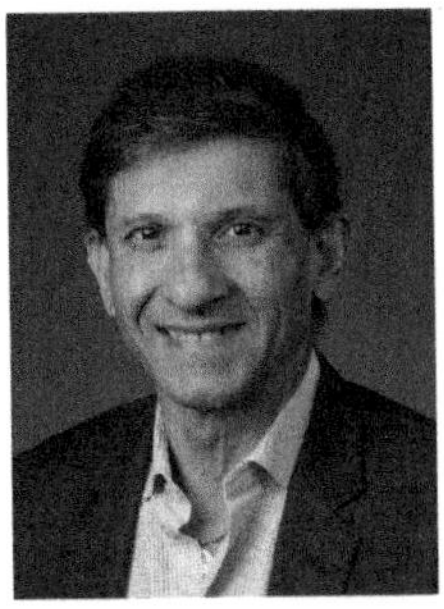

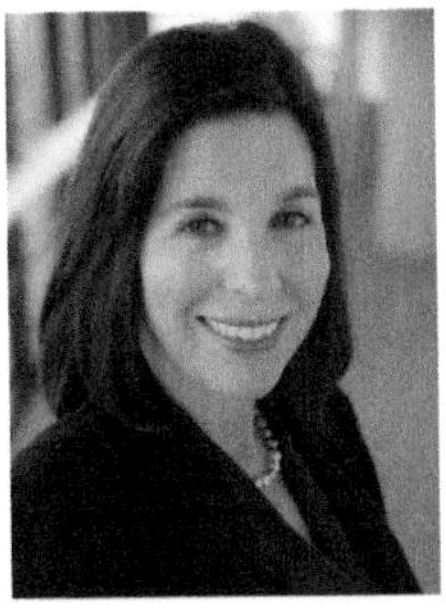

Suresh K. Mukherji, MD, MBA, FACR    Lynne S. Steinbach, MD, FACR

*Consulting Editors*

This issue of *Magnetic Resonance Imaging Clinics of North America* is devoted to Magnetic Resonance Angiography (MRA). We are fortunate to have Drs Prashant Nagpal and Thomas Grist edit this issue. The University of Wisconsin Department of Radiology has always been a leader in the technical developments and clinical applications of MRA, and we were thrilled when they accepted our invitation to be guest editors.

This issue covers MRA from "head to toe," with individual articles devoted to the intracranial and extracranial vasculature, upper and lower extremities, venous system, aorta, and pulmonary vasculature. There are also articles updating techniques for both noncontrast- and contrast-enhanced MRA and 4D-Flow techniques.

A very special thanks to the article authors for their outstanding contributions. All authors are international experts in the field of MR imaging, The articles are comprehensive but concise and beautifully illustrated, which makes this a wonderful issue. Finally, we would like to thank Drs Nagpal and Grist for accepting our invitation to guest edit this wonderful issue, which has clearly reached and surpassed Dr Nagpal's goal of producing a concise reference that will help create and expand an institution's MRA program and answer many routine imaging dilemmas.

Suresh K. Mukherji, MD, MBA, FACR
University of Illinois
ProScan Imaging
Carmel, IN 46032, USA

Lynne S. Steinbach, MD, FACR
University of California San Francisco
505 Parnassus Avenue
San Francisco, CA 94143-0628, USA

*E-mail addresses:*
sureshmukherji@hotmail.com (S.K. Mukherji)
lynne.steinbach@ucsf.edu (L.S. Steinbach)

Magn Reson Imaging Clin N Am 31 (2023) xiii
https://doi.org/10.1016/j.mric.2023.05.005
1064-9689/23/© 2023 Published by Elsevier Inc.

# Preface
# MR Angiography: Current State and Future Directions

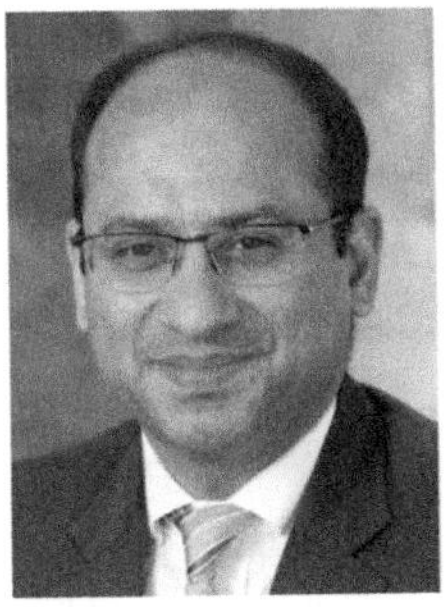
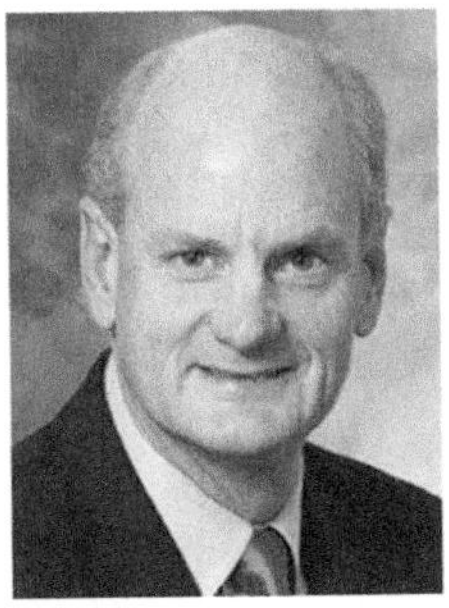

Prashant Nagpal, MD, FSCCT    Thomas M. Grist, MD, FACR
*Editors*

It has been a pleasure and honor to serve as Guest Editors for *Magnetic Resonance Imaging Clinics of North America* for this issue focused on MR Angiography for vascular evaluation. First and foremost, we would like to thank all the authors for their expertise and outstanding contributions to this issue. All contributors are international experts in the field of MR imaging, and we greatly enjoyed reading comprehensive yet succinct reviews by all authors.

MR Imaging, in general, is very rich in methods to exploit contrast mechanisms for assessment of the vascular system. Historically, due to variations in flow velocity, differences in patient-specific physiology, and need for fast imaging to prevent artifacts, the vascular system has been considered challenging to image. In addition, most vascular systems are also affected by respiratory motion. Nevertheless, advances in MR imaging have facilitated very robust anatomic and physiologic imaging of nearly all major vascular systems. While not conventionally considered part of MR Angiography (and hence not part of this issue), microvessel imaging like lymphatic imaging is also now enabled by MR imaging. At one point, the risk of nephrogenic systemic fibrosis (NSF) systemic gadolinium-based contrast agents (GBCA) limited use of gadolinium in patients with renal disease. But even then, noncontrast MR Angiography techniques could be used to provide noninvasive vascular evaluation. Now, as our knowledge regarding safety of GBCA has increased, we know that risk of NSF from macrocyclic and ionic (group II gadolinium agents) is infinitesimal to none. Also, the majority of the implantable devices are now MR imaging safe or conditional. Therefore, the use of MR Angiography continues to expand with very few reasons left that preclude the patient from getting an MR exam.

In this issue, you will find a comprehensive review of noncontrast MR Angiography by Dr Rajiah and colleagues and contrast-enhanced MR Angiography done by the coeditors. MR Angiography, while conventionally thought of as a technique for arterial system evaluation, is also an excellent imaging method for venous evaluation due to its inherent quality of high contrast, including for delayed imaging. Dr Ghoshhajra and colleagues have done an excellent review on the MR Venography technique and its clinical application. Among various arterial organ system MR Angiography reviews, you will find a comprehensive review on extremity vascular evaluation by Dr Steigner and colleagues, aortic evaluation by the coeditors, and pulmonary arterial evaluation by Dr Schiebler and colleagues. Dr Schiebler's group has been leading efforts in the MR imaging of pulmonary vascular imaging, which is an excellent test in young patients with suspicion of pulmonary embolism as well as in patients with contraindication to CT Angiography. Dr Mossa-Basha and colleagues, in their review on MR of extracranial carotid disease, discuss how MR techniques can be used for rapid and comprehensive anatomic evaluation of vasculature along with tissue characterization using structural, diffusion, and perfusion sequences. Dr Eisenmenger and colleagues discuss how vessel wall imaging can be used as

Magn Reson Imaging Clin N Am 31 (2023) xv–xvi
https://doi.org/10.1016/j.mric.2023.05.001
1064-9689/23/© 2023 Published by Elsevier Inc.

a noninvasive method to evaluate vessel wall pathology and depict plaque features, such as intraplaque hemorrhage, lipid-rich necrotic core, and fibrous cap. The breadth of these topics and discussions highlights how MR Angiography is playing a central role in improving anatomic evaluation of multiorgan vascular systems. The discussion in the MR imaging community is evolving from its ability to provide excellent anatomic information to added physiologic information that can be obtained simultaneously to complement clinical decision making. 4D-Flow imaging has championed this trend, and in this issue, Dr Weiben and colleagues discuss the technique and advances in the field of 4D-Flow imaging. This is followed by a brilliant review from Dr Carr and colleagues, in which they discuss the existing clinical applications of this technique using clinical case examples.

We hope that this issue can be of practical value by serving as a quick reference guide to build and advance your MR Angiography program and help answer many routine cardiovascular imaging dilemmas. We also hope that these expert reviews stimulate further debate and research into new areas and the existing controversial areas. Enjoy your reading!

Prashant Nagpal, MD, FSCCT
Cardiovascular Imaging
Department of Radiology
University of Wisconsin–Madison
School of Medicine and Public Health
600 Highland Avenue
Madison, WI 53705, USA

Thomas M. Grist, MD, FACR
Department of Radiology
University of Wisconsin–Madison
School of Medicine and Public Health
600 Highland Avenue
Madison, WI 53705, USA

*E-mail addresses:*
pnagpal@wisc.edu (P. Nagpal)
TGrist@uwhealth.org (T.M. Grist)

# Non-Contrast Magnetic Resonance Angiography: Techniques, Principles, and Applications

Ananya Panda, MBBS, MD, FRCR[a], Christopher J. Francois, MD[b], Candice A. Bookwalter, MD[b], Abhishek Chaturvedi, MD[c], Jeremy D. Collins, MD[b], Tim Leiner, MD, PhD[b], Prabhakar Shantha Rajiah, MBBS, MD, FRCR[b,*]

**KEYWORDS**

- Magnetic resonance • Non-contrast angiography • Magnetic resonance angiography • Renal artery • Peripheral artery • Pulmonary • Cerebral • Flow measurement

**KEY POINTS**

- Various techniques can be used to perform bright-blood (BB) non-contrast magnetic resonance angiography (MRA), each with preferred clinical utility and limitations.
- Balanced steady-state free-precession (b-SSFP) imaging is a rapid technique based on the intrinsically high T2/T1 ratio of blood. It provides simultaneous visualization of arteries and veins.
- Time-of-flight MRA relies on inflow-related enhancement and is most widely used for neurovascular imaging.
- Cardiac phase-dependent, flow-based techniques include subtractive fast spin-echo, Quiescent Interval Steady-State, and three-dimensional b-SSFP with flow-sensitive dephasing, which are typically used for peripheral extremity angiography.
- Phase-contrast MRA are velocity-sensitive techniques and can provide both anatomic information and flow quantification.
- Arterial spin labeling MRA is widely used for renal MRA, and can be further tailored for the evaluation of cerebral, carotid, hepatic, and pulmonary circulations.
- New multi-contrast techniques allow simultaneous evaluation of vessel wall (black-blood) and luminal (BB), and is useful for carotid and cardiovascular imaging.

## INTRODUCTION

Both contrast-enhanced magnetic resonance angiography (CE-MRA) and non-contrast-MRA are widely used in clinical practice to assess the presence, location, and extent of vascular involvement in a variety of conditions. Unlike computed tomography (CT) angiography, delineation of vascular patency is not affected by dense mural calcifications in MRA. Although CE-MRA provides excellent information on vascular anatomy and temporal enhancement kinetics, there has been an increasing focus on developing non-contrast MRA techniques. These developments are motivated by patient comfort, decreased cost as well as the potential risks of nephrogenic systemic fibrosis in patients with acute kidney injury or Grade 4 and Grade 5 chronic kidney disease.[1–3] The clinical need for robust MRA studies

[a] Department of Radiology, All India Institute of Medical Sciences, Jodhpur, India; [b] Department of Radiology, Mayo Clinic, Rochester, MN, USA; [c] Department of Radiology, University of Rochester Medical Center, Rochester, NY, USA
* Corresponding author.
*E-mail address:* radpry3@gmail.com

Magn Reson Imaging Clin N Am 31 (2023) 337–360
https://doi.org/10.1016/j.mric.2023.04.001
1064-9689/23/

is also greatest in patients with chronic kidney disease and related comorbidities (eg, atherosclerosis, diabetes, peripheral vascular disease). In these patient sub-groups, non-contrast MRA can provide a safe, contrast-free, and completely non-invasive imaging workup. Non-contrast MRA may also be preferred in pregnant women and in younger patients who may need repeated CE examinations as MRA exams are not associated with radiation and the long-term effects of gadolinium deposition in brain, bones, and cerebrospinal fluid are not known.[4–6] Although the iron-based contrast agent ferumoxytol is an alternative for CE-MRA, it is more expensive, has a higher anaphylactic risk, and is currently not Food and Drug Adminstration (FDA)-approved for CE-MRA in the United States.[7] Non-contrast MRA avoids all associated costs and adverse risks associated with contrast administration.[8] Non-contrast MRA is also independent of bolus timing, and therefore, can be repeated multiple times, albeit at the cost of increased examination time. Non-contrast MRA may be performed pre- or post-contrast as part of a standard protocol or added on the fly if there are technical issues in the initial CE-MRA acquisition due to contrast bolus mistiming issues. In such cases, non-contrast MRA can provide complementary information to CE-MRA.

Despite the benefits of non-contrast MRA, these techniques have been historically underutilized compared to CE-MRA, due to the lower spatial resolution and signal-to-noise ratio (SNR), longer scan times, and greater artifacts. However, the last few decades have seen multiple developments in scanner hardware, including multi-receiver phased-array coils for parallel imaging, faster and stronger gradients, and higher magnetic field strengths, all of which enable non-contrast MRA with improved SNR in clinically acceptable scan times.[9] Non-Cartesian sampling techniques, compressed sensing, and deep learning for denoising and image reconstruction have the potential to further improve the quality and speed of non-contrast MRA exams.[10,11] Although both bright-blood (BB) and black-blood imaging can be considered non-contrast MRA techniques, this review focuses on various BB non-contrast MRA techniques, their principles, contrast mechanisms, and relevant clinical applications.

**Table 1**
**Mechanisms of non-contrast magnetic resonance angiography techniques**

| Dominant Contrast Mechanism | Non-contrast MRA Technique |
|---|---|
| Intrinsic high T2/T1 ratio of blood (flow-independent MRA) | • b-SSFP (balanced steady-state free precession) |
| Blood-inflow-based | • Time-of-flight (TOF)<br>• Quiescent Interval Slice-Selective (QISS)<br>• Inflow-Dependent Inversion Recovery (IFDIR) |
| Cardiac phase-dependent, flow-based | • Subtractive 3D fast spin-echo (FSE)<br>• 3D-b-SSFP with flow-sensitive dephasing (FSD) |
| Velocity sensitive techniques | • Phase-contrast (PC)-MRA: 3D or 4D flow imaging<br>• Velocity –selective MRA |
| Arterial spin labeling (ASL) | • Flow-in ASL<br>• Flow-out ASL<br>• Alternate tag On/Off subtractive MRA |
| Multi-contrast techniques | • Simultaneous non-contrast angiography (SNAP)<br>• MTC-BOOST |

## NON-CONTRAST MAGNETIC RESONANCE ANGIOGRAPHY TECHNIQUES

Non-contrast MRA techniques can be broadly classified based on the dominant contrast mechanism used to produce images (**Table 1**). In non-contrast MRA, the visualization of blood vessels is based on utilizing the (a) properties of blood flow and velocity or the (b) intrinsic high T1 and T2 relaxation times of blood. These properties are combined with background suppression techniques, flow-encoding or flow-dephasing gradients, and flow-compensated readouts to produce MRA images.[11–13]

## BALANCED STEADY-STATE FREE PRECESSION

### *Principle*

Balanced steady-state free-precession (b-SSFP) MRA is a gradient-echo technique based on the long T1 and T2 relaxation times of blood and its high T2/T1 ratio, which produces BB images with high vessel-to-background contrast.[12] For a three-dimensional (3D)-slab acquisition, imaging is performed by applying a series of equally spaced alternating radiofrequency (RF) pulses in all three axes, such that a coherent steady-state with balanced longitudinal and transverse magnetization is produced after many repetition times (TRs). The signal intensity of the resultant image is dependent on the T2/T1 ratio. The TR is kept as short as possible (typically <5 msec on modern MR systems, but much less than the T2 relaxation time of blood) to minimize signal loss due to the dephasing of transverse magnetization. The readout is acquired such that the time of echo (TE) and free induction decay (FID) coincide in the middle of the TR (TR/2) (**Fig. 1**). Background fat suppression is applied at the time of readout, as fat has a similarly high T2/T1 ratio. For additional background tissue and venous suppression, a T2 prep pulse or DIXON technique may also be used.[9,12,14,15] Because of the symmetric nature of applied gradients, this technique is flow-compensated which is also advantageous for other non-contrast MRA techniques, as described later. Using a breath-hold acquisition or free breathing with navigator gating can mitigate respiratory motion in the thorax and abdomen.[14] For coronary MRA, additional electrocardiogram (ECG)-gating is also used and images are acquired in mid-late diastole to reduce pulsation artifacts (**Fig. 2**).[16,17]

Intrinsic high SNR and lack of reliance on blood flow make this sequence ideal for imaging slow flow (including venous flow), and in areas where background anatomic information is useful (eg, thoracic and abdominal imaging).[18] The sequence can also cover a large field of view with relatively short scan times.[9]

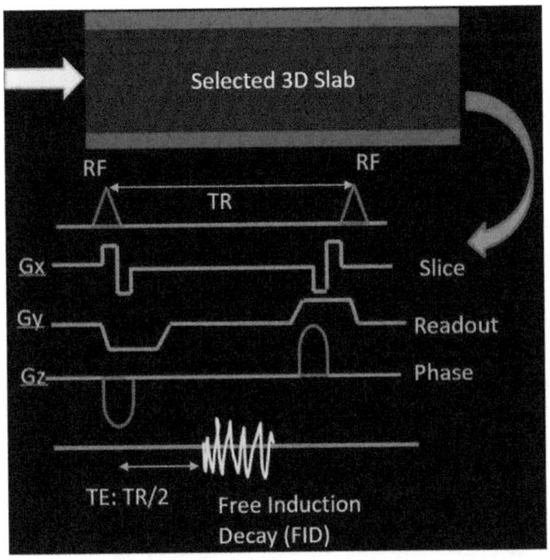


Fig. 1. Schematic of 3D-b-SSFP sequence. Multiple radiofrequency (RF) pulses are applied at short time of repetition (TRs). Balanced gradients are applied in all three axes (x, y, z) such that FID and TE coincide in the middle of TR. Coherent steady-state is attained after many such repetitions and signals are combined from multiple TRs to produce BB MRA images. Due to symmetric gradients, the sequence is flow-compensated and the final bright signal in the vessels is due to the high T2/T1 ratio of blood. Fat suppression techniques or DIXON are used for background fat suppression.

### *Limitations*

Balanced SSFP is very sensitive to off-resonance artifacts often occurring at the ends of a large field of views (Moire' fringe artifacts). It is also prone to susceptibility artifacts due to metallic hardware (eg, vascular stents, clips, hardware, implantable cardiac devices, prosthetic valves) and air-tissue interfaces (eg, bowel, lungs) (**Fig. 3**). These can be partially mitigated by improved shimming, and are less obtrusive at lower field strengths.[9] Due to the short out-of-phase TE, there can be India ink artifacts from chemical shift imaging effect at fat–water interfaces, which can limit the detectability of mural thrombi and plaques.[14] As this sequence is independent of flow velocity, concomitant visualization of venous vasculature may be considered as unwanted venous contamination if the clinical question is only arterial imaging.

### *Common Clinical Applications*

Balanced SSFP MRA is widely used for cardiothoracic, pulmonary, coronary, and abdominal MRA (**Fig. 4**).[19,20] It can also be combined with retrospective ECG-gated cine acquisition to visualize aortic and pulmonary outflow dynamics.[14,21] In body imaging, it has been used for visualization of hepatoportal, renal, and pelvic vasculature.[22–24] This technique has also been applied for lower extremity MRA and MR venograms (MRV) in combination with DIXON-based fat/water separation.[25]

## TIME-OF-FLIGHT

### *Principle*

Time-of-flight (TOF) MRA is the oldest and most widely used non-contrast BB MRA technique. It is based on the principle of inflow-related enhancement, that is, when unsaturated moving spins flow into a pre-selected slice that has been saturated by multiple RF excitations, these moving spins produce a bright signal in contrast to the stationary spins in the background saturated tissue. Additional spatial saturation pulses can be applied below or above the selected slice to suppress unwanted arterial and/or venous flow.[12] The placement of spatial saturation pulse depends on the anatomy and direction of unwanted flow. For example, in head and neck MRA, the spatial saturation pulse is applied above the selected slice to

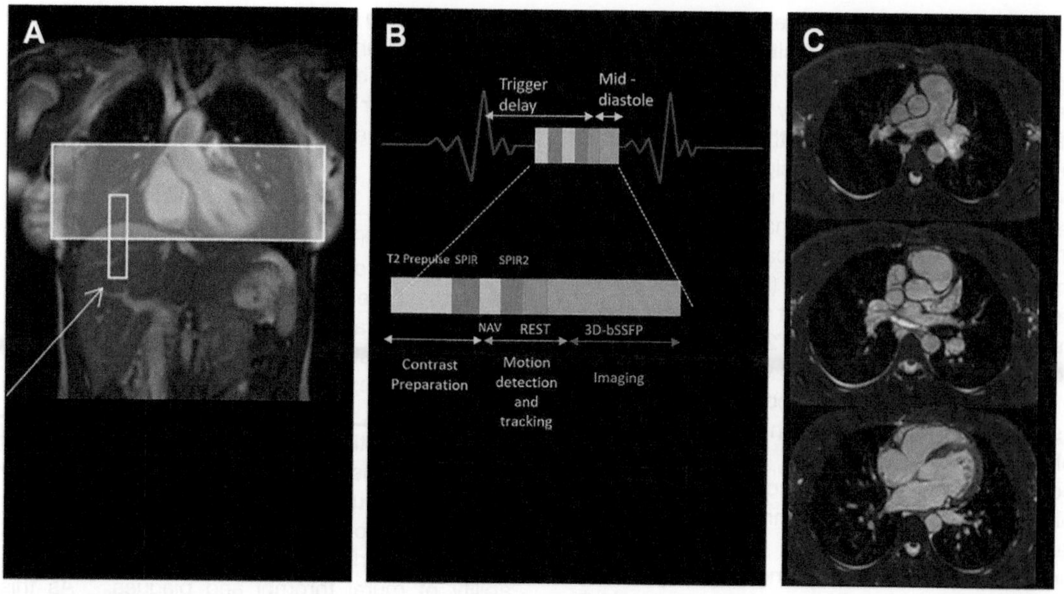


**Fig. 2.** 3D-b-SSFP sequence as modified for cardiac MRA. (*A*) Depicts placement of 3D slab (*white box*) for 3D-cardiac MRA. The yellow box (*yellow arrow*) denotes placement of the navigator gating slab over the right diaphragm for free breathing acquisition. (*B*) Depicts typical sequence design. In this example, a T2 prep pulse is used to saturate myocardium for visualization of coronary arteries. Fat suppression is obtained with Spectral Presaturation with Inversion Recovery (SPIR) technique. ECG-gating is used to reduce cardiac pulsation artifacts. The b-SSFP pulse sequence is applied in mid- to end-diastole. (*C*) Depicts selected three slices from the final 3D-MRA volume, depicting pulmonary arteries, SVC, and aorta (top image), ventricular outflow tracts and left coronary origin (middle image), and four-chamber view and right and left coronary arteries in atrioventricular grooves (bottom image) with a high in-plane spatial resolution (1.3 mm × 1.3 mm).

suppress unwanted venous inflow, or applied below the selected slice to suppress unwanted arterial inflow for MRV (**Fig. 5**). Conversely for thoracoabdominal and peripheral MRA, spatial saturation pulses are placed below the selected slice as the direction of venous flow in the extremities and inferior vena cava (IVC) is caudocranial. For thoracoabdominal and peripheral MRV, the spatial saturation pulses are placed above the selected slice to suppress arterial inflow.

For optimal TOF imaging, the flow needs to be fast and the slice needs to be thin, so that the

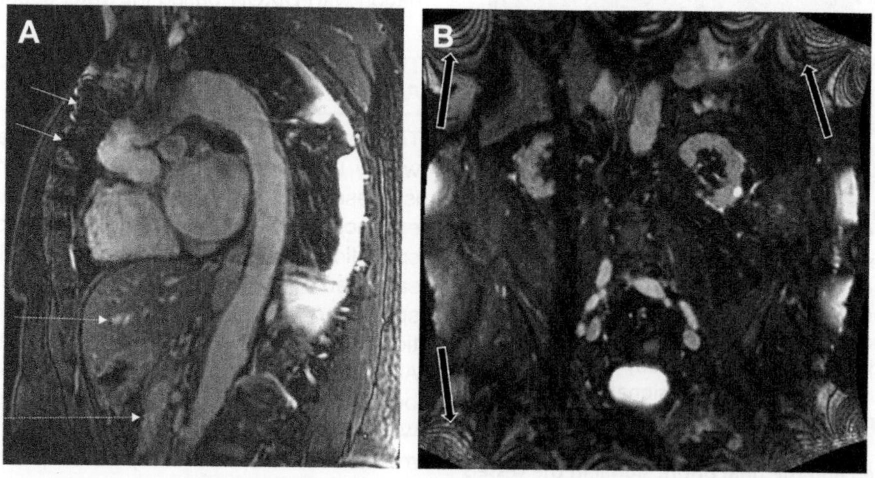


**Fig. 3.** Common pitfalls with b-SSFP MRA. Pitfalls include metallic susceptibility artifacts due to sternotomy wires (*solid white arrows, A*), simultaneous visualization of venous signal from portal vein, hepatic veins, and IVC (*dotted white arrows, B*) and Moire'/fringe artifacts at edges (*block arrow, B*).

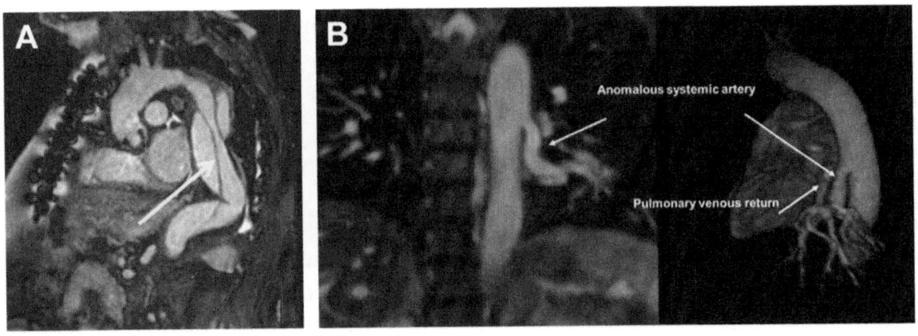


Fig. 4. Clinical applications of 3D-b-SSFP MRA. (*A*) Selected image from 3D acquisition shows aortic dissection in the thoracic aorta (*arrow, A*) (*B*) 3D-b-SSFP in a case of intralobar pulmonary sequestration demonstrated the anomalous systemic artery arising from the descending thoracic aorta and drainage into pulmonary vein.

blood within the selected saturated slice is entirely replaced by fast-inflowing unsaturated spins during acquisition, which produces the maximum signal. Thus this sequence works best when the blood flow velocity is greater than the slice thickness and TR.[12] Another requirement for optimal TOF imaging is that vessels need to be perpendicular to the selected slice. This can be a challenge for 3D-TOF where some of the moving spins are partially saturated through a 3D slab and lose optimal signal. This can be mitigated by the use of multiple overlapping thin slab acquisition technique and spatially variable (ramped) RF pulses, such as spins entering a slab experience less saturation (due to smaller flip angles) compared to spins exiting a slab (due to larger flip angles).[26–28] The use of magnetization transfer RF pulse allows for better background suppression and higher SNR.[28] As with any MRA technique, tradeoffs occur with parameter optimization. For example, longer TR increases vascular signal but also static tissue signal, and thus, TR is kept between 15 and 35 msec. Longer TE increases vascular signal but turbulent flow can also cause loss of signal due to flow dephasing and thus TE is kept between 3 and 7 msec. TOF is also commonly paired with flow-compensated gradient-echo readouts (eg, b-SSFP) to reduce signal loss from spin flow dephasing. Good contrast between static tissue and blood signal is provided when flip angles between 30° and 70° are used for 2D TOF and between 10° and 30° for 3D-TOF. For peripheral extremity MRA, ECG-gating is needed to avoid ghosting from multiphasic flow.[29]

### *Limitations*

TOF is insensitive to in-plane flow, thus, the area imaged must be perpendicular to the image slice. Stenosis can be overestimated and artifacts can be produced by turbulent in-plane flow in segments with non-perpendicular anatomy (eg, at the carotid bulb and intracranial MRV) (**Fig. 6**). In the subclavian steal syndrome, the reversal of flow in the vertebral artery may be mistaken for occlusion when spatial saturation pulses are applied

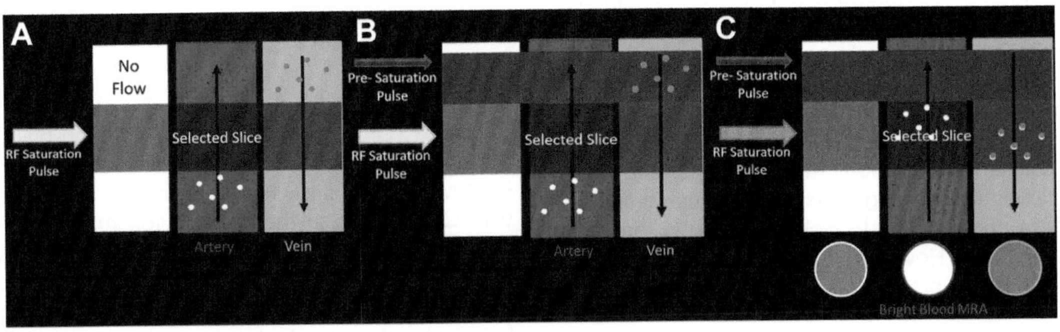


Fig. 5. Schematic of TOF-MRA as applied to head and neck region. The arteries have caudo-cranial flow and veins have cranio-caudal flow (*black arrows*). (*A*) Depicts application of initial multiple slice-selective RF pulses (*yellow block arrow*) to partially saturate background static signal. (*B*) Depicts application of spatial saturation pulse above the slice to be imaged (*purple arrow*) to suppress unwanted signal from the inflowing venous flow. (*C*) Depicts final MRA images at the time of readout such that inflowing unsaturated spins in the artery produce BB images while inflowing saturated signals in the vein appear dark.

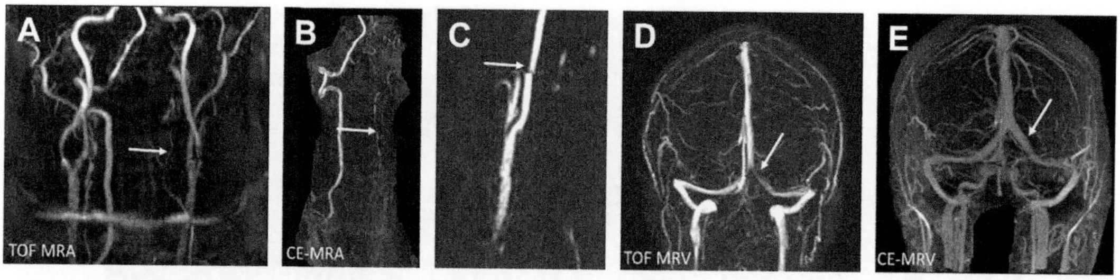


Fig. 6. Schematic and clinical applications of 3D-TOF-MRA in the brain. (*A*) Depicts acquisition of intracranial 3D-TOF-MRA with the selected region of interest and venous saturation pulse. (*B*) Maximum Intensity Projection (MIP) image from 3D-TOF-MRA shows a normal Circle of Willis anatomy. (*C, D*) Axial source (*C*) and MIP (*D*) images from 3D-TOF-MRA in a patient with a right parietal arteriovenous malformation show nidus (*white arrow,* C), prominent draining veins (*dashed arrow, C*), and arterial feeders from the middle cerebral artery (*white arrow, D*) and posterior cerebral artery (*dashed arrow, D*). (*E*) Axial image from 3D-TOF (*E*) in a patient with Moya-Moya disease well demonstrates bilateral lenticulostriate collaterals (*white arrows, E*) when compared with CE-MRA.

above the imaging slice. The correct diagnosis of vertebral artery flow reversal can be confirmed by repeating TOF with spatial saturation pulse applied below the slice or with the PC-MRA technique.[30] TOF is suboptimal for imaging renal and visceral arteries as these arise in an axial or oblique plane from the aorta. In patients with severe peripheral vascular disease, distal arteries with slow flow are poorly visualized. TOF images are also affected by respiratory motion in the abdomen and by swallowing motion in the neck. As 2D-TOF needs separate acquisition for each station, this can lead to stair step artifacts and long imaging times for peripheral vasculature (see **Fig. 6**). Compressed sensing, iterative reconstruction, and acceleration using parallel imaging techniques can be used to minimize scan times for single station at a time, and for 3D-TOF-MRA.[31–33]

### *Common Clinical Applications*

Two-dimensional TOF-MRA is best suited for imaging fast arterial flow of the cervical and carotid vessels. TOF is less preferred than QISS for peripheral vasculature imaging due to the above-mentioned limitations for visualizing slow distal flow and overestimating stenosis. Three-dimensional TOF is best for intracranial MRA and has been widely used for the detection of aneurysms, stenosis, occlusions, arteriovenous malformations, and post-intervention imaging, where longer scan times are not a problem due to lack of motion in the brain (**Fig. 7**).[34,35] However, for MRV, the 3D-TOF technique is less preferred than PC-MRV (see below).

## QUIESCENT INTERVAL SINGLE-SHOT

### *Principle*

Similar to TOF, quiscent interval single-shot (QISS) is also based on the principle of inflow-dependent enhancement in perpendicularly oriented vessels. QISS is traditionally performed using ECG-gating and b-SSFP single-shot technique. In QISS acquisition, shortly after R-wave, a slice-selective pulse is applied along with the application of spatial saturation pulse above or below for arterial or venous flow suppression and followed by a fat suppression pulse. Following a quiescent interval of ~ 230 msec (range 200–300 msec) timed to systole, such that maximum systolic-inflow occurs into the selected slice, a b-SSFP readout gradient is applied and images are acquired at end-diastole (**Fig. 8**).[36]

QISS offers several advantages over TOF for peripheral vascular imaging. In QISS, as the QI is much longer than TR used in TOF, it allows a greater time for arterial inflow and is better suited for detecting residual flow in diseased peripheral segments with a slow flow (which can be overestimated on TOF as absent flow).[36] QISS is more rapidly acquired than TOF with a single-shot acquisition per slice. QISS can also be tailored for peripheral venous imaging by increasing the duration of the quiescent interval to allow more venous inflow and reversing the location of spatial saturation pulse.[37]

### *Limitations*

Similar to TOF, QISS is sensitive to through-plane flow and is best suited for perpendicular vessels in the lower extremities. However, newer advances with QISS optimize the method for imaging the vasculature in other body regions too.[38] QISS is sensitive to inhomogeneity and susceptibility artifacts related to the b-SSFP readout. Using a fast low-angle shot readout can mitigate b-SSFP-related artifacts. However, tradeoffs include lower SNR and greater flow saturation.[39] Like all ECG-gated MRA sequences, QISS is suboptimal in patients with arrhythmias. To overcome this, Edelman, and colleagues and Koktzoglou and colleagues,

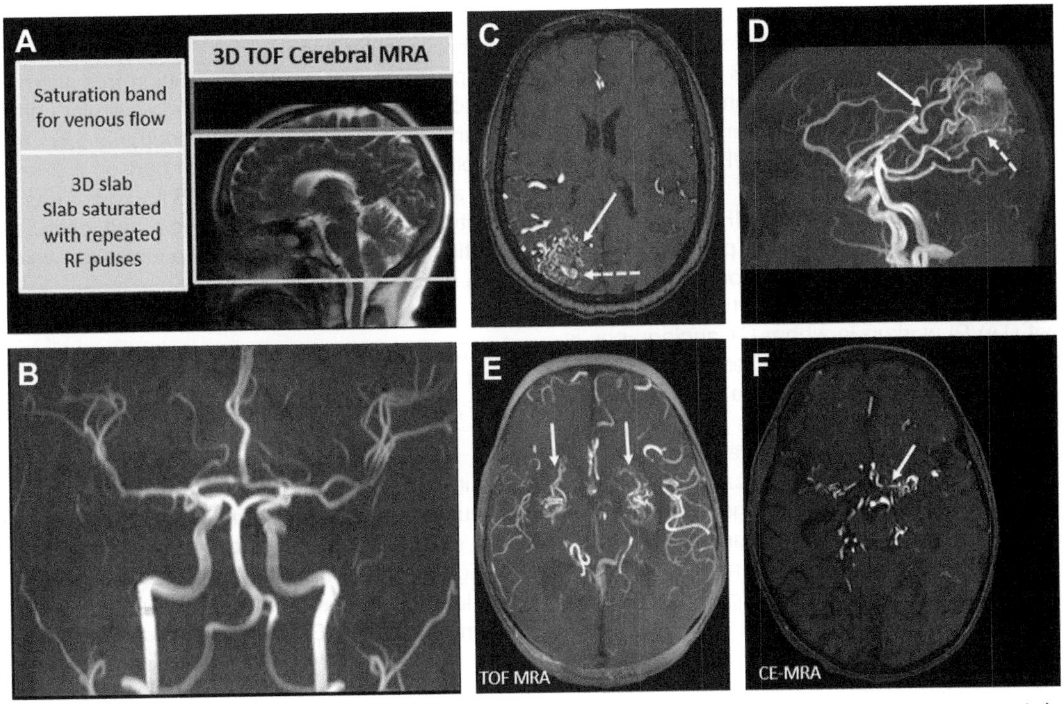


**Fig. 7.** Common pitfalls with TOF-MRA technique. (*A, B*) TOF-MRA overestimated left vertebral artery stenosis (*arrow, A*) compared to CE-MRA (*arrow, B*). This is due to turbulent flow causing loss of signal. (*C*) Swallowing and neck motion between slabs can lead to stair-steps artifacts (*arrow*) in the carotid MRA. (*D–F*) There is a partial loss of signal in left transverse venous sinus due to through-plane flow on TOF-MRV (*arrow, D*), corresponding CE-MRV shows widely patent left transverse sinus (*arrow, E*).

have recently developed ungated-QISS (unQISS) and fast interrupted steady-state (FISS)-MRA.[40,41] Although both these "second-generation QISS"-MRA sequences do not require ECG-gating, due to longer scan times, these are better suited for imaging body regions unaffected by respiratory motion including the peripheral veins and extracranial carotid arteries.[38,42,43]

## *Common Clinical Applications*

Since its initial description, QISS has been widely adopted for imaging peripheral arterial disease in lower extremities given the ease of acquisition and its high accuracy for detecting diseased segments when compared with CE-MRA or digital subtraction angiograms (DSA) in multiple studies

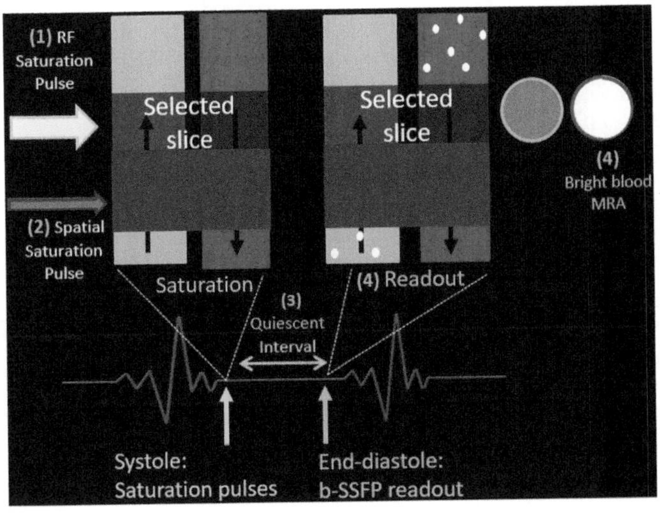


**Fig. 8.** Schematic of QISS sequence as applied to peripheral limb MRA. The direction of flow in the artery and vein is denoted by black arrows. The sequence is ECG-gated. (1) Shortly after R-wave in systole, slice-selective saturation pulse (*yellow block arrow*) is applied in the region of interest. (2) Application of spatial saturation pulses (*purple arrow*) above selected slice for suppression of venous signal and fat saturation pulses. (3) After a quiescent interval, fresh blood washes in the selected slice. (4) Single-shot b-SSFP readout is applied at end diastole for the final BB MRA images.

(**Fig. 9**).[29,44,45] A meta-analysis including 17 studies demonstrated that QISS has a pooled sensitivity, specificity, and accuracy of 0.88 (95% CI: 0.85–0.91), 0.94 (95% CI: 0.92–0.96), and 0.96 (95% CI: 0.94–0.98), respectively, on a per-segment basis when compared with DSA/CE-MRA as reference for peripheral arterial disease.[44] QISS has also been used for upper extremity MRA with detailed visualization of distal arteries and palmar arches.[46]

Recently, QISS has been applied to patients undergoing pre-transcatheter aortic valve replacement (TAVR) workup in whom CT angiography is contraindicated due to impaired renal function.[47,48] QISS can be acquired along with a proton-density-weighted in-phase stack-of-stars pulse sequence that can simultaneously identify vascular calcifications comparable to CTA. Identification of vascular calcifications can be useful to guide the site of percutaneous arterial puncture during TAVR.[49]

QISS can be performed with breath-hold imaging or free breathing with navigator-respiratory gating for mesenteric, thoracic, and pulmonary MRA.[38,50,51] QISS can also be combined with non-Cartesian radial sampling for coronary and cerebrovascular imaging.[50,52–55] Radial QISS can also provide a non-contrast, radiation-free alternative to CTA for follow-up after endovascular aortic aneurysm repair (EVAR) procedures in the abdomen. In a head-to-head comparison between CTA and radial QISS, radial QISS had good image quality near the EVAR prosthesis and detected additional slow-flow type II endoleaks which were not seen on CTA.[56]

## CARDIAC-GATED SUBTRACTIVE 3D-FAST SPIN-ECHO- MRA

### *Principle*

Fast spin-echo (FSE) sequences are extremely sensitive to spin dephasing with fast-flowing blood producing a signal void. This flow-related sensitivity of FSE is harnessed for MRA by using ECG-gating to acquire two successive coronal oblique 3D slabs of images; one at peak systole and one at end diastole. During peak systole, arteries have the fastest flow, which produces flow voids

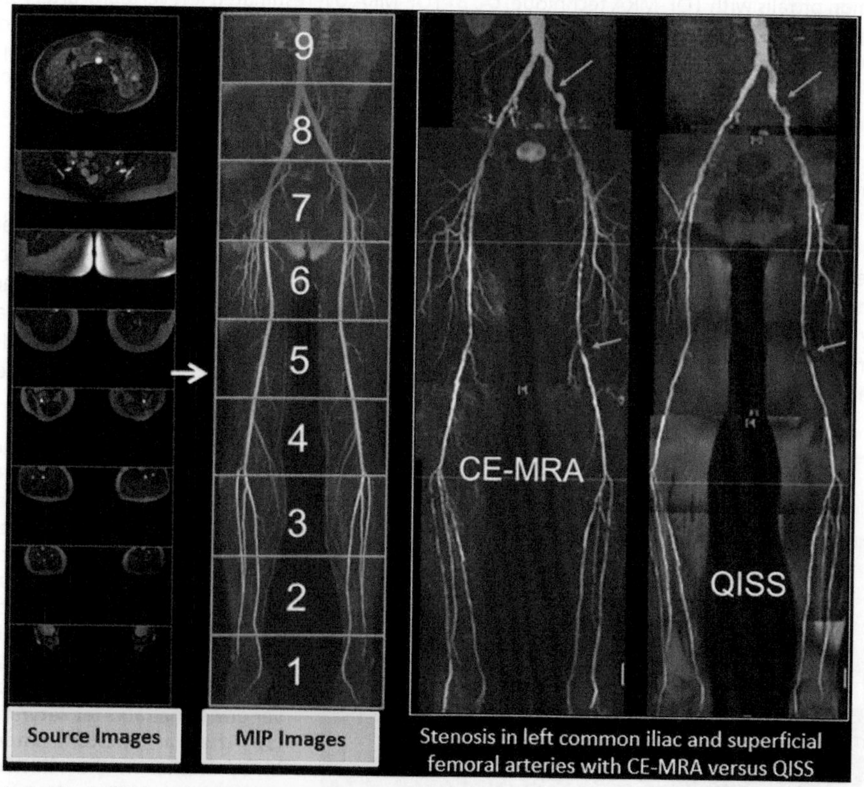


**Fig. 9.** Peripheral limb MRA with QISS denoting peripheral artery disease. The acquisition is a multi-station acquisition such that a series of 2D slabs are acquired from the abdomen to feet. The axial source images are used to generate MIP images per slab which are fused to create a peripheral run-off MRA. The final fused image derived from the QISS-MRA depicts short segment stenosis in the left common iliac artery (*top arrow*) and left superficial femoral artery (bottom *arrow*), which is concordant with the findings on CE-MRA. The total scan time for this QISS-MRA acquisition was ~12 minutes at 1.5 minutes/slab.

or dark blood (DB) images. During end diastole, there is relatively slower flow in arteries compared to systole with some preservation of signal leading to BB images. Subtraction of systole (S) from diastole (D) images (D-S) demonstrates arterial flow as BB imaging. The venous flow being slower than arterial flow appears bright on both systole and diastole and thus appears dark on the final (D-S) subtracted images (**Fig. 10**). Subtraction also suppresses background static tissue, which can be further suppressed by applying fat suppression techniques during readout. To enable fast imaging, a partial Fourier scheme, long-echo train length, and parallel imaging are used, along with ultra-short echo spacing to prevent complete spin dephasing for creation of BB images.[13,57] Unlike the previously described inflow-enhancement-based sequences, which require vessels to be perpendicular to the imaging slice, this sequence is less sensitive to the orientation partitions relative to vessels.

There are several factors that determine the visualization of vessels in this sequence, which are described in detail in the review by Wheaton, and colleagues.[12] Briefly larger arteries are better demonstrated by the use of higher refocusing flip angles (160° +) and the use of partial flow-compensating readout gradients. Conversely, smaller arteries are better visualized by the use of low refocusing flip angles (<120°) and the use of additional flow-dephasing gradients during readout.[12] An ECG-gated 3D-FSE with variable flip angles and flow-dephasing gradients has also been described for visualization of distal arteries in hands.[58] This sequence with 3D-FSE readout is also more immune to B0 inhomogeneity compared to QISS with b-SSFP readout and is better suited for large volumes of coverage and thoracoabdominal MRA.

### *Limitations*

As an ECG-gated sequence, it is affected by cardiac arrhythmias. Due to its subtractive nature and acquisition of two scans over multiple R-R intervals, scan times are longer for extremity MRA. Even though both systolic and diastolic scans are acquired successively, artifacts due to patient motion and incomplete subtraction can still occur. This sequence also requires multiple ECG-prep scans at different trigger delays with manual selection of the correct ECG-trigger delays for systolic and diastolic images. Additionally, this sequence is not suitable for carotid MRA due to rapid flow in internal jugular veins which also shows similar flow-related dephasing effects. In cases of severe stenosis with increased turbulent flow, 3D-FSE-MRA can overestimate stenosis as even diastolic phase images now appear dark, and subtracted images show flow voids instead of the expected bright signals. Thus, it is necessary to review both subtracted images and diastolic images together to detect critical stenosis.[12,59]

### *Common Clinical Applications*

Given its robustness to susceptibility effects, 3D-FSA-MRA can be used for the assessment of the thoracoabdominal aorta and pulmonary arteries with good visualization of pulmonary branches in the lungs and vessels adjacent to metallic devices. For imaging the thoraco-abdominal aorta, a single diastolic acquisition can suffice to produce BB MRA, as there is little venous contamination or background signal in this region (**Fig. 11**).[60] In

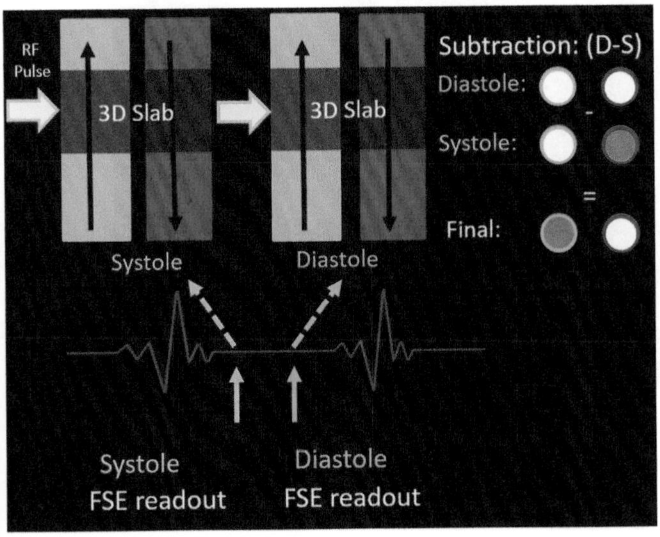


**Fig. 10.** Schematic for 3D-FSE-MRA technique as applied to peripheral limb MRA. The direction of flow in the artery and vein is denoted by black arrows. In this ECG-gated subtractive technique, RF pulses are applied to selected 3D slabs in both systole and diastole with FSE readout. In diastole, both artery and vein produce a bright signal, while in systole artery show a loss of signal due to fast flow-related dephasing while the vein is bright due to slow non-pulsatile flow. Subtraction of systole from diastole (D-S) produces final BB MRA images as venous flow is canceled and arterial flow is accentuated.

pulmonary MRA, subtraction of systolic from diastole images also provides pulmonary perfusion MRA that can be used for detecting perfusion deficits associated with pulmonary embolisms.[61,62]

This sequence can be used for peripheral vascular MRA, but head-to-head comparisons showed a greater proportion of non-diagnostic segments with ECG-gated 3D- FSE compared to QISS-MRA.[63] Sensitivities for 3D-FSE-MRA and QISS, were similar but ECG-gated 3D–FSE showed slightly lower specificity. 3D-FSE-MRA images of proximal pelvic and distal pedal arteries were limited compared to QISS, with greater susceptibility to patient motion.[64] However, given the high negative predictive value, 3D-FSA-MRA can be useful as a screening modality (see **Fig. 11**).[29,65] Other applications include non-contrast peripheral MR venography by additional subtraction of subtracted images from systole images [S-(D-S)] and non-contrast MR portography with good visualization of the intrahepatic and extrahepatic portal circulation.[66] Similar to aortic 3D-FSE-MRA, a single diastolic phase acquisition with an appropriately selected diastolic phase trigger delay depicts the portal circulation as BB while the background signal from the aorta is suppressed.

## 3D- BALANCED STEADY-STATE FREE-PRECESSION WITH FLOW-SENSITIVE DEPHASING

### *Principle*

This is another ECG-gated subtractive technique based on the same principle of DB imaging during peak systole and BB imaging during end diastole. Instead of an FSE readout, flow-sensitive dephasing (FSD) gradients are applied along vessel length with a b-SSFP readout. This sequence uses an FSD pre-pulse along with large bipolar gradients to produce flow-related loss of signal from moving spins.

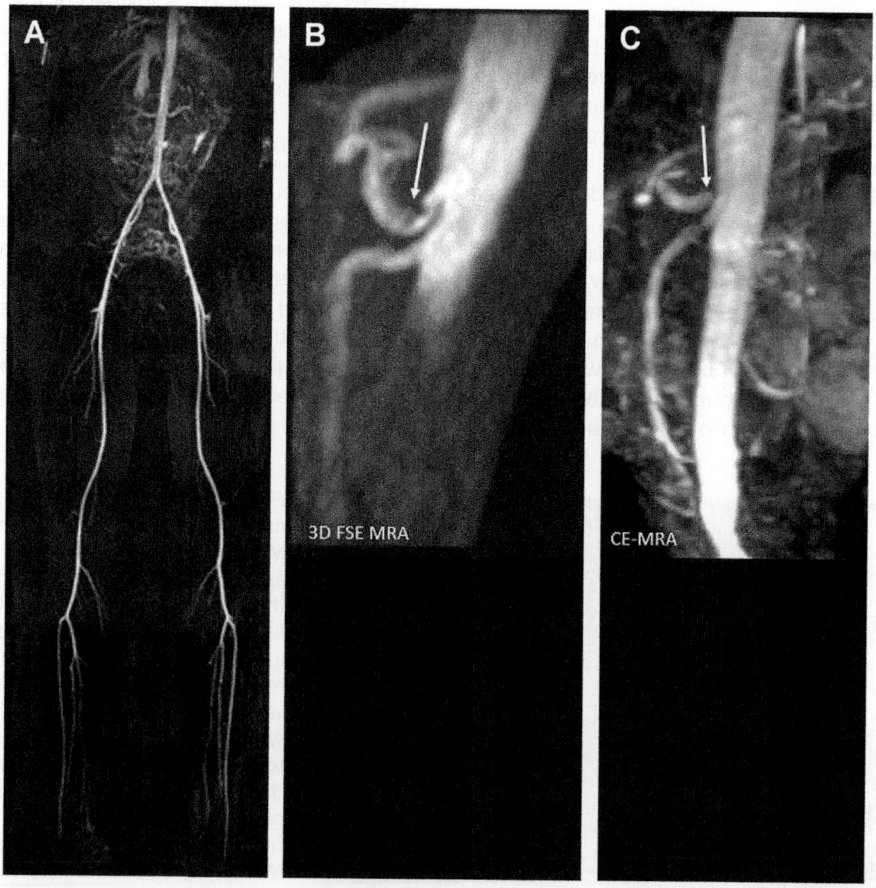


**Fig. 11.** Clinical applications of 3D-FSE-MRA. (*A*) Aorto-iliac and peripheral MRA with 3D-FSE-MRA in the patient shows a good depiction of all vessels thereby excluding atherosclerotic disease. (*B, C*) Median arcuate ligament syndrome. There is severe ostial stenosis of the celiac trunk with hook-like superior indention (*arrow*) seen on non-contrast 3D-FSE-MRA in a patient with post-prandial abdominal pain. This finding is also confirmed on a CE-MRA MRA suggestive of median arcuate ligament syndrome (*arrow*).

The FSD pre-pulse comprises alternate +90°-x, +180°-y, −90°-x pulses and interleaved bipolar gradients on either side of +180°-y pulse. After excitation by the initial +90°-x pulse, spins are dephased by bipolar gradients depending on their velocities. With optimally selected bipolar gradients, a greater degree of spin dephasing occurs in arteries with little effect on veins or background signals. Following the application of bipolar gradients, the −90°-x flip back pulse restores longitudinal magnetization of rephased spins to produce a signal while a spoiler gradient prevents refocusing of dephased spins in later modules (**Fig. 12**). During systole, the FSD pre-pulse is applied with bipolar gradients turned on to produce DB images, while during diastole, the FSD pre-pulse is applied with all bipolar gradients turned off to produce BB images, followed by (D-S) subtraction to accentuate arterial flow and strongly suppress background flow.[67,68]

This sequence produces better DB images in systole compared to 3D-FSE. However, the technical success of this sequence and vessel visibility depends on the strength and duration of bipolar gradients. Large bipolar gradients increase flow-sensitivity and thus may lead to simultaneous visualization of veins as well as background tissue due to the diffusion effect. Smaller bipolar gradients decrease flow-sensitivity with impaired visualization of small arteries with lower velocities, and resultant overestimation of stenosis.[69] The FSD pre-pulses can also be applied in all three orthogonal planes to detect flow in multiple directions in hands and feet.[70]

### *Limitations*

Other limitations are similar to those of ECG-gated subtracted techniques (eg, selection of appropriate triggers for systolic and diastolic images, sensitivity to cardiac arrhythmias, patient motion, and long scan times) and those of b-SSFP readout (eg, susceptibility to B0 inhomogeneity). Additionally, this sequence is not commercially available.

### *Current Clinical Applications*

The initial studies showed utility for visualization of infragenual (below the knee) arteries, and small arteries of feet and hands in patients with diabetes and autoimmune vasculopathies (**Fig. 13**).[71–76]

## PHASE-CONTRAST-MRA (3D AND 4D FLOW IMAGING)

### *Principle*

This is based on the principle that moving spins experience a net shift in the phase when exposed to bipolar gradients, while stationary spins show no net-phase shift. The net shift in the phase is proportional to the velocity of moving spins, thus this is a velocity sensitive technique. In this sequence, three flow-encoding bipolar gradients with pre-determined velocity encoding (Venc) and one flow-compensated bipolar gradient are

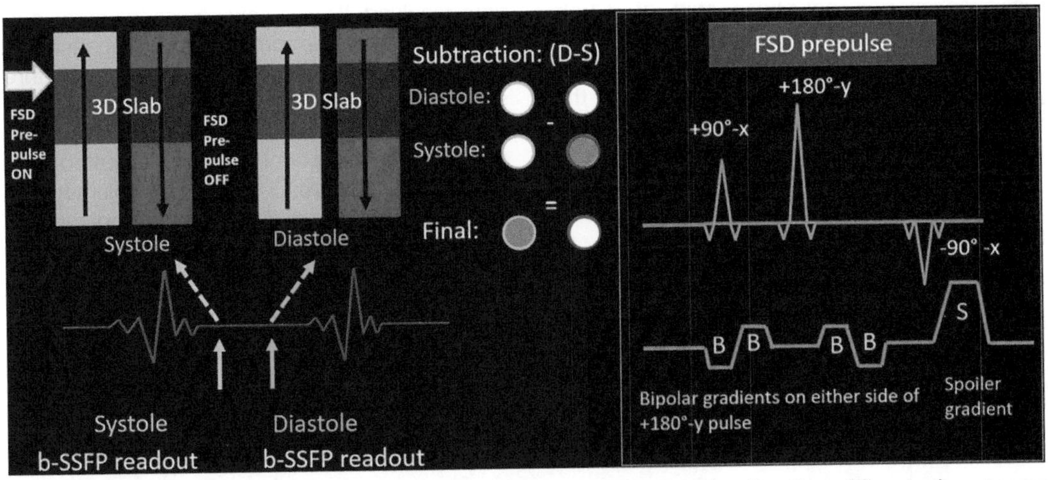


**Fig. 12.** 3D-b-SSFP FSD MRA technique as applied to peripheral limb MRA. The direction of flow in the artery and vein is denoted by black arrows. In this ECG-gated subtractive technique with b-SSFP readout, acquisition in systole is done with the FSD pre-pulse turned on. In diastole, the FSD pre-pulse is turned off. Both artery and vein produce a bright signal in diastole; the artery shows loss of signal due to FSD in systole. Subtraction of systole from diastole (D-S) produces final BB MRA images. The diagram on the right shows FSD pre-pulse comprising +90°-x, +180°-y, −90°-x pulses with interleaved bipolar gradients on either side of +180°-y pulse. Spoiler gradient applied after 90°-x pulse prevents refocusing of dephased spins in later modules. The sensitivity of this sequence to depict arterial flow depends on the strength and duration of these bipolar gradients.

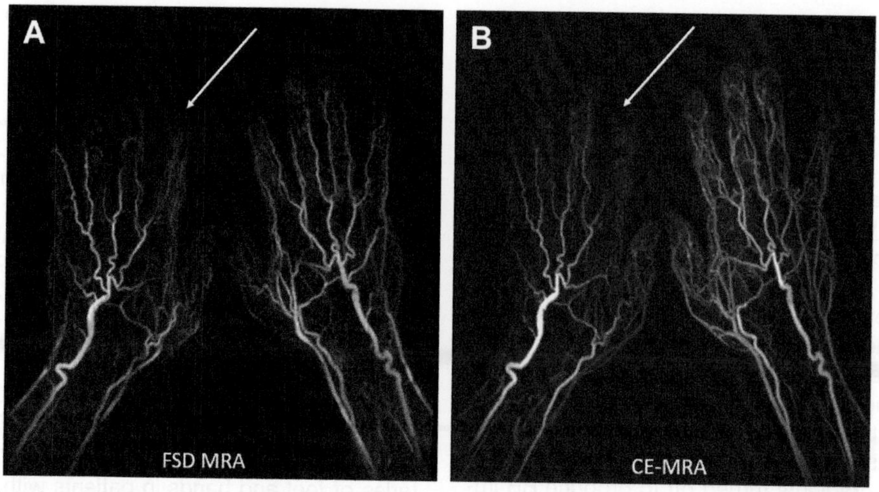


Fig. 13. Clinical application of 3D-b-SSFP FSD MRA in scleroderma. In this patient presenting with ischemia of the right hand index finger, 3D-FSD MRA demonstrates paucity of digital vessels at the tip of the right index finger (*arrow, A*), similar to CE-MRA (*arrow, B*). Also, note the attenuated distal vessels in other digits of the right hand seen on both non-contrast and CE-MRA images.

applied in three orthogonal directions to generate pairs of datasets. These pairs of datasets are subtracted from each other to produce phase (flow information) and magnitude (anatomic information) images. As stationary spins experience no net-phase shift, these are inherently suppressed on subtracted images. The Venc is decided by the operator and is guided by the area of interest. The Venc should be set slightly higher than the maximum expected velocity at the time of scanning, such that at maximum velocities, the moving spins experience a net-phase shift of $\pm 180^\circ$ (**Fig. 14**). If the velocity of blood in the vessel of interest is greater than the pre-selected Venc, aliasing occurs leading to artifactual signal loss. If the Venc is much higher than the maximum velocity, then sensitivity for slow flow is decreased.[77] Typical settings for Venc are 150 to 200 cm/s in the thoracic aorta, 250 to 400 cm/s in the aorta with aortic stenosis or coarctation, 100 to 150 cm/s for intra-cardiac flow, and 50 to 80 cm/s in large vessels of the venous system.[78] To optimize SNR for non-contrast MRA of smaller vessels, a lower Venc can be used, such as 40 cm/second for non-contrast MRA of the renal arteries.[79] For MRA or MRV, a 3D or 4D acquisition is needed, a 2D acquisition may suffice for flow information (eg, for evaluation of valvular stenosis/regurgitation).[77,80]

In 4D-flow imaging, 3D phase-contrast (PC) imaging is used along with ECG-gating to produce time-resolved 3D cine flow across the cardiac cycle. Each 4D volume comprises one magnitude volume and three velocity/flow volumes in three spatial (x, y, z) directions (**Fig. 15**). Multiple display options are possible and additional quantitative analysis can be performed on dedicated post-processing software.[78,81] Due to the volumetric nature of acquisition, specific planning is not required, and any vessel can be evaluated in the included

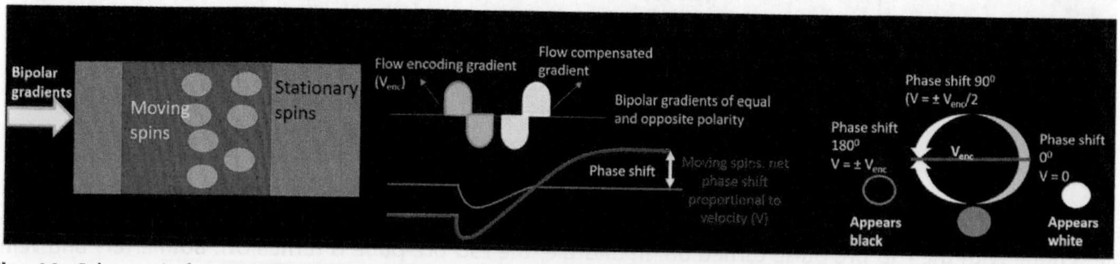


Fig. 14. Schematic for PC MRA. Bipolar flow-encoding gradients with pre-determined velocity (Venc) and flow-compensated gradient are applied in three orthogonal directions to produce pairs of images which are subtracted to produce BB images. The net-phase shift ranges from 00 to 1800, depending on the velocity (V) in relation to Venc. Stationary spins (V = 0) experience no phase shift and appear white. Moving spins ($V \leq$ Venc) show phase shift of up to 1800. Spins with V > Venc show aliasing as these experience phase shift greater than 1800.

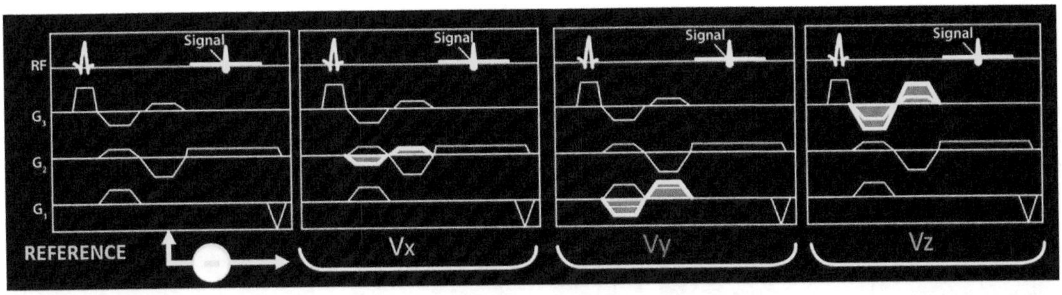


**Fig. 15.** 4D flow MR imaging. 4D flow MR acquisition comprises 3D PC imaging in three directions (x,y,x) using ECG-gating to provide time-resolved flow information across the cardiac cycle. Each 4D volume is comprised of one reference magnitude volume and three velocity/flow volumes in three spatial (Vx,Vy,Vz) directions.

field of view. The technical details of 4D-flow are beyond the scope of this review, and have been described in other comprehensive reviews.[82,83]

### *Limitations*

The scan time of PC-MRA depends on the specific sequence used and could be long. Some of the commercially available sequences could be performed more rapidly than the 3D-SSDP sequence. 3D-PC-MRA is also prone to signal losses of turbulence and tortuosity. Parallel imaging, radial sampling, and compressed sensing have all been used to decrease scan times of 4D-flow imaging by a factor of four to six times, with preserved anatomic resolution and accurate flow quantification.[84,85]

### *Current Clinical Applications*

Clinically, 3D-PC-MRA has been limited to the evaluation of mesenteric and native and transplant renal arteries. For renal artery imaging, significant flow-dephasing and signal loss in areas of turbulence indicates hemodynamically significant stenosis.[86] In the brain, 3D-PC-MRA can be used as an alternative to 3D-TOF-MRA in the presence of hemorrhage or subacute thrombosis to avoid diagnostic pitfalls induced by artifactual T1 shine-through effect on TOF-MRA. In the brain, 3D-PC-MR venogram remains popular for the detection of cerebral venous sinus stenosis or thrombosis. A low-resolution PC-MRA is also commonly used as a scout image for identifying carotid arteries (**Fig. 16**).[13]

Multiple novel clinical applications of 4D flow imaging have been described in dedicated reviews.[78,83,87] The most common application of 4D-flow imaging lies in cardiovascular imaging to depict blood flow patterns in complex congenital cardiac diseases and aortopathies.[88,89] 4D-flow imaging is also being applied for abdominal imaging for evaluation of portal circulation as well as the abdominal aorta and its major branches (**Fig. 17**).[90] In, neurovascular imaging, 4D flow imaging can be useful for the evaluation of complex arteriovenous malformations and fistulas, intracranial aneurysms, and Moya-Moya disease.[87]

## VELOCITY SELECTIVE MRA

### *Principle*

In this technique, a velocity selective magnetization preparation pulse is applied at peak systole using ECG-gating which sensitizes the sequence to arterial flow while suppressing background stationary and venous flow. The velocity selective preparation pulse comprises multiple RF pulses of small flip angles, with interleaved repeated bipolar gradients.[91,92] This is usually combined with b-SSFP readout, although alternatively gradient-echo readout can also be used to reduce the banding artifacts associated with b-SSFP (**Fig. 18**).

As the sequence is only applied in systole and diastolic acquisition is not needed, it is faster than the previously described ECG-gated subtractive MRA techniques and is insensitive to motion and cardiac arrhythmias. The sequence also has high spatial resolution and large coverage when used with 3D-b-SSFP readout.

### *Limitations and Current Clinical Applications*

This sequence is not available commercially, however, it has been shown to be feasible for cerebral MRA, abdominal MRA, and peripheral artery MRA.[93–95] The main clinical application lies in the evaluation of peripheral arterial disease in patients without stents or prostheses and with known cardiac disease.[95]

## ARTERIAL SPIN LABELING MRA

### *Principle*

Arterial spin labeling (ASL)-MRA techniques can be of three types: flow-in, flow-out, or alternate

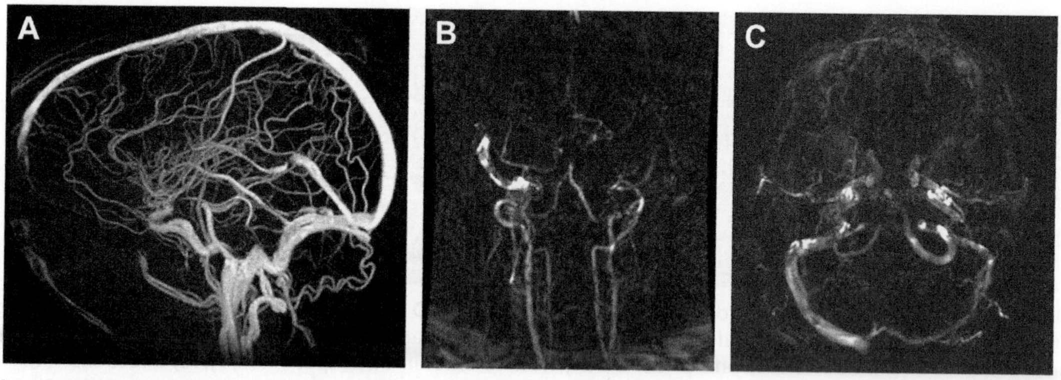


Fig. 16. Clinical applications of PC technique. (*A*) Example of 3D-phase-contrast cerebral MR venogram (MRV) showing excellent visualization of the patent cerebral venous sinuses. (*B*, *C*) Phase-contrast technique can also be used for scout images before TOF-MRA (*B*) and TOF-MRV (*C*).

tag on-off/subtracted ASL-MRA. This sequence is based on the principle of selectively "tagging" the longitudinal magnetization of flowing blood using a selective inversion recovery pulse, such that a difference is created in the longitudinal magnetization between flowing blood and stationary tissue. Following tagging and an appropriately selected inversion time (TI) such that background tissue reaches the null point, blood flowing into (flow-in) or flowing out of (flow-out) of the tagged slab can be read out by either half-Fourier FSE or b-SSFP sequence with or without additional fat suppression sequences (**Fig. 19**).[13] In the "alternate tag on-off sequence", two alternate datasets are acquired with "tag on" and "tag off" which are subtracted from each other to generate BB images from the tagged region. Thus, in the "alternate tag on-off technique", background suppression relies on subtraction and is independent of the selected TI (see **Fig. 19**).[96] Between the two readout options, b-SSFP readout provides better resolution and the flow-compensated nature of b-SSFP sequence makes it preferable for most regions, except for distal pulmonary and subclavian vessels near air–tissue interfaces where half-Fourier FSE is preferred. Half-Fourier FSE readout may be suitable for imaging vessels with slow flow like hepatic veins, portal veins, and small vessels of hands and feet where the flow-related spin dephasing effect associated with FSE sequences is not so pronounced.[13]

### *Flow-in arterial spin labeling -magnetic resonance angiography: considerations and clinical applications*

In this sequence, tagging is applied to the entire imaging slab such that both moving spins in blood and stationary spins in the background are inverted. After a certain TI, such that all spins (moving and stationary) in the tagged slab are at a null point, untagged blood flowing into the tagged slab with preserved longitudinal magnetization produces

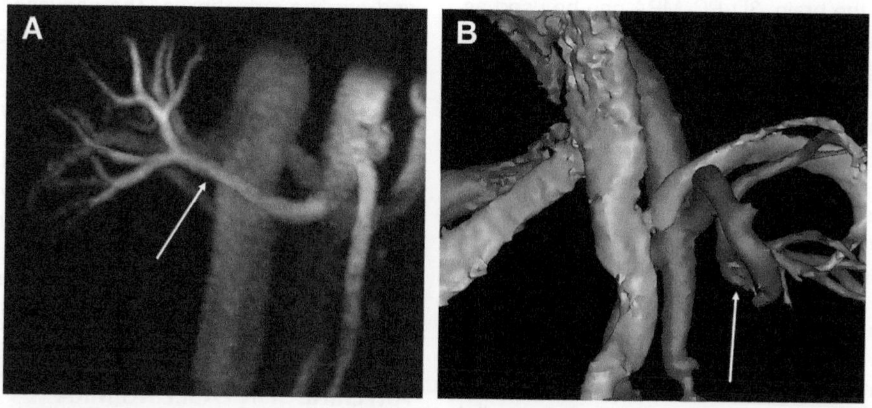


Fig. 17. Clinical application of 4D flow MRA. MIP (*A*) and volume rendered (*B*) reconstructions from non-contrast PC-MR angiographic images from a 4D flow acquisition. This provides good anatomical information on renal vessel arteries (*arrow*) without the need for intravenous contrast, which is beneficial in patients with severe renal dysfunction or contrast allergies.

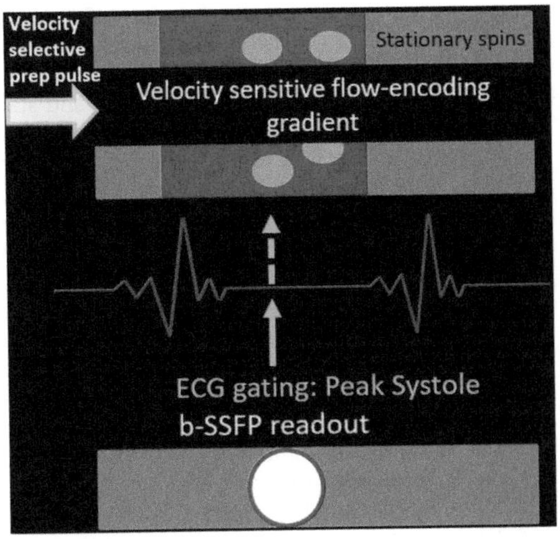


Fig. 18. Schematic for velocity selective MRA. In this ECG-gated sequence, a velocity selective preparation pulse that sensitizes to arterial flow and suppresses background stationary and venous flow is applied in peak systole with readout to produce BB images. No diastolic acquisition is performed.

BB images.[13] Thus, in this sequence, the tagged slab overlaps with the imaging volume of interest (see **Fig. 19**). As all untagged blood flowing into the slab can produce a signal, individual contributions cannot be determined, such as superior mesenteric vein and splenic vein for portal circulation.[13] As venous flow can also be seen, an additional presaturation slab is needed.

This technique is most widely validated for renal MRA for the detection of renal artery stenosis in both native and transplant kidneys (**Fig. 20**). For renal artery imaging, the sequence can be done with breath-hold or with navigator-gated respiratory gating. A thick axial band of RF pulses is applied in the region of renal vessels to invert background tissue. Following a long waiting interval (typical T1: 1200–1800 msec at 1.5 T), the readout is performed with 3D-b-SSFP sequence (see **Fig. 19**). Just before the readout, fat suppression is applied. Imaging is typically done in the axial plane for maximum inflow effect and greater signal in arteries, but this is at the expense of decreased coverage for missing accessory renal arteries. The coronal plane can cover the entire abdomen to see accessory renal arteries, but there is signal loss inferiorly in the slab. This technique has shown high accuracy for the detection of renal artery stenosis in comparison with CTA, CE-MRA, or DSA.[97–102] In a multicenter study, ASL-MRA had sensitivity of 74%, specificity of 93%, and accuracy of 90% for the detection of stenosis in comparison with CTA.[100] In a study by Parienty and colleagues, the sensitivity, specificity, and accuracy of ASL-MRA were 93%, 88%, and 91%, respectively, for the diagnosis of a stenosis of 50% or greater when compared with DSA.[101,103] In a head-to head comparison between NC-MRA and CE-MRA, both techniques showed similar detection rates for diagnosis of renal artery stenosis but NC-MRA achieved better technical success rates, feasibility, and image quality in motion artifacts than CE-MRA.[102]

### *Flow-out arterial spin labeling -magnetic resonance angiography: considerations and clinical applications*

In this sequence, first a non-selective inversion pulse is applied in the desired imaging volume to invert all magnetization (moving as well as stationary spins). This is followed by a selective inversion recovery pulse immediately upstream of the volume of interest which restores longitudinal magnetization of upstream tagged blood. At TI, stationary tissue in the imaging volume reaches the null point and the original blood in the imaging volume flows out. The tagged blood with fully restored longitudinal magnetization flows out of the tagged slab into the imaging volume to produce BB images.[13] In contrast to the flow-in technique, it is possible to select vessels with the flow-out technique as only vessels with tagged blood upstream of imaging volume will produce BB images (see **Fig. 19**).

This technique can be used for hepatic arteries, hepatic veins, and portal veins.[104–107] Double-tag techniques are used for hepatic veins with one inversion pulse (tag) on the upper liver to suppress inflowing blood from the aorta and another inversion pulse below the liver to suppress inflowing blood from portal veins.[105] Similarly for portal venograms, one inversion pulse is applied over the liver and thorax to suppress the liver, myocardium, and inflowing blood from hepatic arteries, and another inversion pulse is applied below the liver to suppress the inflowing blood from IVC.[107] Multiple tagged segments can also be used for acquisitions over a larger area of coverage for abdominopelvic MRA.[108] This technique has also been used for selective visualization of the external carotid artery and its branches.[109], and for separate visualization of pulmonary arteries and pulmonary veins by selectively placing an inversion pulse on the aorta and heart.[110]

### *Alternate tag on-off arterial spin labeling-magnetic resonance angiography: considerations and clinical applications*

As this technique relies on subtractive effects between two datasets acquired with "tag on" and "tag off" (control), this is less reliant on the precise timing of TI. Unlike flow-in and flow-out

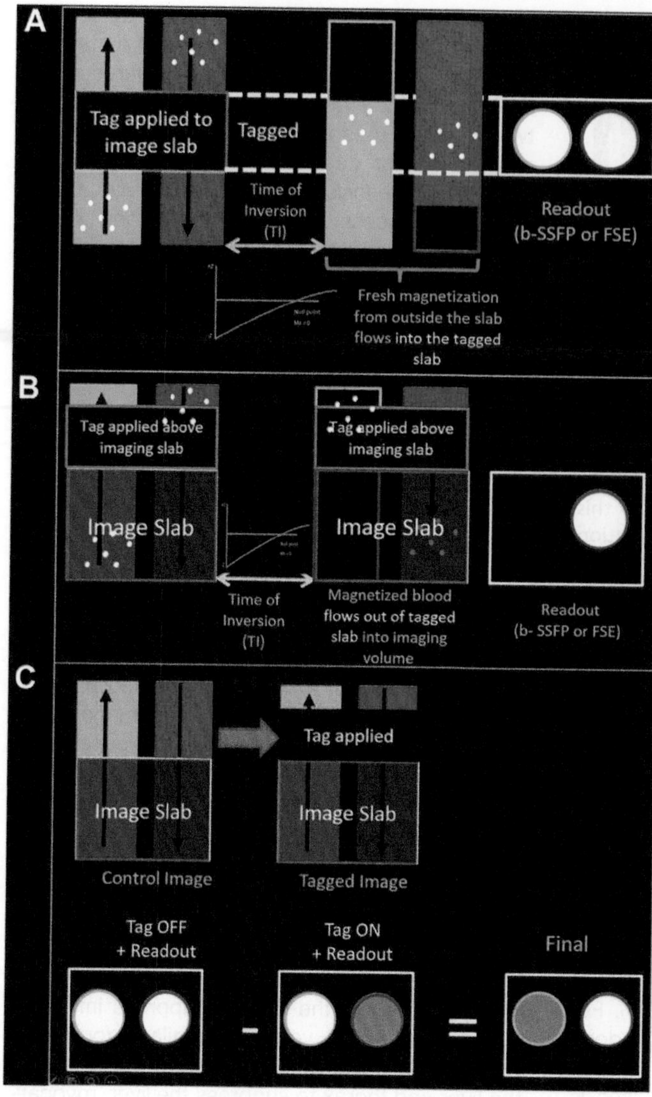


**Fig. 19.** Schematic for ASL-MRA techniques. (*A*) Flow-in ASL-MRA: Tag pulse applied to the entire image slab inverting both flowing spins (blood) and stationary spins in the slab. At the time of inversion (TI), spins in the imaging slab reach a null point and fresh inflowing blood with fully preserved longitudinal magnetization produces a bright signal at the readout. (*B*) Flow-out ASL-MRA: Initially, a non-selective inversion pulse is applied everywhere inverting both flowing spins (blood) and stationary spins in the slab. A selective tag pulse is applied on the vessel of interest upstream of imaging volume, thereby, restoring magnetization of tagged blood. At TI, stationary spins in the image slab reach a null point and the original blood in the image slab flows out. The freshly tagged blood upstream of image slab flows out of the tagged slab into the imaging volume and produces a bright signal at the readout. (*C*) Tag On/Off Subtractive ASL-MRA: In this subtractive technique, first a "tag on" image is acquired with tagging of arterial blood followed by the acquisition of a control "tag off" image. Subtraction removes stationary signal and only tagged spins produce BB images.

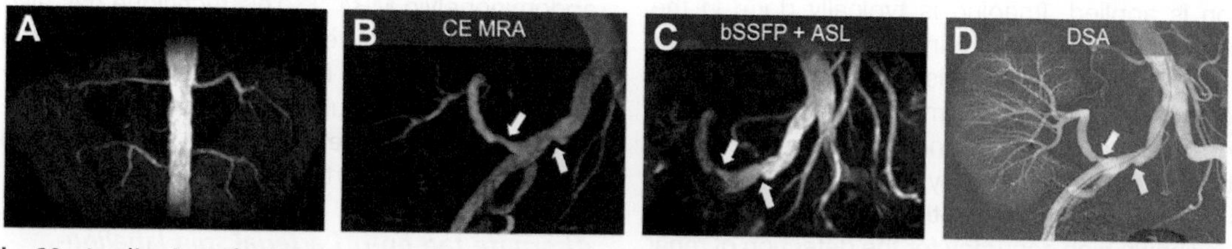


**Fig. 20.** Application of ASL-MRA in renal imaging. (*A*) ASL-MRA in a patient with a horseshoe kidneys and renovascular hypertension shows two renal arteries on each side without stenosis. (*B–D*) ASL-MRA in a patient with suspected transplant renal artery stenosis. Both CE-MRA (*B*) and ASL-MRA (*C*) show stenosis in the right common artery (*proximal yellow arrow*) and at the origin of the transplant renal artery (*white arrow*). These findings were confirmed on DSA (*D*). The gradient across the right common artery was greater than 10 mm Hg and angioplasty was performed. The gradient across the transplant renal artery was less than 10 mm Hg and no treatment was needed.

**Table 2**
**Summary of non-contrast bright blood MRA techniques**

| | TOF | QISS | 3D-B-SSFP | 3D-FSE | 3D-FSD | Phase- Contrast | VS-MRA | ASL-MRA |
|---|---|---|---|---|---|---|---|---|
| Gating | ECG-gating for peripheral MRA | ECG-gating | ECG-gating needed for cardiac, thorax, abdomen<br>Breath-hold or respiratory gated | ECG-gating | ECG-gating | ECG-gating for 4D flow MRA | ECG-gating | Breath-hold or respiratory gated for thorax, abdomen |
| Subtraction required | No | No | No | Yes | Yes | No | No | For alternate tag technique |
| Preferred vasculature | Brain, carotid, less preferred for peripheral MRA | Lower extremity<br>Newer QISS techniques: Additional regions | Coronary, aorta, great vessels of thorax, renal MRA | Large vessels of thorax, abdomen, pelvis<br>Less preferred for extremities | Distal extremities, hands, and feet | Cardiac, renal, abdomen, brain<br>4D PC: Any vessel can be imaged | Lower extremity.<br>Also feasible for cerebral MRA | Brain, carotid, renal, hepatic, portal, pulmonary |
| *Vendor names* Siemens | TOF | QISS | TrueFISP | NATIVE SPACE | Not commercially available | PC | Not commercially available | ASL-MRA |
| GE | TOF | - | FIESTA | Inhance Deltaflow | | PC, Inhance Velocity | | Inhance Inflow/ IFDIR |
| Philips | TOF | - | Balanced FFE | TRANCE | | PC, Q-Flow | | 4D-TRANCE |
| Toshiba | TOF | - | True SSFP/FFE 3D | Fresh Blood Imaging | | PS | | mASTAR |
| Hitachi | TOF | VASC | Balanced SARGE | VASC-FSE | | PC | | VASL-ASL |

*Abbreviations:* 3D: three-dimensional; ASL: arterial spin labeling; b-SSFP: balanced steady-state free precession; ECG: electrocardiogram; FSD: flow-sensitive dephasing; FSE: fast spin-echo; MRA: magnetic resonance angiography; QISS: Quiescent Interval Slice-Selective (QISS); TOF: time-of-flight ; VS: velocity selective.

ASL, where TI needs to be carefully selected to suppress background tissue, subtraction in alternate tag on-off ASL provides excellent background suppression. However, this is slower as at least two separate scans are required for subtraction. Multiple TIs can also be selected in an incremental manner for successive acquisitions to provide time-resolved MRA (or 4D-MRA). In time-resolved ASL-MRA too, the scan time increases proportionately to the number of TI increments.[12] However, with recent advances in MRI technology, 4D-MRA can capture dynamic information with comparable temporal and spatial resolution than dynamic CE-MRA and DSA.[111]

This technique is most widely used for carotid and intracranial MRA.[112] Time-resolved ASL/4D-MRA can act as a radiation-free alternative to DSA for non-invasive alternative to DSA dynamic assessment of arteriovenous malformations or arteriovenous fistula in the brain.[113–115] In the brain, ASL with pseudo-continuous labeling can be modified to provide simultaneous MRA and perfusion information.[116] This technique can also be used for imaging of vascular malformations in the pelvis and peripheral extremities, pulmonary arteries in patients with chronic pulmonary thromboembolic disease, and regions with slower flow, for example, in pedal and digital arteries of the foot.[13,117]

## MULTI-CONTRAST TECHNIQUES

Several groups of investigators have proposed multi-contrast techniques for simultaneous depiction of the vascular or cardiac chamber lumen with BB as well as the vessel and cardiac walls using DB contrast. The two most widely used techniques are Simultaneous Non-Contrast Angiography and Intra-Plaque Hemorrhage (SNAP), primarily used for carotid and cerebrovascular imaging[118] and inversion recovery prepared Magnetization Transfer Contrast Bright blOOD phase SensiTive (MTC-BOOST) that simultaneously generates co-registered 3D-BB and black-blood whole-heart images, which has been applied to the anatomical assessment of the pulmonary veins and left atrium as well in patients with congenital heart disease.[119]

### *Simultaneous Non-Contrast Angiography and Intra-Plaque Hemorrhage*

The SNAP technique was developed for the assessment and characterization of carotid atherosclerosis and utilizes a phase-sensitive reconstruction that generates images with a negative signal corresponding to MRA and a positive signal corresponding to intra-plaque hemorrhage (IPH). By displaying only the negative signals, a non-contrast MRA is rendered with no contamination from background tissues. Alternatively, displaying only the positive signals yields a highly T1-weighted image suitable for IPH detection.[118] Several proof-of-concept studies have demonstrated the clinical feasibility of the SNAP technique with high accuracy for carotid stenosis grading as well as for the detection of carotid IPH.[120,121]

### *Magnetization Transfer -BOOST*

The underlying principle of MTC-BOOST is a magnetization transfer prepared BB and black-blood phase-sensitive inversion recovery (PSIR) acquisition with two differently weighted BB volumes in an interleaved fashion. The two data sets are then combined in a PSIR-like reconstruction to obtain a complementary black-blood volume which can be used for visualization of the vessel wall or cardiac chamber walls. Image-based navigation and non-rigid respiratory motion correction are exploited for 100% scan efficiency and predictable acquisition time.[119]

Although both SNAP and MTC-BOOST can be considered investigational techniques, their dual contrast mechanism approach within a single acquisition generates high spatial resolution images with nearly perfect co-registration.

## SUMMARY

There are multiple options for non-contrast MR angiography as described in this review. **Table 2** provides a summary of the available techniques, preferred clinical applications, and various vendor-specific trade names. Understanding the principles and the relative advantages and limitations of various non-contrast MRA techniques can enable appropriate sequence selection in various clinical scenarios where contrast administration is not preferred or contraindicated.

## DISCLOSURE

Dr P.S. Rajiah—Royalties from Elsevier.

## REFERENCES


1. Schieda N, Maralani PJ, Hurrell C, et al. Updated Clinical Practice Guideline on Use of Gadolinium-Based Contrast Agents in Kidney Disease Issued by the Canadian Association of Radiologists. Can Assoc Radiol J 2019;70(3):226–32.
2. Gallo-Bernal S, Patino-Jaramillo N, Calixto CA, et al. Nephrogenic Systemic Fibrosis in Patients

with Chronic Kidney Disease after the Use of Gadolinium-Based Contrast Agents: A Review for the Cardiovascular Imager. Diagnostics 2022; 12(8):1816.

3. Mathur M, Jones JR, Weinreb JC. Gadolinium Deposition and Nephrogenic Systemic Fibrosis: A Radiologist's Primer. Radiographics 2020;40(1): 153–62.
4. Runge VM. Critical Questions Regarding Gadolinium Deposition in the Brain and Body After Injections of the Gadolinium-Based Contrast Agents, Safety, and Clinical Recommendations in Consideration of the EMA's Pharmacovigilance and Risk Assessment Committee Recommendation for Suspension of the Marketing Authorizations for 4 Linear Agents. Invest Radiol 2017;52(6):317–23.
5. Murata N, Murata K, Gonzalez-Cuyar LF, et al. Gadolinium tissue deposition in brain and bone. Magn Reson Imaging 2016;34(10):1359–65.
6. McDonald JS, McDonald RJ. MR Imaging Safety Considerations of Gadolinium-Based Contrast Agents: Gadolinium Retention and Nephrogenic Systemic Fibrosis. Magn Reson Imaging Clin N Am 2020;28(4):497–507.
7. Jalili MH, Yu T, Hassani C, et al. Contrast-enhanced MR Angiography without Gadolinium-based Contrast Material: Clinical Applications Using Ferumoxytol. Radiol Cardiothorac Imaging 2022;4(4):e210323.
8. Available at: contrast_media.pdf. https://www.acr.org/-/media/acr/files/clinical-resources/contrast_media.pdf. Accessed February 27, 2023.
9. Edelman RR, Koktzoglou I. Non-contrast MR angiography: An update. J Magn Reson Imaging 2019; 49(2):355–73.
10. Kato Y, Ambale-Venkatesh B, Kassai Y, et al. Non-contrast coronary magnetic resonance angiography: current frontiers and future horizons. Magma N Y N 2020;33(5):591–612.
11. Navot B, Hecht EM, Lim RP, et al. MR Angiography Series: Fundamentals of Non–Contrast-enhanced MR Angiography. Radiographics 2021. https://doi.org/10.1148/rg.2021210141.
12. Wheaton AJ, Miyazaki M. Non-contrast enhanced MR angiography: Physical principles. J Magn Reson Imaging 2012;36(2):286–304.
13. Miyazaki M, Akahane M. Non-contrast enhanced MR angiography: Established techniques. J Magn Reson Imaging 2012;35(1):1–19.
14. Ludwig DR, Shetty AS, Broncano J, et al. Magnetic Resonance Angiography of the Thoracic Vasculature: Technique and Applications. J Magn Reson Imaging 2020;52(2):325–47.
15. Kourtidou S, Jones MR, Moore RA, et al. mDixon ECG-gated 3-dimensional cardiovascular magnetic resonance angiography in patients with congenital cardiovascular disease. J Cardiovasc Magn Reson 2019;21(1):52.
16. Heerfordt J, Stuber M, Maillot A, et al. A quantitative comparison between a navigated Cartesian and a self-navigated radial protocol from clinical studies for free-breathing 3D whole-heart bSSFP coronary MRA. Magn Reson Med 2020;84(1):157–69.
17. Fotaki A, Munoz C, Emanuel Y, et al. Efficient non-contrast enhanced 3D Cartesian cardiovascular magnetic resonance angiography of the thoracic aorta in 3 min. J Cardiovasc Magn Reson 2022; 24(1):5.
18. François CJ, Tuite D, Deshpande V, et al. Pulmonary vein imaging with unenhanced three-dimensional balanced steady-state free precession MR angiography: initial clinical evaluation. Radiology 2009;250(3):932–9.
19. François CJ, Tuite D, Deshpande V, et al. Unenhanced MR Angiography of the Thoracic Aorta: Initial Clinical Evaluation. Am J Roentgenol 2008; 190(4):902–6.
20. Potthast S, Mitsumori L, Stanescu LA, et al. Measuring aortic diameter with different MR techniques: comparison of three-dimensional (3D) navigated steady-state free-precession (SSFP), 3D contrast-enhanced magnetic resonance angiography (CE-MRA), 2D T2 black blood, and 2D cine SSFP. J Magn Reson Imaging JMRI 2010;31(1): 177–84.
21. Amano Y, Takahama K, Kumita S. Non-contrast-enhanced MR angiography of the thoracic aorta using cardiac and navigator-gated magnetization-prepared three-dimensional steady-state free precession. J Magn Reson Imaging JMRI 2008;27(3): 504–9.
22. Herborn CU, Watkins DM, Runge VM, et al. Renal Arteries: Comparison of Steady-State Free Precession MR Angiography and Contrast-enhanced MR Angiography. Radiology 2006;239(1):263–8.
23. Maki JH, Wilson GJ, Eubank WB, et al. Steady-state free precession MRA of the renal arteries: breath-hold and navigator-gated techniques vs. CE-MRA. J Magn Reson Imaging JMRI 2007; 26(4):966–73.
24. Tao W, Shen Y, Guo L, et al. Role of non-contrast balanced steady-state free precession megnetic resonance angiography compared to contrast-enhanced megnetic resonance angiography in diagnosing renal artery stenosis: a meta-analysis. Chin Med J (Engl). 2014;127(19):3483–90.
25. Helyar VG, Gupta Y, Blakeway L, et al. Depiction of lower limb venous anatomy in patients undergoing interventional deep venous reconstruction-the role of balanced steady state free precession MRI. Br J Radiol 2018;91(1082):20170005.
26. Parker DL, Yuan C, Blatter DD. MR angiography by multiple thin slab 3D acquisition. Magn Reson Med 1991;17(2):434–51.

27. Davis WL, Blatter DD, Harnsberger HR, et al. Intracranial MR angiography: comparison of single-volume three-dimensional time-of-flight and multiple overlapping thin slab acquisition techniques. AJR Am J Roentgenol 1994;163(4):915–20.
28. Goodrich KC, Blatter DD, Parker DL, et al. A quantitative study of ramped radio frequency, magnetization transfer, and slab thickness in three-dimensional time-of-flight magnetic resonance angiography in a patient population. Invest Radiol 1996;31(6):323–32.
29. Cavallo AU, Koktzoglou I, Edelman RR, et al. Non-contrast Magnetic Resonance Angiography for the Diagnosis of Peripheral Vascular Disease. Circ Cardiovasc Imaging 2019;12(5):e008844.
30. Drutman J, Gyorke A, Davis WL, et al. Evaluation of subclavian steal with two-dimensional phase-contrast and two-dimensional time-of-flight MR angiography. AJNR Am J Neuroradiol 1994;15(9):1642–5.
31. Hutter J, Grimm R, Forman C, et al. Highly undersampled peripheral Time-of-Flight magnetic resonance angiography: optimized data acquisition and iterative image reconstruction. Magma N Y N 2015;28(5):437–46.
32. Fushimi Y, Okada T, Kikuchi T, et al. Clinical evaluation of time-of-flight MR angiography with sparse undersampling and iterative reconstruction for cerebral aneurysms. NMR Biomed 2017;30(11). https://doi.org/10.1002/nbm.3774.
33. Sakata A, Fushimi Y, Okada T, et al. Evaluation of cerebral arteriovenous shunts: a comparison of parallel imaging time-of-flight magnetic resonance angiography (TOF-MRA) and compressed sensing TOF-MRA to digital subtraction angiography. Neuroradiology 2021;63(6):879–87.
34. HaiFeng L, YongSheng X, YangQin X, et al. Diagnostic value of 3D time-of-flight magnetic resonance angiography for detecting intracranial aneurysm: a meta-analysis. Neuroradiology 2017; 59(11):1083–92.
35. Ahmed SU, Mocco J, Zhang X, et al. MRA versus DSA for the follow-up imaging of intracranial aneurysms treated using endovascular techniques: a meta-analysis. J Neurointerventional Surg 2019; 11(10):1009–14.
36. Edelman RR, Sheehan JJ, Dunkle E, et al. Quiescent-interval single-shot unenhanced magnetic resonance angiography of peripheral vascular disease: Technical considerations and clinical feasibility. Magn Reson Med 2010;63(4):951–8.
37. Lombardi P, Carr JC, Allen BD, et al. Updates in Magnetic Resonance Venous Imaging. Semin Interv Radiol 2021;38(2):202–8.
38. Edelman RR, Carr M, Koktzoglou I. Advances in non-contrast quiescent-interval slice-selective (QISS) magnetic resonance angiography. Clin Radiol 2019;74(1):29–36.
39. Varga-Szemes A, Aherne EA, Schoepf UJ, et al. Free-Breathing Fast Low-Angle Shot Quiescent-Interval Slice-Selective Magnetic Resonance Angiography for Improved Detection of Vascular Stenoses in the Pelvis and Abdomen: Technical Development. Invest Radiol 2019;54(12):752–6.
40. Edelman RR, Giri S, Murphy IG, et al. Ungated radial quiescent-inflow single-shot (UnQISS) magnetic resonance angiography using optimized azimuthal equidistant projections: Ungated Quiescent-Inflow Single-Shot MRA. Magn Reson Med 2014;72(6):1522–9.
41. Koktzoglou I, Edelman RR. Radial Fast Interrupted Steady-State (FISS) Magnetic Resonance Imaging. Magn Reson Med 2018;79(4):2077–86.
42. Koktzoglou I, Huang R, Ong AL, et al. Feasibility of a sub-3-minute imaging strategy for ungated quiescent interval slice-selective MRA of the extracranial carotid arteries using radial k-space sampling and deep learning-based image processing. Magn Reson Med 2020;84(2):825–37.
43. Koktzoglou I, Gupta N, Edelman RR. Nonenhanced extracranial carotid MR angiography using arterial spin labeling: Improved performance with pseudo-continuous tagging. J Magn Reson Imaging 2011; 34(2):384–94.
44. Verma M, Pandey NN, Singh V, et al. A meta-analysis of the diagnostic performance of quiescent-interval-single-shot magnetic resonance angiography in peripheral arterial disease. Eur Radiol 2022;32(4):2393–403.
45. Lam A, Perchyonok Y, Ranatunga D, et al. Accuracy of non-contrast quiescent-interval single-shot and quiescent-interval single-shot arterial spin-labelled magnetic resonance angiography in assessment of peripheral arterial disease in a diabetic population. J Med Imaging Radiat Oncol 2020;64(1):35–43.
46. Salehi Ravesh M, Lebenatus A, Bonietzki A, et al. High-resolution, non-contrast-enhanced magnetic resonance angiography of the wrist, hand and digital arteries using optimized implementation of Cartesian quiescent interval slice selective (QISS) at 1.5 T. Magn Reson Imaging 2021;78:58–68.
47. LaBounty TM, Bhave N, Giri S, et al. Comparison of ileofemoral arterial access size between noncontrast 3T MR angiography and contrast-enhanced computed tomographic angiography in patients referred for transcatheter aortic valve replacement. J Magn Reson Imaging 2017;46(6):1847–50.
48. Cannaò PM, Muscogiuri G, Schoepf UJ, et al. Technical Feasibility of a Combined Noncontrast Magnetic Resonance Protocol for Preoperative Transcatheter Aortic Valve Replacement Evaluation. J Thorac Imaging 2018;33(1):60–7.
49. Ferreira Botelho MP, Koktzoglou I, Collins JD, et al. MR imaging of iliofemoral peripheral vascular

calcifications using proton density-weighted, in-phase three-dimensional stack-of-stars gradient echo: MRI of Iliofemoral Peripheral Vascular Calcifications. Magn Reson Med 2017;77(6):2146–52.
50. Edelman RR, Silvers RI, Thakrar KH, et al. Nonenhanced MR angiography of the pulmonary arteries using single-shot radial quiescent-interval slice-selective (QISS): a technical feasibility study. J Cardiovasc Magn Reson 2017;19(1):48.
51. Salehi Ravesh M, Tesch K, Lebenatus A, et al. Clinical Value of Noncontrast-Enhanced Radial Quiescent-Interval Slice-Selective (QISS) Magnetic Resonance Angiography for the Diagnosis of Acute Pulmonary Embolism Compared to Contrast-Enhanced Computed Tomography and Cartesian Balanced Steady-State Free Precession. J Magn Reson Imaging 2020;52(5):1510–24.
52. Edelman RR, Giri S, Pursnani A, et al. Breath-hold imaging of the coronary arteries using Quiescent-Interval Slice-Selective (QISS) magnetic resonance angiography: pilot study at 1.5 Tesla and 3 Tesla. J Cardiovasc Magn Reson 2015;17:101.
53. Koktzoglou I, Murphy IG, Giri S, et al. Quiescent interval low angle shot magnetic resonance angiography of the extracranial carotid arteries: QLASH MRA of the Carotid Arteries. Magn Reson Med 2016;75(5):2072–7.
54. Koktzoglou I, Edelman RR. Super-resolution intracranial quiescent interval slice-selective magnetic resonance angiography. Magn Reson Med 2018; 79(2):683–91.
55. Shen D, Edelman RR, Robinson JD, et al. Single-Shot Coronary Quiescent-Interval Slice-Selective Magnetic Resonance Angiography Using Compressed Sensing: A Feasibility Study in Patients With Congenital Heart Disease. J Comput Assist Tomogr 2018;42(5):739–46.
56. Mostafa K, Pfarr J, Langguth P, et al. Clinical Evaluation of Non-Contrast-Enhanced Radial Quiescent-Interval Slice-Selective (QISS) Magnetic Resonance Angiography in Comparison to Contrast-Enhanced Computed Tomography Angiography for the Evaluation of Endoleaks after Abdominal Endovascular Aneurysm Repair. J Clin Med 2022;11(21):6551.
57. Miyazaki M, Sugiura S, Tateishi F, et al. Non-contrast-enhanced MR angiography using 3D ECG-synchronized half-Fourier fast spin echo. J Magn Reson Imaging JMRI 2000;12(5):776–83.
58. Lim RP, Storey P, Atanasova IP, et al. Three-dimensional electrocardiographically gated variable flip angle FSE imaging for MR angiography of the hands at 3.0 T: initial experience. Radiology 2009; 252(3):874–81.
59. Nakamura K, Miyazaki M, Kuroki K, et al. Noncontrast-enhanced peripheral MRA: Technical optimization of flow-spoiled fresh blood imaging for screening peripheral arterial diseases. Magn Reson Med 2011;65(2):595–602.
60. Urata J, Miyazaki M, Wada H, et al. Clinical evaluation of aortic diseases using nonenhanced MRA with ECG-triggered 3D half-Fourier FSE. J Magn Reson Imaging 2001;14(2):113–9.
61. Suga K, Ogasawara N, Okada M, et al. Lung perfusion impairments in pulmonary embolic and airway obstruction with non-contrast MR imaging. J Appl Physiol Bethesda Md 1985 2002;92(6):2439–51.
62. Ogasawara N, Suga K, Zaki M, et al. Assessment of lung perfusion impairment in patients with pulmonary artery-occlusive and chronic obstructive pulmonary diseases with noncontrast electrocardiogram-gated fast-spin-echo perfusion MR imaging. J Magn Reson Imaging JMRI 2004; 20(4):601–11.
63. Ward EV, Galizia MS, Usman A, et al. Comparison of quiescent inflow single-shot and native space for nonenhanced peripheral MR angiography. J Magn Reson Imaging JMRI 2013;38(6):1531–8.
64. Haneder S, Attenberger UI, Riffel P, et al. Magnetic resonance angiography (MRA) of the calf station at 3.0 T: intraindividual comparison of non-enhanced ECG-gated flow-dependent MRA, continuous table movement MRA and time-resolved MRA. Eur Radiol 2011;21(7):1452–61.
65. Lim RP, Hecht EM, Xu J, et al. 3D nongadolinium-enhanced ECG-gated MRA of the distal lower extremities: Preliminary clinical experience. J Magn Reson Imaging 2008;28(1):181–9.
66. Ono A, Murase K, Taniguchi T, et al. Deep vein thrombosis using noncontrast-enhanced MR venography with electrocardiographically gated three-dimensional half-Fourier FSE: preliminary experience. Magn Reson Med 2009;61(4):907–17.
67. Fan Z, Saouaf R, Liu X, et al. Non-Contrast MR Angiography: Flow-Sensitive Dephasing (FSD)-Prepared 3D Balanced SSFP. MAGNETOM Flash 2013;4:2–7.
68. Fan Z, Sheehan J, Bi X, et al. 3D noncontrast MR angiography of the distal lower extremities using flow-sensitive dephasing (FSD)-prepared balanced SSFP. Magn Reson Med 2009;62(6):1523–32.
69. Fan Z, Zhou X, Bi X, et al. Determination of the optimal first-order gradient moment for flow-sensitive dephasing magnetization-prepared 3D noncontrast MR angiography. Magn Reson Med 2011;65(4):964–72.
70. Fan Z, Hodnett PA, Davarpanah AH, et al. Noncontrast Magnetic Resonance Angiography of the Hand: Improved Arterial Conspicuity by Multidirectional Flow-Sensitive Dephasing Magnetization Preparation in 3D Balanced Steady-State Free Precession Imaging. Invest Radiol 2011;46(8):515.
71. Lim RP, Fan Z, Chatterji M, et al. Comparison of Nonenhanced MR Angiographic Subtraction

Techniques for Infragenual Arteries at 1.5 T: A Preliminary Study. Radiology 2013;267(1):293–304.
72. Sheehan JJ, Fan Z, Davarpanah AH, et al. Nonenhanced MR Angiography of the Hand with Flow-Sensitive Dephasing-prepared Balanced SSFP Sequence: Initial Experience with Systemic Sclerosis. Radiology 2011;259(1):248–56.
73. Zhang N, Fan Z, Luo N, et al. Noncontrast MR angiography (MRA) of infragenual arteries using flow-sensitive dephasing (FSD)-prepared steady-state free precession (SSFP) at 3.0 Tesla: Comparison with contrast-enhanced MRA. J Magn Reson Imaging 2016;43(2):364–72.
74. Liu J, Zhang N, Fan Z, et al. Image Quality and Stenosis Assessment of Non-Contrast-Enhanced 3-T Magnetic Resonance Angiography in Patients with Peripheral Artery Disease Compared with Contrast-Enhanced Magnetic Resonance Angiography and Digital Subtraction Angiography. PLoS One 2016;11(11):e0166467.
75. Liu X, Fan Z, Zhang N, et al. Unenhanced MR angiography of the foot: initial experience of using flow-sensitive dephasing-prepared steady-state free precession in patients with diabetes. Radiology 2014;272(3):885–94.
76. Liu X, Zhang N, Fan Z, et al. Detection of infragenual arterial disease using non–contrast-enhanced MR angiography in patients with diabetes. J Magn Reson Imaging 2014;40(6):1422–9.
77. Wymer DT, Patel KP, Burke WF, et al. Phase-Contrast MRI: Physics, Techniques, and Clinical Applications. Radiographics 2020;40(1):122–40.
78. Stankovic Z, Allen BD, Garcia J, et al. 4D flow imaging with MRI. Cardiovasc Diagn Ther 2014; 4(2):173–92.
79. François CJ, Lum DP, Johnson KM, et al. Renal arteries: isotropic, high-spatial-resolution, unenhanced MR angiography with three-dimensional radial phase contrast. Radiology 2011;258(1):254–60.
80. Hom JJ, Ordovas K, Reddy GP. Velocity-encoded Cine MR Imaging in Aortic Coarctation: Functional Assessment of Hemodynamic Events. Radiographics 2008;28(2):407–16.
81. Roldán-Alzate A, Francois CJ, Wieben O, et al. Emerging Applications of Abdominal 4D Flow MRI. AJR Am J Roentgenol 2016;207(1):58–66.
82. Azarine A, Garçon P, Stansal A, et al. Four-dimensional Flow MRI: Principles and Cardiovascular Applications. Radiographics 2019;39(3):632–48.
83. Markl M, Schnell S, Barker AJ. 4D flow imaging: current status to future clinical applications. Curr Cardiol Rep 2014;16(5):481.
84. Neuhaus E, Weiss K, Bastkowski R, et al. Accelerated aortic 4D flow cardiovascular magnetic resonance using compressed sensing: applicability, validation and clinical integration. J Cardiovasc Magn Reson 2019;21(1):65.
85. Pathrose A, Ma L, Berhane H, et al. Highly accelerated aortic 4D flow MRI using compressed sensing: Performance at different acceleration factors in patients with aortic disease. Magn Reson Med 2021;85(4):2174–87.
86. de Boer A, Villa G, Bane O, et al. Consensus-Based Technical Recommendations for Clinical Translation of Renal Phase Contrast MRI. J Magn Reson Imaging 2022;55(2):323–35.
87. Youn SW, Lee J. From 2D to 4D Phase-Contrast MRI in the Neurovascular System: Will It Be a Quantum Jump or a Fancy Decoration? J Magn Reson Imaging 2022;55(2):347–72.
88. Dyverfeldt P, Bissell M, Barker AJ, et al. 4D flow cardiovascular magnetic resonance consensus statement. J Cardiovasc Magn Reson 2015;17(1): 72.
89. Zhong L, Schrauben EM, Garcia J, et al. Intracardiac 4D Flow MRI in Congenital Heart Disease: Recommendations on Behalf of the ISMRM Flow & Motion Study Group. J Magn Reson Imaging 2019;50(3):677–81.
90. Oechtering TH, Roberts GS, Panagiotopoulos N, et al. Abdominal Applications of Quantitative 4D Flow MRI. Abdom Radiol N Y 2022;47(9):3229–50.
91. Shin T, Hu BS, Nishimura DG. Off-resonance-robust velocity-selective magnetization preparation for non-contrast-enhanced peripheral MR angiography. Magn Reson Med 2013;70(5): 1229–40.
92. de Rochefort L, Maître X, Bittoun J, et al. Velocity-selective RF pulses in MRI. Magn Reson Med 2006;55(1):171–6.
93. Qin Q, Shin T, Schär M, et al. Velocity-Selective Magnetization-Prepared Non-Contrast-Enhanced Cerebral MR Angiography at 3T: Improved Immunity to B0/B1 Inhomogeneity. Magn Reson Med 2016;75(3):1232–41.
94. Zhu D, Li W, Liu D, et al. Non-contrast-enhanced abdominal MRA at 3 T using velocity-selective pulse trains. Magn Reson Med 2020;84(3): 1173–83.
95. Shin T, Menon RG, Thomas RB, et al. Unenhanced Velocity-Selective MR Angiography (VS-MRA): Initial Clinical Evaluation in Patients With Peripheral Artery Disease. J Magn Reson Imaging 2019;49(3): 744–51.
96. Edelman RR, Siewert B, Adamis M, et al. Signal targeting with alternating radiofrequency (STAR) sequences: application to MR angiography. Magn Reson Med 1994;31(2):233–8.
97. Zhang LJ, Peng J, Wen J, et al. Non-contrast-enhanced magnetic resonance angiography: a reliable clinical tool for evaluating transplant renal artery stenosis. Eur Radiol 2018;28(10):4195–204.
98. Sebastià C, Sotomayor AD, Paño B, et al. Accuracy of unenhanced magnetic resonance angiography

for the assessment of renal artery stenosis. Eur J Radiol Open 2016;3:200–6.
99. Braidy C, Daou I, Diop AD, et al. Unenhanced MR angiography of renal arteries: 51 patients. AJR Am J Roentgenol 2012;199(5):W629–37.
100. Albert TSE, Akahane M, Parienty I, et al. An international multicenter comparison of time-SLIP unenhanced MR angiography and contrast-enhanced CT angiography for assessing renal artery stenosis: the renal artery contrast-free trial. AJR Am J Roentgenol 2015;204(1):182–8.
101. Parienty I, Rostoker G, Jouniaux F, et al. Renal artery stenosis evaluation in chronic kidney disease patients: nonenhanced time-spatial labeling inversion-pulse three-dimensional MR angiography with regulated breathing versus DSA. Radiology 2011;259(2):592–601.
102. Liang KW, Chen JW, Huang HH, et al. The Performance of Noncontrast Magnetic Resonance Angiography in Detecting Renal Artery Stenosis as Compared With Contrast Enhanced Magnetic Resonance Angiography Using Conventional Angiography as a Reference. J Comput Assist Tomogr 2017;41(4):619–27.
103. Bley TA, François CJ, Schiebler ML, et al. Non-contrast-enhanced MRA of renal artery stenosis: validation against DSA in a porcine model. Eur Radiol 2016;26(2):547–55.
104. Shimada K, Isoda H, Okada T, et al. Non-contrast-enhanced MR portography with time-spatial labeling inversion pulses: Comparison of imaging with three-dimensional half-fourier fast spin-echo and true steady-state free-precession sequences. J Magn Reson Imaging 2009;29(5):1140–6.
105. Shimada K, Isoda H, Okada T, et al. Non-contrast-enhanced MR angiography for selective visualization of the hepatic vein and inferior vena cava with true steady-state free-precession sequence and time-spatial labeling inversion pulses: Preliminary results. J Magn Reson Imaging 2009;29(2):474–9.
106. Shimada K, Isoda H, Okada T, et al. Non-contrast-enhanced hepatic MR angiography with true steady-state free-precession and time spatial labeling inversion pulse: optimization of the technique and preliminary results. Eur J Radiol 2009;70(1):111–7.
107. Ohno T, Isoda H, Furuta A, et al. Non-contrast-enhanced MR portography and hepatic venography with time-spatial labeling inversion pulses: comparison at 1.5 Tesla and 3 Tesla. Acta Radiol Open 2015;4(5). 2058460115584110.
108. Atanasova IP, Kim D, Lim RP, et al. Noncontrast MR angiography for comprehensive assessment of abdominopelvic arteries using quadruple inversion-recovery preconditioning and 3D balanced steady-state free precession imaging. J Magn Reson Imaging JMRI 2011;33(6):1430–9.
109. Satogami N, Okada T, Koyama T, et al. Visualization of external carotid artery and its branches: non-contrast-enhanced MR angiography using balanced steady-state free-precession sequence and a time-spatial labeling inversion pulse. J Magn Reson Imaging JMRI 2009;30(3):678–83.
110. Okuaki T, Ishimoto T, Miyati T, et al. Separate pulmonary artery and vein magnetic resonance angiography by use of an arterial spin labeling method. Radiol Phys Technol 2014;7(2):352–7.
111. Eddleman CS, Jeong HJ, Hurley MC, et al. 4D radial acquisition contrast-enhanced MR angiography and intracranial arteriovenous malformations: quickly approaching digital subtraction angiography. Stroke 2009;40(8):2749–53.
112. Suzuki Y, Fujima N, van Osch MJP. Intracranial 3D and 4D MR Angiography Using Arterial Spin Labeling: Technical Considerations. Magn Reson Med Sci 2020;19(4):294–309.
113. Rojas-Villabona A, Pizzini FB, Solbach T, et al. Are Dynamic Arterial Spin-Labeling MRA and Time-Resolved Contrast-Enhanced MRA Suited for Confirmation of Obliteration following Gamma Knife Radiosurgery of Brain Arteriovenous Malformations? AJNR Am J Neuroradiol 2021;42(4):671–8.
114. Jensen-Kondering U, Lindner T, van Osch MJP, et al. Superselective pseudo-continuous arterial spin labeling angiography. Eur J Radiol 2015;84(9):1758–67.
115. Fujima N, Osanai T, Shimizu Y, et al. Utility of noncontrast-enhanced time-resolved four-dimensional MR angiography with a vessel-selective technique for intracranial arteriovenous malformations. J Magn Reson Imaging JMRI 2016;44(4):834–45.
116. Suzuki Y, Helle M, Koken P, et al. Simultaneous acquisition of perfusion image and dynamic MR angiography using time-encoded pseudo-continuous ASL. Magn Reson Med 2018;79(5):2676–84.
117. Altes TA, Mai VM, Munger TM, et al. Pulmonary embolism: comprehensive evaluation with MR ventilation and perfusion scanning with hyperpolarized helium-3, arterial spin tagging, and contrast-enhanced MRA. J Vasc Interv Radiol JVIR 2005;16(7):999–1005.
118. Wang J, Börnert P, Zhao H, et al. Simultaneous noncontrast angiography and intraplaque hemorrhage (SNAP) imaging for carotid atherosclerotic disease evaluation. Magn Reson Med 2013;69(2):337–45.
119. Ginami G, Lòpez K, Mukherjee RK, et al. Non-contrast enhanced simultaneous 3D whole-heart bright-blood pulmonary veins visualization and

black-blood quantification of atrial wall thickness. Magn Reson Med 2019;81(2):1066–79.

120. Li D, Qiao H, Han Y, et al. Histological validation of simultaneous non-contrast angiography and intraplaque hemorrhage imaging (SNAP) for characterizing carotid intraplaque hemorrhage. Eur Radiol 2021;31(5):3106–15.

121. Li D, Zhao H, Chen X, et al. Identification of intraplaque haemorrhage in carotid artery by simultaneous non-contrast angiography and intraPlaque hemorrhage (SNAP) imaging: a magnetic resonance vessel wall imaging study. Eur Radiol 2018;28(4):1681–6.

# Magnetic Resonance Angiography of the Arteries of the Upper and Lower Extremities

Ayaz Aghayev, MD*, Michael Steigner, MD

**KEYWORDS**

• Magnetic resonance angiography • Upper extremity artery • Lower extremity artery

**KEY POINTS**

- Magnetic resonance angiography (MRA) can provide high temporal and relatively high spatial resolution images of both upper and lower extremity arteries.
- Contrast-enhanced (CE)-MRA with gadolinium-based contrast agents (GBCA) is the most utilized technique for assessing ischemic and non-ischemic arterial pathologies.
- Non-contrast MRA is an alternative option for patients with chronic kidney disease or contraindication to GBCA.
- An alternative off-label contrast agent, such as ferumoxytol, can be used in specific clinical scenarios when CE-MRA is necessary and GBCA is contraindicated.

## INTRODUCTION

Arterial pathologies can be diagnosed using various imaging modalities, including ultrasound (US), computed tomography angiography (CTA), magnetic resonance angiography (MRA), and diagnostic catheter angiography (DCA).[1] Although each modality has its advantages and disadvantages, DCA utilization has substantially decreased due to its invasiveness and has been replaced by other modalities. However, DCA has the highest spatial and temporal resolutions compared with other modalities and is still considered the standard of reference in extremity artery imaging. Meanwhile, with both B-mode and Doppler techniques, US is the first-line imaging modality for screening and diagnosing extremity artery pathologies.[1] US has high spatial resolution that can provide dynamic/flow information on the vasculature. However, limitations of US include limited access to the proximal segments of extremity arteries, particularly upper extremity (UE) vessels, lack of global capture of the arteries, and dependence on sonographer experience. Data from the national Medicare claims database showed that utilization of non-invasive angiography techniques have substantially increased over the last two decades due to the adoption of CTA.[2] CTA can provide high spatial resolution images and can be easily performed on arteries of the extremities. However, disadvantages of CTA include radiation exposure and administration of nephrotoxic contrast agents that may pose a risk in patients with acute kidney injury. Moreover, dense vessel wall calcifications (ie, blooming artifacts) limits the luminal assessment of small vessels. However, novel technologies in CT, including dual-energy or photon-counting CT, can resolve the latter limitation.

An alternative for extremity artery imaging is MRA, which can provide dynamic imaging with high soft tissue contrast. Although MRA has the lowest spatial resolution among the abovementioned imaging

Cardiovascular Imaging Program, Department of Radiology, Brigham and Women's Hospital, Harvard Medical School, Boston, MA, USA
* Corresponding author. Harvard Medical School.
*E-mail address:* AAGHAYEV@BWH.HARVARD.EDU

Magn Reson Imaging Clin N Am 31 (2023) 361–372
https://doi.org/10.1016/j.mric.2023.04.002

modalities, recent advances in hardware, pulse sequences, and image reconstruction algorithms have enabled extremity artery imaging with high spatial resolution and signal-to-noise ratio (SNR). Extremity artery imaging is usually performed with a gadolinium-based contrast agent (GBCA), which is known as contrast-enhanced MRA (CE-MRA). However, the use of GBCA in patients with chronic kidney disease (CKD) has been traditionally limited due to the risk for nephrogenic systemic fibrosis (NSF) or accumulation of gadolinium in the brain and bones.[3,4] In contrast, data demonstrated that not all GBCAs lead to similar side effects. An alternative to GBCA, ferumoxytol has been safely used as an off-label contrast agent in MRA to diagnose vascular pathologies.[5] Ferumoxytol was originally approved to treat iron-deficiency anemia in patients with CKD; however, given its unique features, including a long intravascular half-time, less immunogenicity, and ideal MR relaxometry, it has been utilized in MR imaging since 2009. Non-contrast MRA (NC-MRA) techniques have been developed in recent years to replace CE studies in arteries of the extremities; however, the utilization of these techniques remains limited due to spatial resolution issues and difficulties in imaging small vessels of the extremities.

In this article, we will review the available MRA imaging techniques, protocols, and utilization of MRA in assessing extremity artery pathologies.

## MAGNETIC RESONANCE ANGIOGRAPHIC IMAGING TECHNIQUES FOR ARTERIES OF THE EXTREMITIES

Extremity artery imaging can be performed with CE-MRA and NC-MRA to assess both ischemic and non-ischemic pathologies. The goal of extremity MRA is to obtain the highest possible image resolution with sufficient vessel contrast intensity to visualize arteries without venous contamination.

### *Contrast-Enhanced Magnetic Resonance Angiography*

CE-MRA is predominantly performed to visualize arteries of the extremities as it has high temporal resolution, which allows the capture of early arterial flow and real-time flow dynamics in vessels. Additionally, recent technological advances have resulted in high spatial resolution images from CE-MRA, allowing visualization of small vessels in the hands or feet. Compared to NC-MRA, CE-MRA produces fewer artifacts and is less dependent on vessel orientation as it mostly depends on (1) injected contrast agents (mostly GBCA), (2) timing of contrast injection and image acquisition, and (3) sequences.

#### *1. Contrast agents*

Most are gadolinium-based; however, off-label non-gadolinium-based medications (ferumoxytol) have been safely used in MRA. A detailed discussion of GBCA is out of the scope of this article, but it is imperative to mention important nuances that the American College of Radiology (ACR) has implemented in recent guidelines. GBCA has been divided into three groups depending on the risk of NSF[6]: group I (gadodiamide, gadopentetate dimeglumine, gadoversetamide); group II (gadobenate dimeglumine, gadobutrol, gadoterate meglumine, gadoteridol); and group III (gadoxetate disodium). Of note, not all GBCAs have similar side effects. A recent meta-analysis has shown that the risk for NSF with group II GBCAs is <0.07% in patients with stage 4/5 CKD.[3] Therefore, the ACR manual on contrast agents has recommended that if administration of a contrast agent is necessary, only group II GBCAs should be used and at the lowest dose possible to obtain a diagnosis under the supervision of radiologists.[6] Meanwhile, group I contrast agents are contraindicated in patients with CKD. Although the risk for NSF following use of group III GBCAs is extremely low in patients with CKD, the role of this group in vascular imaging is limited. The off-label contrast agent ferumoxytol has been used in multiple institutions, especially in patients with CKD. However, one complication of ferumoxytol includes acute hypersensitivity-related adverse events (79 events/1.2 million injections) that prompted the Food and Drug Administration to issue black box warnings. Per the updated therapeutic prescription recommendation, ferumoxytol can only be injected in diluted form over 15 minutes and requires 30 minutes of hemodynamic monitoring.[5]

#### *2. The timing of contrast injection and image acquisition*

CE-MRA does not directly visualize contrast agents. Instead, the paramagnetic effects of contrasts shorten the T1 signal of adjacent water molecules, which makes blood appear brighter on T1-weighted images. This effect is dose-dependent; therefore, an extremely high concentration of gadolinium can create a T2-shortening effect, which overwhelms the T1 signal effects and results in signal loss similar to a metal artifact.[7] After peak contrast opacification of arteries, GBCA wanes off from the vessel and opacifies the extracellular space of solid organs; the average intravascular half-time of GBCAs is 90 seconds. Therefore, the timing of contrast injection and

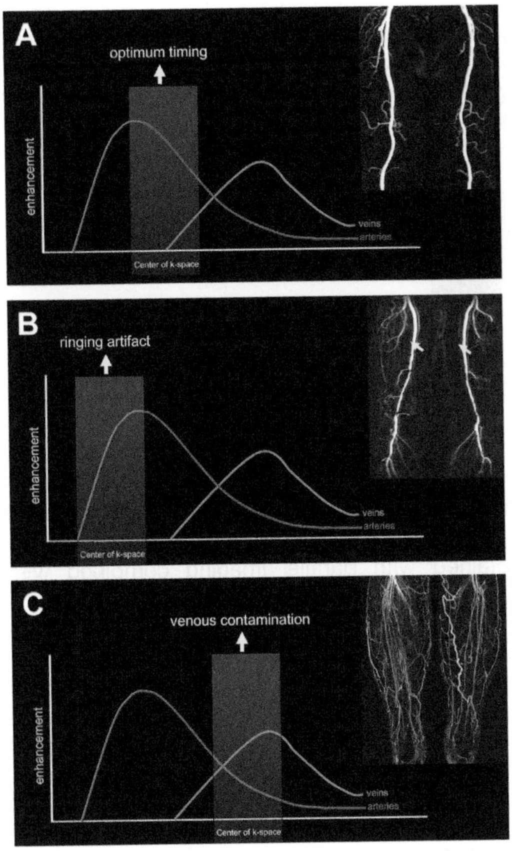


Fig. 1. (*A*) For the ideal images, the timing of contrast injection and image acquisition should be synchronized to obtain images when the contrast media is at its peak concentration. (*B*) Early image acquisition will result in ringing artifacts (*yellow arrows*). (*C*) Late image acquisition will result in venous contamination.

image acquisition should be synchronized to obtain images when the contrast media is at its peak concentration in the artery of interest (**Fig. 1**A). In other words, arterial opacification of gadolinium must be synchronized with the center of k-space acquisition.[8] Early image acquisition will result in poor opacification of the arteries and ringing artifacts, while late acquisition will cause venous contamination (**Fig. 1**B, C). Another parameter is the contrast injection rate, which for arteries is 2 to 3 mL/sec with power injectors, followed by 40 to 50 mL of saline flushing in the same injection parameters. A higher injection rate will produce a higher SNR and contrast–noise ratio (CNR) in images; on the other hand, an injection rate of 1.5 mL/sec or lower will result in a broader plateau, thus a lower SNR and CNR, and results in increased risk of venous contamination (**Fig. 2**). The timing of contrast injection can be achieved via (a) test bolus timing, (b) bolus chasing (fluoroscopic triggering), and (c) time-resolved (TR) imaging. In extremity imaging, a hybrid technique, which is a combination of bolus chasing and TR imaging, is performed to prevent venous contamination in arteries of the calves or hands. In the time bolus technique, a small amount of contrast (2 mL) is administered with two-dimensional image acquisition of the vessel of interest. Owing to background contamination, this technique is not often used. Meanwhile, bolus chasing or fluoroscopic triggering is more frequently used in extremity imaging. In this technique, injection of contrast and rapid imaging with 2D-gradient-echo sequences (Canon–Visual prep; GE–SmartPrep, Fluoro Trigger; Hitachi–FLUTE; Philips–Bolus track; Siemens–CareBolus) allows demonstration of contrast arrival to the artery of interest. The last technique for contrast timing is TR imaging, which is a unique technique to image arteries at the highest temporal resolution and is used for arteries below the knees and in the hands.[9] TR imaging obtains data from the center of the k-space every few seconds after contrast injection, providing dynamic (flow) information in the extremity arteries without venous contamination. Obtaining NC (mask) images is essential as it allows subtraction from post-contrast images to create maximum intensity projection images of the arteries.

### *3. Sequences*

Detailed CE-MRA sequences have been discussed elsewhere in this volume. Briefly, the T1-weighted spoiled gradient echo sequence is mainly utilized to obtain high spatial and contrast resolution images (Canon–RF-Spoiled FE; GE–SPGR, MPSPGR; Hitachi–RSSG; Philips–T1-FFE; Siemens–FLASH). As mentioned above, the second most utilized sequence in extremity imaging is the TR-MRA sequence, particularly for small distal vessels (Canon–Freeze frame; GE–TRICKS; Hitachi–TRAQ; Philips–4D-TRAK; Siemens–TWIST).

## *Non-Contrast Magnetic Resonance Angiography*

For patients who cannot receive GBCA, NC-MRA is an alternative for imaging arteries of the extremities. Multiple sequences are available to visualize arteries, which will be discussed in the first article of this volume. In clinical practice, extremity arterial imaging is performed with quiescent interval slice-selective (QISS), three-dimensional fast (turbo) spin echo (3D-FSE), and time-of-flight (TOF).[10]

*TOF* is an inflow-based technique that depends on the differences in magnetization between the presaturated stationary tissue and radio frequency pulse-excited protons in blood. TOF is the oldest

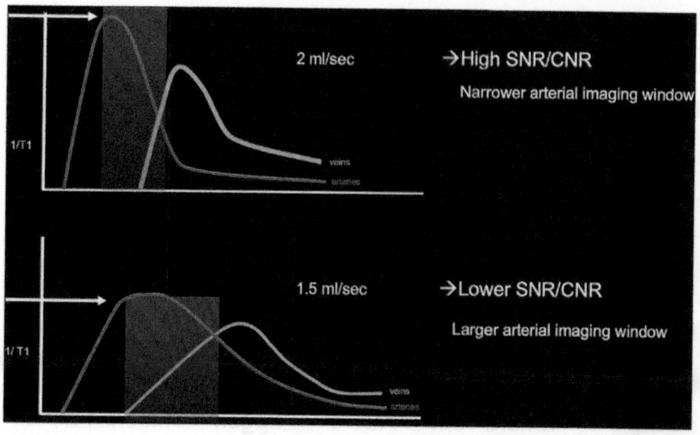


**Fig. 2.** Higher injection rate (>2 mL/sec) will produce a higher SNR and CNR but a narrower arterial imaging window. However, a lower injection rate (<1.5 mL/sec) will result in lower SNR and CNR, but larger arterial imaging window.

NC-MRA technique; however, its role in extremity artery imaging remains limited, and it is mostly used on head/neck arteries. Selective venous blood flow suppression should be performed using parallel saturation bands/pulses to obtain arterial-only images. TOF can be performed as 2D or 3D, and imaging readouts are on the axial plane approximately perpendicular to the arterial flow. One of the most important limitations in extremity TOF MRA studies is that the saturation band can prohibit signal acquisition in in-plane and retrograde directions, which can artifactually mimic occlusion (**Fig. 3**). In contrast, 2D-TOF images of arteries of the extremities are acquired with cardiac gating to prevent ghosting artifacts.[11] To minimize the scan time and improve image quality, lower extremity (LE) TOF images can be obtained with parallel imaging combined with compressed sensing reconstruction.[12]

*QISS* is a cardiac-gated inflow-based technique developed to visualize vessels of lower extremities.[13] It uses bright blood imaging sequence single-shot 2D balanced steady-state free precession (bSSFP) readout. During an R–R cardiac cycle, three steps occur: (1) radiofrequency pulses for background/in-plane and venous saturation; (2) waiting time (quiescent interval) for magnetized arterial spins to flow to

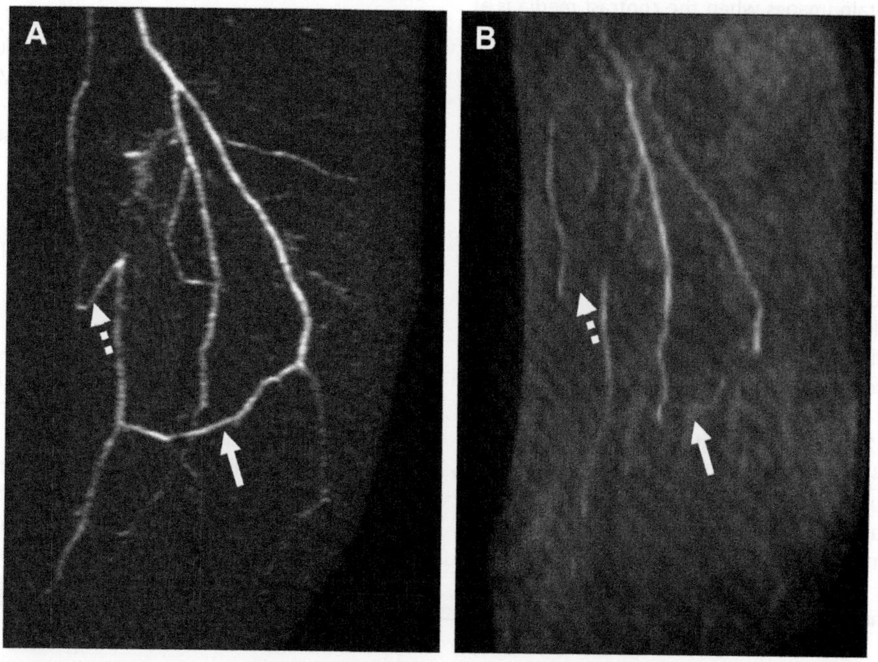


**Fig. 3.** TR-MRA image (*A*) of the foot demonstrates patent arch vessel (*arrow*) and retrograde collateral flow (*dashed arrow*) to the distal anterior tibial artery. Correlative 3D-TOF image (*B*), however, is lacking to demonstrate in-plane (*arrow*) or retrograde (*dashed arrow*) flow in the patent vessels.

the imaging slice; and (3) at diastole, the bSSFP readout creates bright arteries on a dark background. QISS is highly sensitive and specific for >50% stenosis in the lower extremities when compared with DSA (91.4% and 96.4%, respectively) or CE-MRA (89.2% and 96.0%, respectively).[11] In a study where QISS and CTA were compared with DSA as a standard reference, both sensitivity and specificity were higher in QISS and with high interobserver agreement.[14] QISS performance is also better on 3T MR imaging compared with 1.5 T. QISS is ideal for visualizing vessels that are straight and orthogonal to the imaging plane and has limited in-plane-oriented segments with retrograde flow.

*3D-FSE* is a cardiac-gated flow-dependent technique based on the subtraction of signals between arteries and veins at different phases of the cardiac cycle. During systole, the arterial blood flow is fast, and it dephases and yields no signal; veins, on the other hand, remain bright due to slow blood flow. However, in diastole, both veins and arteries demonstrate high signal intensity, termed as bright blood effect. Hence, subtraction datasets in diastole and systole create arterial images. Commercially available sequence images (Canon–FBI, CIA; GE–Inhance Deltaflow; Hitachi–VASC-FSE; Philips–TRANCE; Siemens–NATIVE SPACE) have been used to visualize arteries of the extremities.[15,16] 3D-FSE has high diagnostic accuracy (>90%) and a high negative predictive value (>95%) in LE arteries when compared to DSA.[16] A study (20 patients) compared 3D-FSE with CE-MRA in visualizing foot (small caliber) vessels using DSA as a reference standard and showed that NC-MRA had high diagnostic accuracy; however, the proportions of non-diagnostic vessel segments were considerably higher in 3D-FSA compared to CE-MRA studies.[17] Studies comparing 3D-FSE to QISS have shown that 3D-FSE is inferior to QISS in patients with chronic limb ischemia.[18,19] Although it is an alternative to NC-MRA, 3D-FSE has limitations, including its assessment of small vessels and its longer scan time when multiple areas need to be covered.

## PATIENT POSITIONING AND IMAGE ACQUISITION

Extremity artery MRA is challenging and should be tailored based on clinical findings. For example, arterial occlusion due to atherosclerosis-related disease versus dynamic compression of the thoracic outlet or popliteal arteries is assessed differently. The most important aspect is placing the patient in a comfortable position since some studies can take a long time. Phased-array coils are utilized in most studies; however, 16-element extremity wrap and foot coils should be used for smaller areas.

### Upper Extremity

From the subclavian artery to the tip of the fingers, all vascular abnormalities can be visualized with CE-MRA sequences using phased-array coils. Stents in arteries will cause a signal dropout; therefore, prior clinical information regarding the intervention is important.

#### Subclavian artery

For subclavian artery assessment, the arms are placed either at the sides (adduction) or at a hyperabducted position (Superman position). In suspected thoracic outlet syndrome (TOS), imaging of the arms in both positions should be performed to assess dynamic compression. GBCA should be administered to the asymptomatic arm so that the susceptibility artifact from the T* effect of gadolinium in the veins does not obscure the artery (pseudo-stenosis; **Fig. 4**). If symptoms are bilateral, saline flushing should be performed. Finally, gadolinium must be injected in both arm positions in suspected TOS to obtain good arterial opacification.

#### Brachial artery

Assessment is performed in two positions: (1) translated anatomic position to image the brachial artery with the subclavian/axillary artery; the arms are at the sides, and the body is positioned

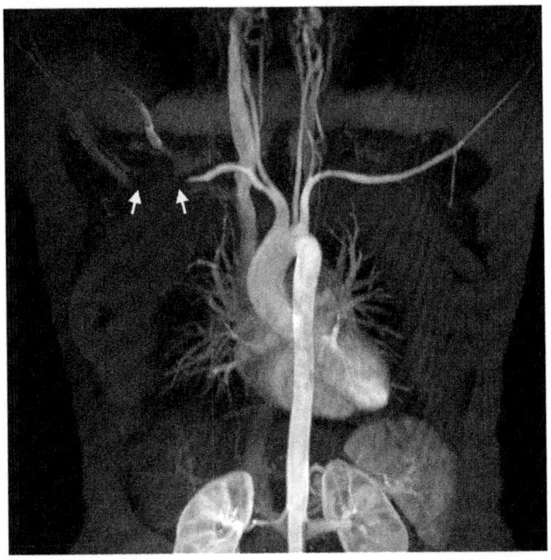

**Fig. 4.** Coronal maximum intensity projection of 3D-MRA of the chest in arms up position to assess for TOS. Pseudostenosis (*arrows*) of the right subclavian artery in a patient with suspected left-sided thoracic outlet syndrome resulting from T2* susceptibility artifacts due to high concentration gadolinium.

laterally so that the location of the arm of interest is near the isocenter of the magnet,[20] and (2) Superman position to visualize the brachial artery and forearm.

#### *Forearm and hand*

Forearm and hand imaging is usually performed in the Superman position for the vessels to be in the isocenter of the magnet. Obtaining TR-MRA images of the forearm and hand is crucial to obtain ideal arterial opacification. Subsequently, two first-phase 3D-SPGR arterial images should be acquired. Some institutions acquire NC-MRA sequences, such as QISS, along with CE-MRA images.

### *Lower Extremity*

LE artery imaging begins from the aortoiliac arteries to the tip of the toes. A dedicated peripheral MRA coil (36-element matrix coil) should be utilized for most of the arteries in a supine position, and a dedicated foot coil is ideal for smaller foot vessels. In patients with critical limb ischemia, TR-MRA images of the foot should be obtained with low-dose contrast (3 mL GBCA) injection. Similarly, TR-MRA should be performed with 3 mL of GBCA beginning from the bilateral calves to assess vessels below the knees.[9] TR-MRA will allow imaging of anterograde arterial flow without venous contamination. Lastly, 3-station (or 4-station) bolus chase MRA images should be acquired (**Fig. 5**). As discussed above, LE arteries can be visualized with NC-MRA sequences such as QISS. Metallic stents will create an abrupt signal void in the vessels (pseudo-stenosis). Hence, in certain clinical scenarios, such as suspected popliteal entrapment syndrome, dynamic imaging is required.

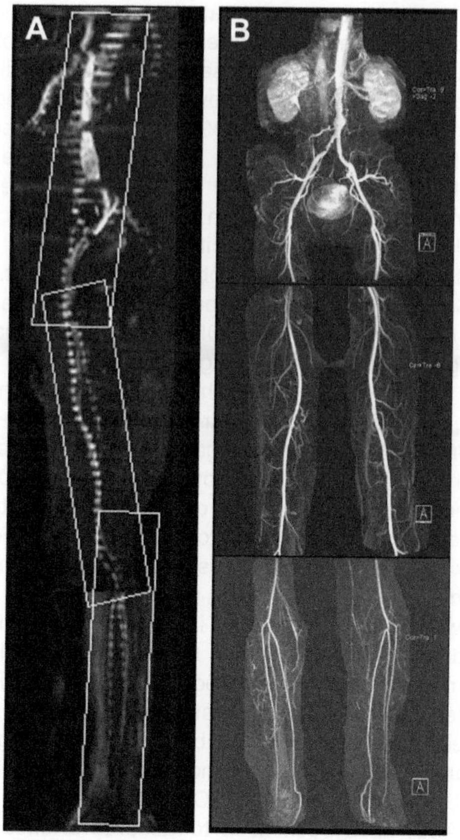


**Fig. 5.** (*A*) Prescription of 3D MRA slabs from 2D TOF locator, and (*B*) 3-station coronal maximum intensity projection reconstruction of 3D-MRA images of the lower extremity.

## EXTREMITY ARTERY PATHOLOGIES

### *Atherosclerotic Disease*

It is the most common cause of UE or LE ischemia. Patients with UE atherosclerotic disease could be asymptomatic or present with exertional pain, gangrene, and ulceration in severe cases. Atherosclerotic disease is relatively easy to diagnose in symptomatic patients; however, for asymptomatic individuals, two important physical examination findings can help identify an atherosclerotic etiology: (1) presence of LE arterial disease and (2) blood pressure difference of 15 mm Hg between the arms. Similarly, patients with LE atherosclerotic disease can be asymptomatic or present with symptoms, including claudication, ulcers, or gangrene. Doppler US is the first-line imaging modality as it is easy to perform; images show a blunted waveform signal distal to the stenotic segment. Although CTA is often utilized, MRA has proven to be an alternative technique. During imaging, it is essential to assess the entire extremity, particularly proximal segments such as the brachiocephalic or common iliac arteries. CE-MRA is often utilized; however, in patients with CKD and low eGFR, NC-MRA or an alternative off-label contrast agent (ferumoxytol) can be used. A recent meta-analysis assessing the diagnostic performance of QISS with CE-MRA demonstrated that QISS has high accuracy in detecting and excluding peripheral arterial disease in symptomatic patients.[21] Imaging findings include focal stenosis or occlusion of the proximal segments of the arteries, and the presence of tortious collateral arteries indicates hemodynamically significant stenosis or occlusion (**Fig. 6**).

### *Thromboembolism*

Thromboembolism is another etiology that can cause UE and LE ischemia and is common in the elderly, especially among those with underlying

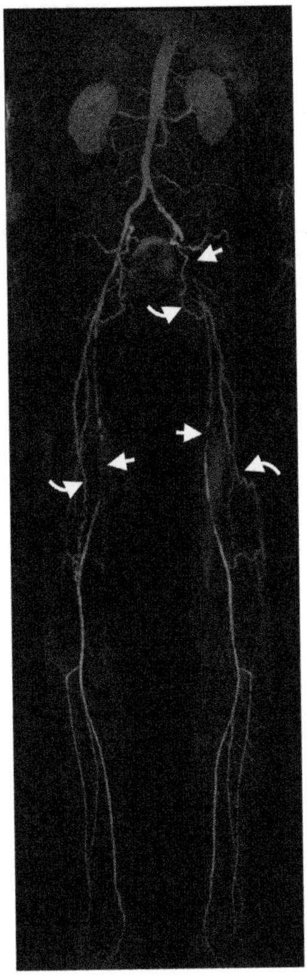

Fig. 6. Three-station coronal maximum intensity projection reconstruction of 3D-MRA images of the lower extremity demonstrates multifocal occlusion of the vessels (*arrows*) and associated collaterals (curved *arrows*).

etiologies such as atrial fibrillation, degenerative valvular diseases and thrombus formation from ischemic heart disease.[22,23] In LE arteries, large aortic plaque can cause emboli. Rare etiologies, such as infective endocarditis or cardiac masses, can also cause thromboembolism. When the clinical presentation and physical findings are highly suspicious for thromboembolism, Doppler US or CTA are performed in acute settings to evaluate the arteries. Alternatively, when the patient cannot receive an iodine-based contrast agent or for interventional planning, MRA of the UE and lower extremities can be performed. Images of thromboembolism include an abrupt cutoff of the distal arteries, particularly at the branching level (**Fig. 7**). Meanwhile, perivascular enhancement is seen in acute embolic events, especially in delayed images.

### *Compression syndromes/repetitive trauma*

**Thoracic outlet syndrome** Subclavian artery compression in the thoracic outlet is rare but results in high morbidity. Chronic compression or repetitive trauma can damage the vessels and induce stenosis, aneurysms, or thrombosis of the distal arteries. The underlying cause could be hypertrophy of the scalene muscles or cervical ribs. Dynamic imaging with MRA is an essential part of the examination and should be performed in hyperabducted and adducted positions to demonstrate vessel compression. In arteries, more than 50% stenosis during hyperabduction should be considered significant (**Fig. 8**). Additionally, post-stenotic dilatation, aneurysm formation, or intraluminal thrombus are seen in arterial TOS.[24]

**Hypothenar hammer syndrome** Repetitive trauma in the hand/hypothenar eminence can result in damage to the distal ulnar artery at the level of the hook of the hamate. The clinical presentation of individuals with hypothenar hammer syndrome is finger ischemia on the ulnar aspect. MRA imaging of the forearm and hand should include TR-MRA sequences. At the initial stages of the condition, the ulnar artery can develop a corkscrew appearance; subsequently, it can form an aneurysm/pseudoaneurysm and thrombosis (**Fig. 9**).

**Popliteal entrapment syndrome** Compression of the popliteal artery at the knee by adjacent structures can cause claudication, particularly in younger individuals. Meanwhile, it can also be caused by an abnormal course of the popliteal artery, abnormal insertion of the gastrocnemius muscles, or additional fibrotic bands/muscles in the popliteal fossa.[25] Dynamic imaging with MRA is the preferred technique (with TR-MRA and T1-SPGR sequences), which can be utilized with a small amount of GBCA in dorsiflexion, plantarflexion, and neutral position. Abrupt cutoff of the vessel at the knee during dorsiflexion and plantarflexion with a resolution during the neutral phase (**Fig. 10**) can help diagnose this entity.

**Vasculitis** Large vessel vasculitides (LVV), such as Takayasu's arteritis (TAK) and giant cell arteritis (GCA), can involve both the UE and LE. Per guidelines, the first imaging modality performed in patients with suspected vasculitis is US/Doppler US, which allows assessment of the head and neck vasculature and proximal extremities.[26] US is also beneficial for patients with cranial involvement, particularly in GCA. However, in TAK, aortic involvement with extension to the proximal branches is common. Therefore, in patients highly suspected of vasculitis and with negative US results, MRA can be performed. Imaging findings of active LVV are circumferential wall thickening and enhancement on post-contrast images (**Fig. 11**). In the chronic phase,

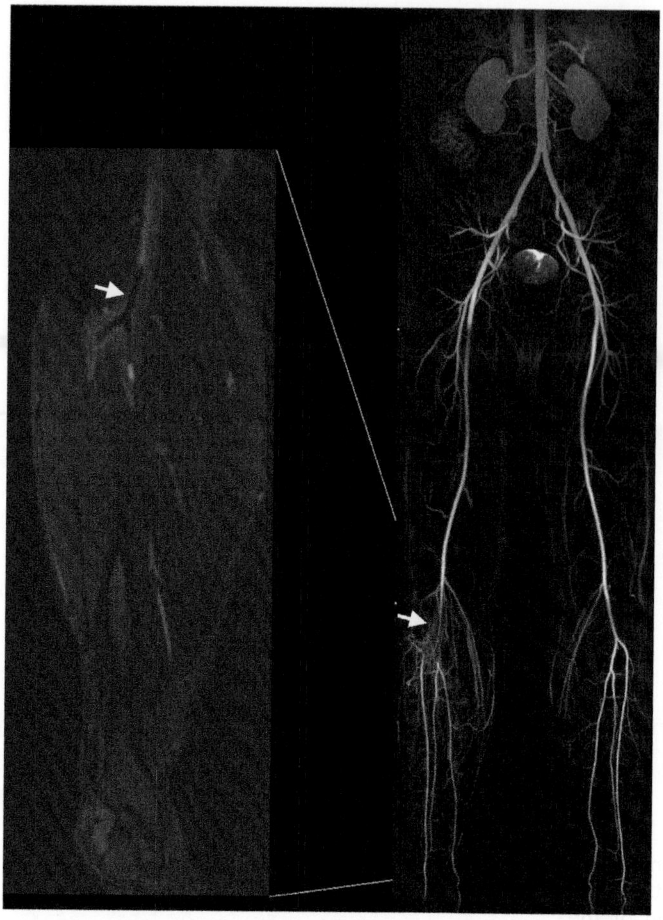

Fig. 7. Coronal 3D-MRA and coronal maximum intensity projection of 3D-MRA images of the lower extremity demonstrate abrupt cutoff and occlusion of the distal popliteal artery, anterior tibial artery, and tiboperoneal trunk due to a thrombus (*arrows*), most likely due to an embolic phenomenon, given the location and absence of atherosclerotic disease elsewhere.

damaged vessels can evolve into high-grade stenosis or occlusion. A recent study by Quin and colleagues[27] has shown that MRA can detect greater extent of LVV vascular involvement than FDG-PET/CT due to the detection of wall thickening/enhancement and luminal abnormalities; however, FDG-PET/CT was superior to detecting disease activity.

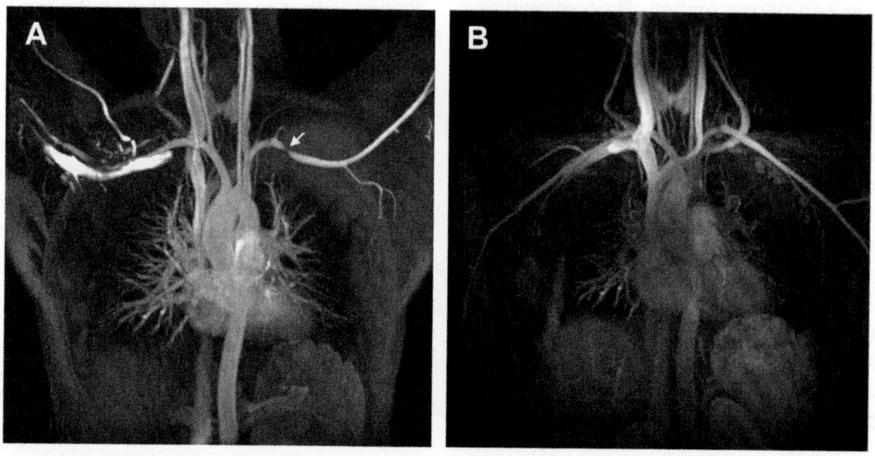


Fig. 8. Coronal 3D-MRA image (*A*) of the chest in hyperabduction of the arms in a patient with suspected arterial thoracic outlet syndrome demonstrates short segment severe stenosis (*arrow*), which resolves in the neutral position of the arms (*B*).

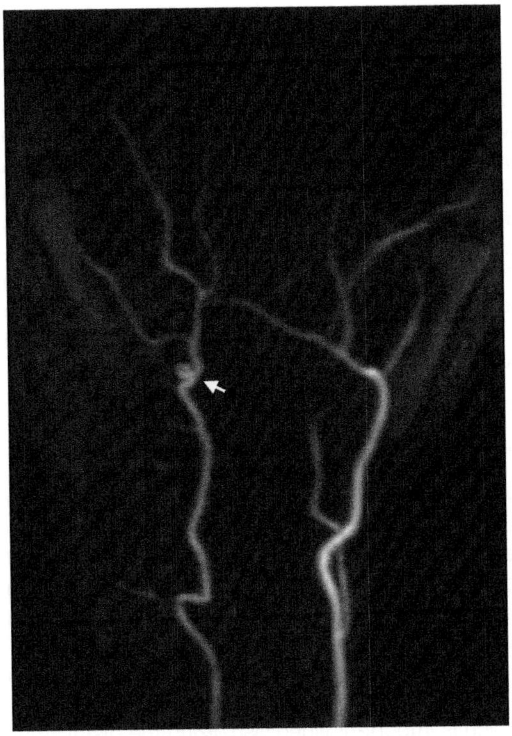

Fig. 9. Coronal 3D-MRA of the hand shows the corkscrew appearance (*arrow*) of the distal ulnar artery at the level of the hook of the hamate, consistent with a hypothenar hammer syndrome.

### *Vasospasms*

**Raynaud's phenomenon** Raynaud's phenomenon or syndrome is localized vasculopathy that involves the distal extremities, particularly the fingers, due to cold temperatures or emotional stress.[28] These patients present with significant discoloration (white) of the distal fingers, pain, and numbness resulting from diffuse vasospasm of the distal arteries. The phenomena can be a primary disease, also known as idiopathic or Raynaud's disease, or secondary to other etiologies, such as scleroderma.[28] Although clinical diagnosis is sufficient for classic Raynaud's disease, imaging can help exclude other etiologies such as embolic events. Hand and forearm MRA show diffuse narrowing and tapering of the distal vessels. Thus, it is important to warm the hands before image acquisition.

**Thromboangiitis obliterans** Thromboangiitis obliterans (TAO) or Buerger's disease is a non-atherosclerotic inflammatory disease involving the medium- and small-sized vessels of the extremities. Commonly seen in young men, TAO is strongly associated with tobacco use. At the early stages of the disease, TAO can mimic Raynaud's phenomenon, with the difference being that TAO involves the unilateral extremity in half of the cases. In advanced stages, patients present with symptoms of ischemia. Clinical findings are usually sufficient to diagnose TAO; however, imaging

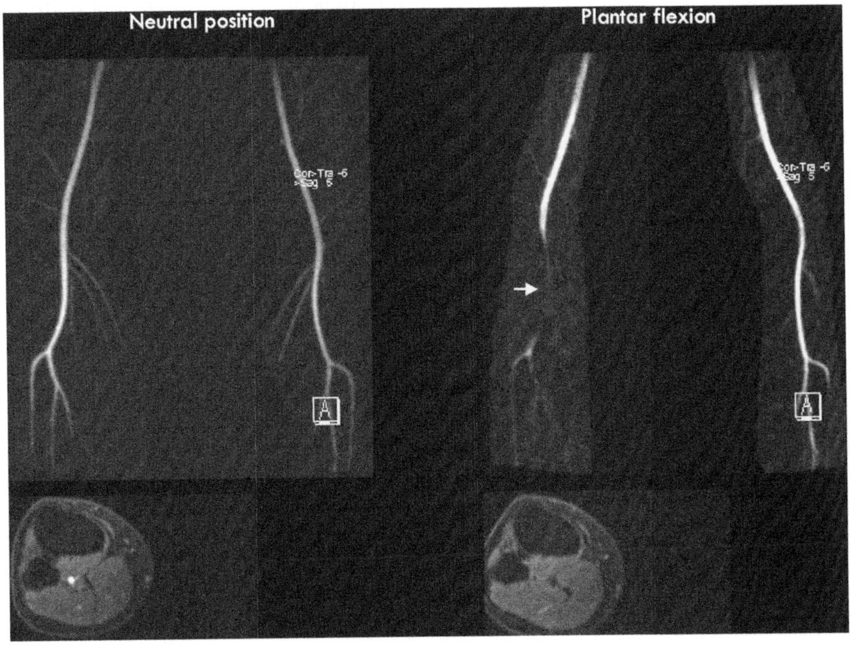


Fig. 10. Coronal maximum intensity projection 3D-MRA and corresponding axial 3D-MRA images of the lower extremities in neutral and plantar flexion demonstrate severe stenosis (*arrow*) of the popliteal artery during plantar flexion in a young athlete patient.

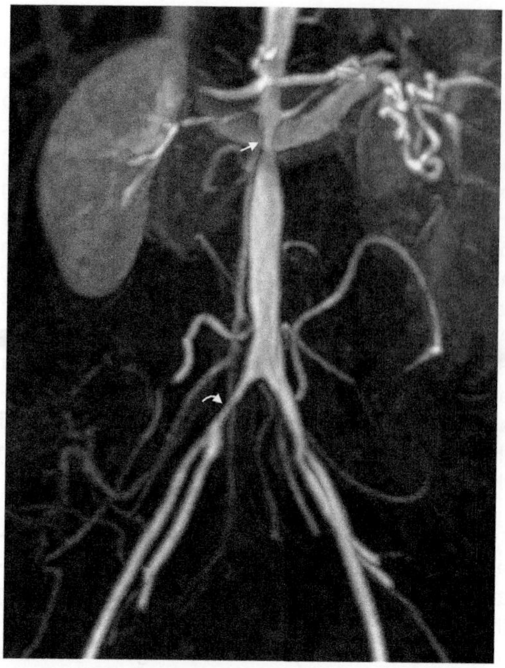

Fig. 11. Coronal maximum intensity projection 3D-MRA image of the abdominal aorta and iliac arteries shows focal narrowing of the abdominal aorta (*arrow*) and right common iliac artery (*curved arrow*) due to known sequela of prior Takayasu's vasculitis.

can exclude other etiologies such as embolism. Although there are no pathognomonic imaging features for TAO, extremity MRA can show segmental occlusion due to thrombosis of the arteries with corkscrew collaterals. TR-MRA sequences can help assess occluded segments and collaterals, while SPGR images can show filling defects/thrombus in the lumen.

### *Arteriovenous fistula for hemodialysis*

Arteriovenous fistula (AVF) is a permanent surgical hemodialysis access for patients with end-stage renal failure. It results in better outcomes, is usually created in the non-dominant arm, and has three types: (1) radiocephalic AVF, (2) brachiocephalic AVF, and (3) brachiobasilic transposition. Non-surgical percutaneous endovascular AVF creation was introduced and has comparable outcomes to those of the surgical method.[29] Imaging plays a role in assessing AVF-associated complications/dysfunction, which is classified as (a) thrombotic flow-related complications, (b) nonthrombotic flow-related complications (such as aneurysms/pseudoaneurysms), and (c) infections; MRA with TR-MRA and 3D-SPGR sequences are utilized to diagnose these complications. Li and colleagues[30] demonstrated that MRA had a sensitivity of 95.4% and specificity of 96.1% when evaluating AVFs. CE-MRA is mostly used for better AVF visualization and to avoid potential flow-related artifacts. However, the major limitation of CE-MRA is the utilization of GBCA in patients with renal failure. Off-label contrast agents, such as ferumoxytol, could be an alternative to GBCA and can also demonstrate the AVF anatomy and associated complications.[31] AVF imaging includes assessment of the UE arteries from their respective origins. The preferred MRA imaging technique requires the arms positioned at the sides to include vessels from the aortic arch to the level of the anastomosis/fistula.

## SUMMARY

MRA is a powerful imaging tool to assess extremity artery pathologies. In addition to the classic advantages of MRA, such as the absence of radiation and iodinated contrast exposure, it can provide high temporal resolution/dynamic images of the arteries with high soft tissue contrast. Although it has a relatively lower spatial resolution than CTA, MRA does not produce blooming artifacts from calcification, which is important when visualizing the distal small arteries. CE-MRA is the most preferred technique to assess ischemic and nonischemic extremity arterial pathologies. TR-MRA sequences are extremely valuable in assessing small vessels of the hands and feet. Recent advances in NC-MRA protocols provide an alternative imaging technique for patients with CKD. Furthermore, off-label contrast agents, such as ferumoxytol, are useful in certain clinical scenarios.

## CLINICS CARE POINTS

- Magnetic Resonance Angiography (MRA) is a non-invasive imaging technique that provides high temporal resolution images of upper and lower extremity arteries with excellent soft tissue contrast.
- Contrast-enhanced MRA (CE-MRA) using gadolinium-based contrast agents (GBCA) is the most commonly used technique for assessing arterial pathologies. However, in patients with chronic kidney disease (CKD), non-contrast MRA (NC-MRA) or alternative contrast agents like ferumoxytol can be utilized.
- CE-MRA offers better spatial resolution and fewer artifacts compared to NC-MRA, but NC-MRA is an alternative option for patients who cannot receive GBCA.

- Timing of contrast injection and image acquisition is crucial in CE-MRA to achieve optimal arterial opacification without venous contamination.

## DISCLOSURE

None.

## REFERENCES


1. Aboyans V, Ricco JB, Bartelink MEL, et al. 2017 ESC guidelines on the diagnosis and treatment of peripheral arterial diseases, in collaboration with the european society for vascular surgery (ESVS): document covering atherosclerotic disease of extracranial carotid and vertebral, mesenteric, renal, upper and lower extremity arteriesEndorsed by: the European Stroke Organization (ESO)The Task Force for the Diagnosis and Treatment of Peripheral Arterial Diseases of the European Society of Cardiology (ESC) and of the European Society for Vascular Surgery (ESVS). Eur Heart J 2018;39(9):763–816.
2. Guichet PL, Duszak R Jr, Chaves Cerdas L, et al. Changing national medicare utilization of catheter, computed tomography, and magnetic resonance extremity angiography: a specialty-focused 16-year analysis. Curr Probl Diagn Radiol 2021;50(3): 308–14.
3. Woolen SA, Shankar PR, Gagnier JJ, et al. Risk of nephrogenic systemic fibrosis in patients with stage 4 or 5 chronic kidney disease receiving a group ii gadolinium-based contrast agent: a systematic review and meta-analysis. JAMA Intern Med 2020; 180(2):223–30.
4. Kanda T, Ishii K, Kawaguchi H, et al. High signal intensity in the dentate nucleus and globus pallidus on unenhanced T1-weighted MR images: relationship with increasing cumulative dose of a gadolinium-based contrast material. Radiology 2014;270(3): 834–41.
5. Nguyen KL, Yoshida T, Kathuria-Prakash N, et al. Multicenter safety and practice for off-label diagnostic use of ferumoxytol in MRI. Radiology 2019; 293(3):554–64.
6. ACR Committee on Drugs and Contrast Media. ACR manual on contrast media, version 10.3. 2022. Available at: https://www.acr.org/-/media/ACR/Files/Clinical-Resources/Contrast_Media.pdf.
7. Primrose CW, Hecht EM, Roditi G, et al. MR angiography series: fundamentals of contrast-enhanced MR angiography. Radiographics 2021;41(4): E138–9.
8. Kramer JH, Grist TM. Peripheral MR angiography. Magn Reson Imaging Clin N Am 2012;20(4):761–76.
9. Raczeck P, Fries P, Massmann A, et al. Diagnostic performance of a lower-dose contrast-enhanced 4D dynamic MR angiography of the lower extremities at 3 T using multisegmental time-resolved maximum intensity projections. J Magn Reson Imaging 2021;54(3):763–74.
10. Navot B, Hecht EM, Lim RP, et al. MR angiography series: fundamentals of non-contrast-enhanced MR angiography. Radiographics 2021; 41(5):E157–8.
11. Cavallo AU, Koktzoglou I, Edelman RR, et al. Noncontrast magnetic resonance angiography for the diagnosis of peripheral vascular disease. Circ Cardiovasc Imaging 2019;12(5):e008844.
12. Hutter J, Grimm R, Forman C, et al. Highly undersampled peripheral Time-of-Flight magnetic resonance angiography: optimized data acquisition and iterative image reconstruction. Magma 2015; 28(5):437–46.
13. Edelman RR, Sheehan JJ, Dunkle E, et al. Quiescent-interval single-shot unenhanced magnetic resonance angiography of peripheral vascular disease: Technical considerations and clinical feasibility. Magn Reson Med 2010;63(4): 951–8.
14. Wu G, Yang J, Zhang T, et al. The diagnostic value of non-contrast enhanced quiescent interval single shot (QISS) magnetic resonance angiography at 3T for lower extremity peripheral arterial disease, in comparison to CT angiography. J Cardiovasc Magn Reson 20 2016;18(1):71.
15. Nakamura K, Miyazaki M, Kuroki K, et al. Noncontrast-enhanced peripheral MRA: technical optimization of flow-spoiled fresh blood imaging for screening peripheral arterial diseases. Magn Reson Med 2011;65(2):595–602.
16. Gutzeit A, Sutter R, Froehlich JM, et al. ECG-triggered non-contrast-enhanced MR angiography (TRANCE) versus digital subtraction angiography (DSA) in patients with peripheral arterial occlusive disease of the lower extremities. Eur Radiol 2011; 21(9):1979–87.
17. Schubert T, Takes M, Aschwanden M, et al. Non-enhanced, ECG-gated MR angiography of the pedal vasculature: comparison with contrast-enhanced MR angiography and digital subtraction angiography in peripheral arterial occlusive disease. Eur Radiol 2016;26(8):2705–13.
18. Ward EV, Galizia MS, Usman A, et al. Comparison of quiescent inflow single-shot and native space for nonenhanced peripheral MR angiography. J Magn Reson Imaging 2013;38(6):1531–8.
19. Altaha MA, Jaskolka JD, Tan K, et al. Non-contrast-enhanced MR angiography in critical limb ischemia: performance of quiescent-interval single-shot (QISS) and TSE-based subtraction techniques. Eur Radiol 2017;27(3):1218–26.

20. Dhaliwal J, Hecht EM, Roditi G, et al. MR angiography series: MR angiography of the extremities. Radiographics 2022;42(4):E132–3.
21. Verma M, Pandey NN, Singh V, et al. A meta-analysis of the diagnostic performance of quiescent-interval-single-shot magnetic resonance angiography in peripheral arterial disease. Eur Radiol 2022;32(4):2393–403.
22. Andersen LV, Lip GY, Lindholt JS, et al. Upper limb arterial thromboembolism: a systematic review on incidence, risk factors, and prognosis, including a meta-analysis of risk-modifying drugs. J Thromb Haemost 2013;11(5):836–44.
23. Gerhard-Herman MD, Gornik HL, Barrett C, et al. 2016 AHA/ACC guideline on the management of patients with lower extremity peripheral artery disease: a report of the American College of Cardiology/American Heart Association Task Force on Clinical Practice Guidelines. Circulation 2017;135(12):e726–79.
24. Aghayev A, Rybicki FJ. State-of-the-art magnetic resonance imaging in vascular thoracic outlet syndrome. Magn Reson Imaging Clin N Am 2015;23(2):309–20.
25. Macedo TA, Johnson CM, Hallett JW Jr, et al. Popliteal artery entrapment syndrome: role of imaging in the diagnosis. AJR Am J Roentgenol 2003;181(5):1259–65.
26. Dejaco C, Ramiro S, Duftner C, et al. EULAR recommendations for the use of imaging in large vessel vasculitis in clinical practice. Ann Rheum Dis 2018;77(5):636–43.
27. Quinn KA, Ahlman MA, Malayeri AA, et al. Comparison of magnetic resonance angiography and (18)F-fluorodeoxyglucose positron emission tomography in large-vessel vasculitis. Ann Rheum Dis 2018;77(8):1165–71.
28. Wigley FM, Flavahan NA. Raynaud's Phenomenon. N Engl J Med 2016;375(6):556–65.
29. Jones RG, Morgan RA. A review of the current status of percutaneous endovascular arteriovenous fistula creation for haemodialysis access. CVIR (Cardiovasc Interventional Radiol) 2019;42(1):1–9.
30. Li B, Li Q, Chen C, et al. Diagnostic accuracy of computer tomography angiography and magnetic resonance angiography in the stenosis detection of autologuous hemodialysis access: a meta-analysis. PLoS One 2013;8(10):e78409.
31. Li Y, Memon AA, Aghayev A, et al. Potential role of 3-dimensional printed vascular models in maintenance hemodialysis care. Kidney Med 2021;3(6):1095–8.

# MR Angiography for Aortic Diseases

Ishan Garg, MD[a], Thomas M. Grist, MD[b], Prashant Nagpal, MD[c,*]

**KEYWORDS**

• Aorta • Aortic diseases • Acute aortic syndrome • Aortic dissection • Aneurysm
• Computed tomography angiography (CTA) • MR imaging • Magnetic resonance angiography (MRA)

**KEY POINTS**

- Aortic diseases range from acute life-threatening emergencies to chronic nonemergent conditions. The choice of imaging depends on the disease, patient factors, and technical expertise.
- MR angiography primarily plays a vital role in nonemergent diseases and repeated follow-up. However, it also serves as an excellent alternative to CT if there is a contraindication to its use.
- Knowledge of aortic disease pathogenesis and a consistent, reliable imaging and measurement method is critical for a successful aortic imaging program.
- Techniques such as 4-dimensional-flow imaging provide anatomic and physiologic information that can be critical for patient management.

**Video content accompanies this article at http://www.mri.theclinics.com.**

## INTRODUCTION

Aortic diseases comprise a broad spectrum of pathologic conditions with varied clinical presentations and urgency of therapeutic interventions.[1–5] Acute aortic pathologic conditions such as aneurysm rupture and aortic dissection present as acute emergencies and are often associated with catastrophic outcomes. The reported mortality rate of acute aortic syndromes (AASs) such as high-grade TAI and ruptured abdominal aortic aneurysm (AAA) are 80% and 80% to 90%, respectively.[3,5,6] One of the critical components toward improving outcomes for aortic diseases is early diagnosis and treatment. Chronic aortic pathologic conditions such as aneurysms and atherosclerosis are usually asymptomatic and are often detected incidentally or on surveillance imaging. Imaging modalities such as ultrasound, computed tomography (CT), MR imaging, and angiography play a critical role in diagnosis, risk stratification, guiding therapeutic interventions, and postintervention surveillance of aortic diseases.[2,7,8] Recent advances in imaging technology such as 4D-flow MR imaging and therapeutic interventions may provide a new paradigm for the management of aortic pathologic conditions and optimizing clinical outcomes.[9–12] The purpose of this article is to review the management of common aortic pathologic conditions using multimodality imaging with a focus on MR imaging.

## AORTIC ANATOMY

The aorta is the largest and main artery in the body, extending from the aortic valve annulus to the pelvis (fourth lumbar vertebra, L4), where it divides into the right and left common iliac arteries. There are various systems used for the classification of aortic anatomy.

Statement of conflict: All authors do not have any relevant disclosures.
[a] Department of Internal Medicine, University of New Mexico Health Sciences Center, 1 University Of New Mexico, Albuquerque, NM 87131, USA; [b] Department of Radiology, University of Wisconsin-Madison, E3/366 Clinical Science Center 600 Highland Avenue Madison, WI 53792, USA; [c] Cardiovascular and Thoracic Radiology, University of Wisconsin School of Medicine and Public Health, E3/366 Clinical Science Center, 600 Highland Avenue, Madison, WI 53792, USA
* Corresponding author.
*E-mail address:* pnagpal@wisc.edu

Magn Reson Imaging Clin N Am 31 (2023) 373–394
https://doi.org/10.1016/j.mric.2023.05.002

## Embryologic Segments: Morphologic Classification

Based on embryologic development, the aorta can be morphologically divided into the aortic root, ascending aorta, aortic arch, descending thoracic aorta, and abdominal aorta (**Fig. 1**).

- The aortic root extends from the aortic valve annulus to the sinotubular junction and includes the aortic valve, sinuses of Valsalva, and the origin of the coronary arteries.[13]
- The ascending aorta extends from the sinotubular junction of the aortic valve upward and to the right before curving posteriorly into the aortic arch (at the origin of the brachiocephalic trunk).[2,13]
- The aortic arch extends from the origin of the brachiocephalic trunk to the ligamentum arteriosum. The aortic arch gives rise to 3 major arterial branches, the brachiocephalic trunk (divided into the right common carotid and right subclavian arteries), the left common carotid artery, and the left subclavian artery in 70% of individuals. It is important to note that there can be several normal variants in aortic arch anatomy, including the common origin of the brachiocephalic and left common carotid arteries (seen in 20%–30% of the population) and the separate origin of the left vertebral artery from the aortic arch (seen in approximately 5% of the population).[2,14]
- Descending thoracic aorta extends from ligamentum arteriosum to the hiatus of the diaphragm, beyond which it continues as the abdominal aorta.
- The abdominal aorta is a retroperitoneal segment extending from the hiatus of the diaphragm to the pelvis (fourth lumbar vertebra, L4), where it divides into the right and left common iliac arteries.

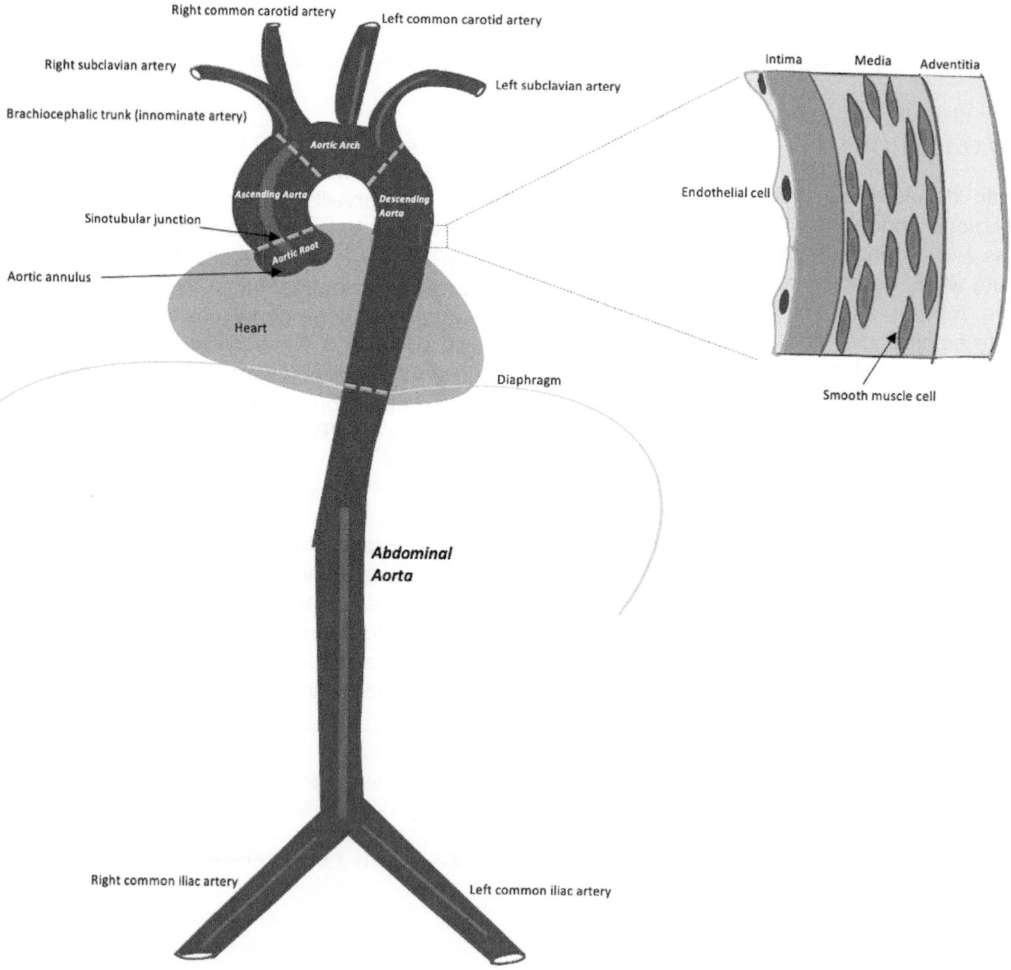


Fig. 1. The anatomy and histology of the aorta.

### *Aortic Wall Anatomy: Histologic Classification*

The aortic wall is composed of 3 layers (see **Fig. 1**).[1]

- Intima is a thin innermost layer. It consists of a layer of endothelial cells within a matrix of connective tissue.
- Media is a thick center layer. It consists of smooth muscle cells, elastic fibers, collagen, and proteins.
- Adventitia is a thin outermost layer. It consists of connective tissue, fibroblasts, nerves, and the vasa vasorum that provides support and perfusion to the artery, respectively.

## IMAGING OF THE AORTA

Various imaging modalities are available for the visualization of aortic anatomy and pathologic condition, including ultrasound (transthoracic and transesophageal echocardiogram and abdominal ultrasound), CT, MR imaging, and angiography. Although chest radiograph may frequently be the first test in acute clinical scenario such as trauma, specific aortic pathologic condition is rarely (if ever) diagnosed on radiograph in modern times. The choice of imaging modality is often dictated by a combination of following factors.[15]

- Modality-specific factors: availability, portability, speed of acquisition, and spatial and temporal resolution.
- Patient-specific factors: acuity of the disease, hemodynamic stability, comorbidities, contrast allergy, renal function, and contraindication to specific modalities such as MR imaging or procedures requiring contrast agents.
- Disease-specific factors: suspected aortic pathologic condition, evaluation of branched vessels, and cardiac and valvular function.
- User-specific factors: level of expertise and familiarity of interpreting radiologists and physicians with different imaging modalities.

### *Ultrasound*

Transthoracic echocardiogram (TTE) is commonly used imaging modality for cardiac evaluation. It can also be used as a screening tool for aortic root and ascending aortic sizing as aortic size can be routinely measured on left ventricular outflow tract views. The primary advantages of echocardiogram are wide availability, real-time dynamic imaging, simultaneous valve imaging, lack of ionizing radiation, and relatively low cost.[16]

Different imaging axis can be used in TTE to help provide a more comprehensive visualization of the aortic and cardiac anatomy, including parasternal long-axis, parasternal short-axis view, apical 4-chamber view, subcoastal view.

Transesophageal echocardiography (TEE), however, is a relatively invasive procedure that provides a more detailed evaluation of thoracic aorta and aortic valve pathologic conditions. It is worth noting that part of the distal ascending aorta, just proximal to the innominate artery, is hidden under acoustic shadowing from the trachea and may not be visually accessible on TEE.

Intravascular ultrasound is used for intraluminal imaging of localized vascular pathologic condition. It is often used intraoperatively for guiding endovascular procedures such as a stent placement and thrombectomy and helps distinguish between true and false lumen (FL) in aortic dissection.[17,18] However, its routine clinical use is limited and not discussed in this review.

Abdominal ultrasound is often used as a diagnostic tool in the screening and surveillance of AAA.[18] Recent advances in ultrasound techniques, including 3D TEE and contrast-enhanced Doppler, have shown promising results in the evaluation of various aortic pathologic conditions such as atheroma, stenosis, thrombus, dissection, aneurysm, rupture, and even surveillance for endoleaks after endovascular repair of AAA.[19,20] However, the use of abdominal ultrasound is most commonly limited to screening for aortic aneurysm.

The major limitations of ultrasound-based assessment include operator dependence and poor visualization of the aorta in patients with large body habitus (limiting ultrasound penetration) or gas in the abdomen (limiting acoustic windows).

### *Computed Tomography*

Cross-sectional imaging modalities, including multidetector CT (MDCT) and MR imaging, are the preferred modalities for aortic imaging because they provide excellent and superior anatomic details over ultrasound. MDCT/MR imaging is limited to a lesser extent by large body habitus. In addition, MDCT/MR imaging imaging protocols minimize the interoperator variability, making them ideal imaging modalities for serial monitoring and comparative follow-up studies.[21]

MDCT has shown nearly 100% sensitivity and specificity for the diagnosis of aortic pathologic conditions.[22] CT angiography (CTA) provides high temporal and spatial resolution images for the evaluation of both the vascular anatomy and solid organs. Electrocardiogram (ECG)-gating, help minimize motion-induced (cardiac motion) artifacts, seen in as much as 92% of nongated scans.[1] This, in turn, allows relatively motionless aortic root evaluation with improved diagnostic accuracy and reproducibility of aortic size measurements.[23] The ECG-gating can be done either prospectively (lower radiation dose) or retrospectively (higher radiation dose).[24] With technological advances such as improved gantry rotation, high-pitch scanning, and use of dual-source scanners, motionless imaging of the aorta can now be obtained even without ECG-gating.[13] The major limitations of CT include potential side effects related to exposure to a modest amount of ionizing radiation and contrast agent used in CTA.[23,25]

## Magnetic Resonance Angiography

Magnetic resonance angiography (MRA) is the preferred imaging modality for the assessment and follow-up of aortic pathologic condition in the nonemergent setting. If there is sufficient technical and reader expertise, MRA can easily be used in emergent setting as well using abbreviated protocols that allow aortic imaging in less than 10 minutes, which is comparable to CTA. MRA is a powerful imaging modality offering several potential advantages over CT, including (1) lack of ionizing radiation (ideal for patients with known aneurysms who require sequential follow-up examinations), (2) functional information including valve evaluation and quantification of dynamic vascular flow (forward and reverse aortic flow), (3) superior soft tissue characterization, and (4) advances like 4D flow that allow physiologic evaluation and assessment of aortic compliance and wall shear stress.[8] When performed as combined MRA and cardiac MR imaging, it can be used a comprehensive test for combined aortic and cardiac anatomy and function.[26,27]

The major disadvantage of MR imaging includes longer acquisition time (remedied via focused protocols), higher cost, limited availability (remedied by education and technical expertise), lower spatial resolution (compared with CT), claustrophobia (often remedied through sedation), risk of nephrogenic systemic fibrosis (remedied via use of ionic macrocyclic agents), MR imaging-specific contraindications such as non-MR imaging compatible implants, and body habitus (limited gantry diameter of the MR imaging scanners.[2,9,28] As highlighted, most of these limitations can be easily overcome and MRA remains the primary workhorse for aortic evaluation at our program during last 2 decades.

### Imaging protocol on MR imaging

The availability of various pulse sequences allows MR imaging to provide versatile imaging evaluation with functional information and excellent soft tissue characterization. Due to the availability of these sequences, MR imaging can be used even without exogenous contrast for the assessment of the entire aorta and the proximal origins of its branches, unlike noncontrast CT.

Typical MR imaging sequences that are obtained as part of MR imaging protocol for aortic imaging include black blood and bright blood sequences, cine sequences through the aortic valve, flow assessment (2D or 4D flow imaging), and contrast-enhanced MRA sequences. Two-station examination of the thoracic and abdominal aorta can be performed to improve spatial resolution and the contrast-to-noise ratio. However, the newer coil arrays allow wide coverage with high-resolution imaging for chest and abdomen. MRA protocol for aortic evaluation is summarized in **Table 1**. The premise behind use of different MR sequences is as follows:

i. Contrast-enhanced MRA (CE-MRA)—CE-MRA sequences are the most commonly used bright-blood technique for luminal assessment. Most MRA chest protocols have CE-MRA sequences as the primary sequence for vascular evaluation. CE-MRA can be performed as a high-spatial resolution 3D spoiled gradient-echo (SPGR) acquisition or dynamic time-resolved MRA.[29] The choice among these techniques depends upon the clinical indication, 3D-MRA preferred in most protocols due to higher spatial resolution and time-resolved imaging reserved for clinical scenarios in which directionality of flow or dynamic information is needed (**Fig. 2**). In our institution, we perform time-resolved imaging of aorta in patients with aortic stent for dynamic evaluation of endoleak or in patients with suspected or known arterio-venous malformations. High-spatial-resolution CE-MRA can be performed with or without ECG-gating. ECG-gating is usually performed if aortic root or ascending aortic evaluation is needed and to perform accurate measurements of thoracic aorta, especially the aortic root.[2]

Of various strategies that can be used to decrease the dose of GBCA for MRA of the aorta, use of a smaller dose of contrast (than standard), which is however diluted with saline and then injected at a standard rate of 1.5 to 2 mL/s has become routine for MRA protocols. This strategy allows the use of a lower contrast dose, which leads to a slightly lower peak signal intensity while extending the duration of contrast enhancement as compared with standard dose, thus reducing the chance of mistiming or missing the peak

**Table 1**
**Aortic MR Angiography protocol at our institute**

| | |
|---|---|
| Scan Range | Chest, chest and abdomen, or chest, abdomen, and pelvis—depending on the suspected or known aortic pathologic condition |
| Contrast type | Gadobenate dimeglumine (Multihance, Bracco Diagnostic, Princeton, New Jersey, USA) |
| Contrast dose | • 0.1 mmol/kg (Max 20 mL), dilute with 25 mL saline, followed with a saline flush; injected at 1.5 mL/s<br>• If time-resolved MRA added (for poststent endoleak evaluation cases): 8 mL of the diluted contrast; injected at 2 mL/s |
| Gating | Vector ECG-gating (for aortic root and ascending aorta), Respiratory (for all) |
| Sequences | • 3-plane localizers<br>• Axial single shot SSFP (GE: FIESTA)<br>• Single breath-hold ECG-gated 3D MRA: precontrast, peak arterial, immediate delay<br>• Postcontrast 3D FSPGR T1W axial sequence (GE: Lava-Flex)<br>• Optional sequences:<br>○ Time-resolved MRA (GE: TRICKS) (Temporal Resolution ~ 4 s), if stent (for endoleak) or dynamic imaging needed (example AV malformation)<br>○ Axial T1-weighted and T2-weighted sequences for vessel wall evaluation. T1W sequence is done both before and after contrast administration. T2W imaging is preferably done only before contrast administration.<br>○ Gated 3D SSFP with respiratory navigators: if noncontrast MRA protocol or if technical issues with 3D MRA sequence<br>○ 4D Flow: If aortic flow and hemodynamics are desired, ex. Aortic coarctation, aortic valve evaluation |

bolus. Hence, it is strongly encouraged to decrease the dose of GBCA for the MRA aorta and perform the scan with diluted contrast solution because it leads to less contrast use with minimal effect on the quality of the MRA examination. If there is contraindication to the use of GBCA, ferumoxytol can be used, typically in doses of 3 to 5 mg/kg with total dose not to exceed one bottle (510 mg). However, it should be noted that use of ferumoxytol is considered an off-label use.[30]

ii. Black-blood sequences (vessel wall)—These sequences are used for visualization of aortic morphology and are acquired using the spin-echo technique. Multiple radiofrequency pulses are used to suppress the signal from the blood, making it seem dark on imaging, hence the name. For instance, in a double inversion recovery sequence, 2 inversion pulses null the signal from the blood to provide a higher contrast-to-noise ratio of the aortic wall. This, in turn, helps in improved visualization of aortic wall morphology.

Precontrast and postcontrast black-blood sequences can be used for further characterization of aortic wall thickening and enhancement or vascular malformations.[10,11] Various variants of black-blood sequences, including T1-weighted and T2-weighted sequences, allow further tissue characterization. Fast spin echo sequences provide high-resolution images while minimizing motion artifacts.[11] These sequences are particularly useful for morphologic assessment of the aorta in patients with suspected aortic wall pathology such as vasculitis or intramural hematoma (**Fig. 3**).

iii. Steady-state fast precision (SSFP) sequence—SSFP is a frequently used workhorse for precontrast and noncontrast imaging of the aorta. Two-dimensional SSFP sequences can be done in cine mode with images acquired through the cardiac cycle or noncine single-shot mode that can serve as an excellent bright-blood localizer as well as serve as an anatomic review sequence. When done as 3D sequence with ECG and respiratory navigators, the SSFP images provide high-resolution bright blood aortic evaluation, which often are the most useful sequence for noncontrast protocols (**Fig. 4**).

iv. Two-dimensional and 4D-phase contrast flow MR imaging—Phase-contrast (PC) imaging is also a noncontrast MRA technique that allows quantification of blood flow and provides directionality information. In 2D sequences' velocity is encoded in one direction through a 2D plane.

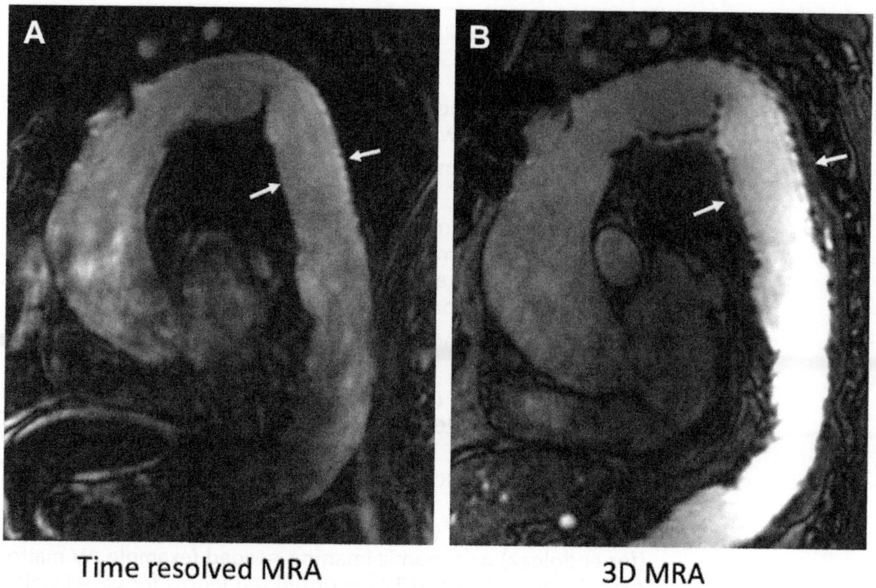


Fig. 2. Sagittal MR angiogram (MRA) images obtained via time-resolved MRA technique (*A*) and 3D-spoiled gradient echo MRA technique (*B*) highlighting the difference in the spatial resolution. The stent details (*arrows*) are much better seen on the 3D MRA (*B*) as compared with time-resolved MRA image (*A*).

Unlike 2D flow mapping (where the velocity vector is encoded in one direction), in 4D flow mapping, the velocity vector is encoded in 3 directions and images are acquired from a 3D spatial volume.[31]

For all PC sequences, operator-selectable parameter known as velocity encoding (VENC) is prescribed before acquisition. Proper setting of VENC estimated based on the velocity of the blood-flow desired to be resolved is critical to the performance of the study. These sequences are ideal for quantitative and qualitative assessment of aortic flow abnormalities, including aortic valvular stenosis or regurgitation (turbulent flow) or flow within the aortic lumen (false or true lumen) (eg, in aortic dissection). This also allows simultaneous evaluation of aortic valvular abnormality, which has direct consequences on treatment planning.[12,32]

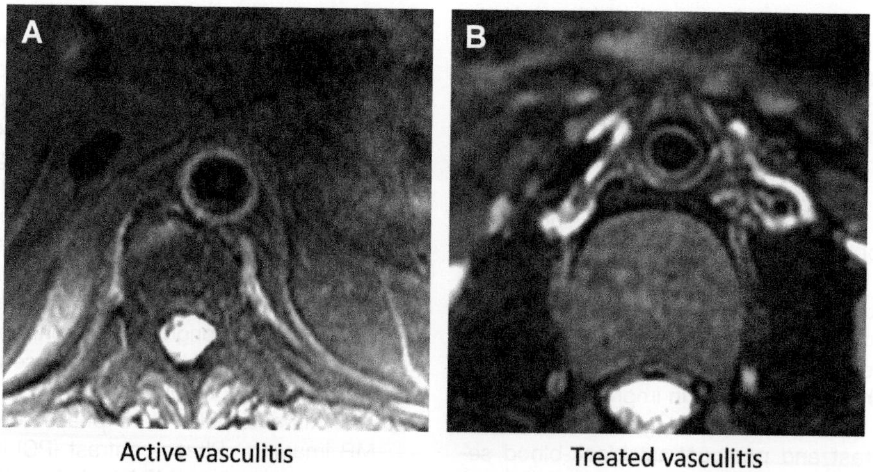


Fig. 3. T2-weighted image in 2 different patients with vasculitis (*A*, *B*). As shown, in patient with acute vasculitis (*A*), the aortic wall shows bright wall signal while aorta seems thickened but does not show bright T2 signal in patients with nonactive or treated vasculitis (*B*). T2-weighted imaging is used for vessel wall evaluation and is typically used to evaluate for edema and disease activity.

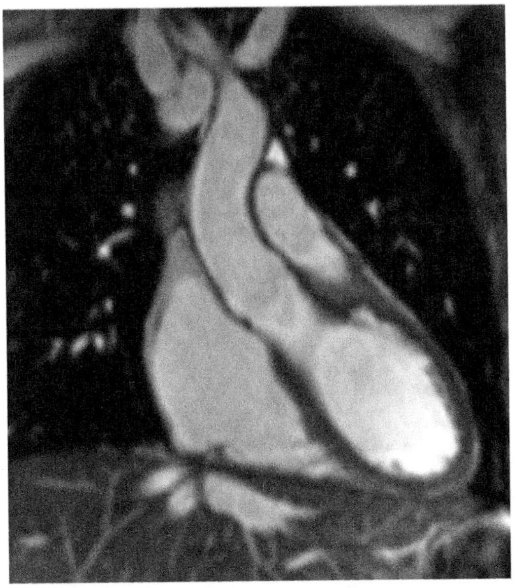

Fig. 4. Noncontrast MRA in a patient with suspected acute aortic emergency. Navigated 3D SSFP images showing high-quality imaging of the aorta without requiring contrast administration.

Four-dimensional-flow MRA can be used for real-time assessment of blood flow patterns. In 4D flow mapping, a series of 3D images are captured over time and converted into a 3D video (Cine-sequence) (Video 1). Four-dimensional-flow mapping has been demonstrated in qualitative and quantitative assessments of hemodynamic consequences of pathologic flow disturbances in diverse cardiovascular regions, including the aorta, ventricles, atria, pulmonary arteries, intracranial arteries, portal, and splanchnic arteries.[33–37] Four-dimensional-flow mapping also offers various advanced hemodynamic measures of pathologic flow disturbances, including vorticity and helicity, wall shear stress, flow displacement, pressure gradients, viscous energy loss, and turbulent kinetic energy. The clinical utility of 4D-flow MR imaging-based metrics remains under investigation, although it is increasingly being recognized.[38,39] Four-dimensional flow mapping is a rapidly evolving technique for the assessment of hemodynamic markers. It may offer several advantages over 2D flow mappings, such as ability retrospective data analysis, improved qualitative assessment, application in diverse cardiovascular regions, and availability of a diverse set of hemodynamic markers with a potential role in the management of aortic diseases.

### *Aortography*

Aortography is an invasive endovascular procedure involving the injection of a contrast agent into the aorta through a catheter. For diagnostic evaluation of aortic diseases, aortography is no longer performed and has been supplanted by less invasive and highly sensitive and specific modalities such as CTA and MRA.[8,40,41] However, aortography is still the preferred modality for guiding endovascular therapeutic interventions.

## AORTIC MEASUREMENT

To define normal ranges (adjusted for age, sex, and body habitus), develop management guidelines, risk stratification, treatment planning, prognostication, and follow-up (treatment response assessment and surveillance) for aortic diseases; it is crucial to first develop an accurate and reproducible system for measurements of the aorta.[12,42] At present, there is no universally accepted standard for aortic diameter measurements (eg, inner edge to the inner edge, outer edge to outer edge) across different imaging modalities.

### *Aortic Measurements Technique*

Measurements of the aortic diameter must be performed perpendicular to the aortic long-axis, as estimation using oblique angles (to vessel long-axis) can lead to overestimation.[8,43] For aortic measurements on CT or MR imaging, the latest (2022) American College of Cardiology and American Heart Association guidelines suggest using double oblique inner-edge-to-inner-edge measurements if the aortic wall is healthy and use outer-to-outer-wall when the aortic wall is diseased in patients with atherosclerotic thickening, aortitis, dissection, or intramural hematoma (IMH)[1] (**Fig. 5**). The aortic root is measured from commissure to the opposite sinus or from sinus to sinus, whichever one is larger at the end-diastole. It is more important to have an institution standard and have consistent method of aortic measurement in every aortic study. Measurement using sinus-to-sinus with inner-edge-to-inner-edge (I-I) on CT and MR imaging has shown high user confidence and lower intraobserver and interobserver variability and better correlation with echocardiogram.[1,16,43] The use of ECG-gated triggered to end-diastole can also help reduce measurement variabilities.[44] In patients with open aortic repair and a replaced aortic graft, the measurement of graft is done from the inner edge to the inner edge (I-I) for the determination of the functional lumen and future treatment planning.

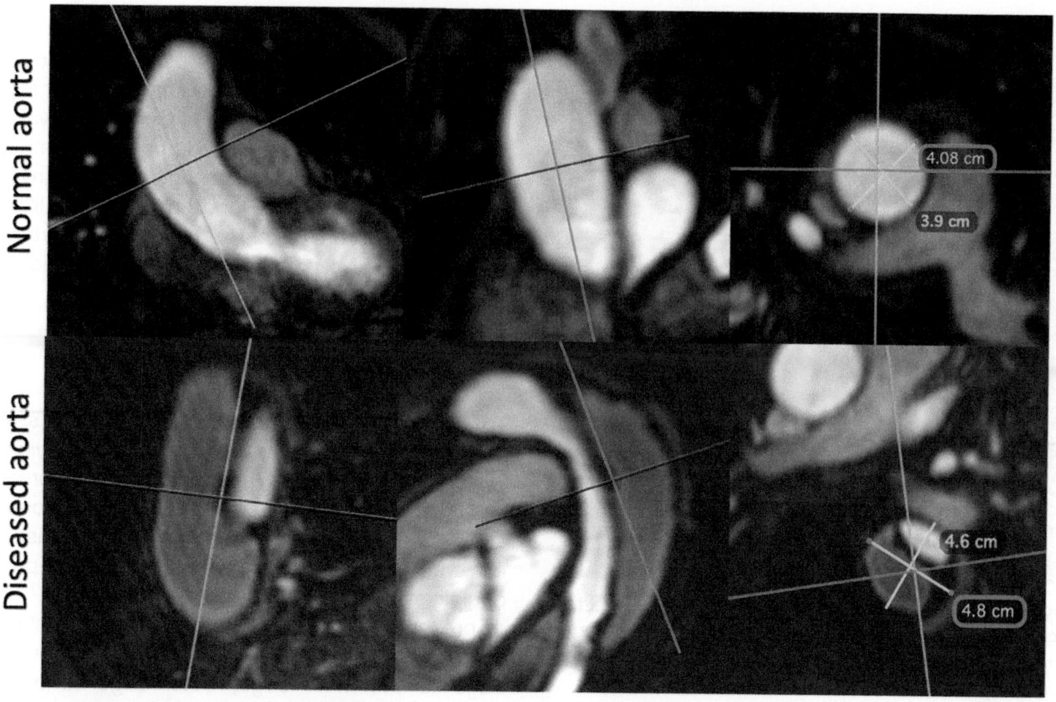


Fig. 5. Double oblique method highlighting the correct technique of measuring aorta from inner-to-inner wall when aortic wall is normal (top row) and measuring from outer diseased wall to outer diseased wall in a patient with aortic aneurysm, mural thrombus, and aortic atherosclerosis (bottom row).

It is worth noting that different imaging techniques may provide slightly different measurements of the aorta. Therefore, to improve the consistency and usability of serial readings, it is advisable to use the same imaging modality for longitudinal monitoring of aortic disease.

### *Normal Aortic Dimensions*

The normal diameter of the aortic root and the ascending aorta is influenced by age, gender, and body surface area. Hence, the use of a single cutoff value is not recommended. Aortic diameter is normalized using a ratio of aortic diameter to body surface area (aortic size index, ASI, centimeter per square meter) or of aortic diameter to the patient's height (aortic height index, AHI, centimeter per centimeter) or ratio of aortic cross-sectional area to the patient's height (cross-sectional area to height ratio, square centimeter per meter) is preferable for clinical use and to use as a predictor of adverse events including rupture, dissection, or death.[45,46] Studies have shown a cross-sectional area-to-height ratio of 10 $cm^2/m$ or greater as a threshold predictive of increased risk of adverse events.[7,16]

## AORTIC DISEASES

Aortic diseases represent a group of diverse pathologic conditions ranging from acute conditions presenting as life-threatening emergencies to chronic conditions, presenting with varied cardiovascular symptoms or as an incidental finding on imaging. Based on the temporal presentation, aortic diseases can be broadly classified as acute or chronic. The most commonly encountered aortic pathologic conditions include AAS, aneurysm, aortitis (inflammatory and infectious), atherosclerosis, and congenital anomalies.

### *Acute Aortic Syndrome*

AAS represents a group of life-threatening aortic pathologic conditions characterized by a sudden disruption in the integrity of the aortic wall. The most common causes of AAS include aortic dissection, IMH, penetrating aortic ulcer (PAU), traumatic aortic rupture, and aortic aneurysm rupture (contained or not contained).[47] These heterogeneous conditions have different underlying causes but they often present with similar clinical features, characterized by acute severe chest (or abdominal) pain that may radiate to the neck or back, hemodynamic instability (shock), and often requiring emergent intervention.[28,47–49]

Given the acute life-threatening nature of AAS, imaging is critical in early and accurate diagnosis, identifying site(s) of involvement and complications to help guide optimum and timely therapeutic interventions. CTA is the preferred imaging modality for the evaluation of AAS due to its widespread availability and speed of acquisition. However, MRA is useful for the evaluation of patients when CTA is contraindicated or for longitudinal follow-up.

### *Aortic dissection*

Aortic dissection is the most common cause of AAS. It is characterized by a tear in the intima, the innermost layer of the aortic wall. This tear allows the blood to pass through the tear into the media and thereby creates a dissection flap (filled with blood). This dissection flap can expand in either direction (antegrade or retrograde, along the aortic long-axis). There is an evident entry and exit tear with double barrel appearance of the aorta.

**Etiopathogenesis** The overall incidence of aortic dissection ranges from 0.5 to 3 cases per 100,000 person-years.[1] The usual age at presentation ranges between 50 and 70 years, with people with congenital aortic diseases may present at a younger age. The most common risk factor is hypertension, followed by preexisting aortic diseases (Marfan syndrome, bicuspid aortic valve, Loeys-Dietz syndrome, and Ehlers-Danlos syndrome), aortic valve disease, familial aortic disease, cigarette smoking, direct, blunt chest trauma, and the use of intravenous drugs such as cocaine and amphetamine.[25,50,51]

**Classification** Aortic dissection is classified based on anatomic location (Stanford or DeBakey classification) or time from onset of symptoms.

The DeBakey system divides dissections into types I, II, and III based on the origin of the intimal tear and the extent of the dissection (**Fig. 6**).[52]

- Type I: Dissection tear originating in the ascending aorta and extending distally to the aortic arch.
- Type II: Dissection tear confined to the ascending aorta.
- Type III: Dissection tear originates in the descending thoracic aorta.
  - Type IIIa: confined to descending thoracic aorta.
  - Type IIIb: extending distally below the diaphragm.

The Stanford classification system divides dissections into 2 categories based on the involvement of ascending aorta (see **Fig. 6**).[1]

- Type A: Involving the ascending aorta. More common and managed surgically.
- Type B: Not involving the ascending aorta. Less common, managed conservatively with antihypertensive therapy or by endovascular stent repair unless complicated by end-organ ischemia or persistent symptoms.[53] Endovascular stent treatment is associated with reduced aorta-specific mortality but no overall mortality benefit when compared with medical management.[2]

In 2019, a new category was published by the European Association for Cardio-Thoracic Surgery and the European Society for Vascular Surgery, Non-A-non-B, in which the proximal dissection flap start in the aortic arch.[54] In 2020, the Society of Thoracic Surgeons and Society for Vascular Surgery proposed a new classification in which aortic dissection was divided based on the location of intimal tears and the proximal and distal extent of the dissection process.[55] Stanford classification remains the most commonly used classification system, although frequently, there is institutional variability.

The aortic dissection is divided into 4 temporal types: hyperacute (within 24 hours), acute (2–7 days), subacute (8–30 days), and chronic (more than 30 days).[56] The hyperacute and acute period carries a high mortality risk, approximately 1% to 2% per hour rupture risk, with 75% of aortic dissection–related deaths reported during the first 2 weeks.[8,57]

**Complications** Aortic regurgitation (AR) is a common complication associated with type A aortic dissection, seen in up to 50% of cases. There are multiple underlying mechanisms, including aortic dilatation, an extension of the dissection flap into the sinuses of Valsalva (thereby detaching the aortic valve commissures from the aortic wall) or prolapse of the dissection flap through aortic leaflet.[58,59] It is important to recognize AR and its underlying mechanisms of AR to allow appropriate surgical intervention (repair vs replacement of aortic valve). Although MR imaging can help with delineation of aortic valve pathologic condition, echocardiogram is faster and superior.

Malperfusion syndrome is characterized by clinical evidence of end-organ ischemia by branch vessel obstruction. The presence of malperfusion syndrome is a poor prognostic sign and is associated with a mortality rate of 30.5% versus 6.2% in patients without malperfusion. Mesenteric malperfusion has an associated mortality rate of 63.2%.[60,61] The branch vessel obstruction can be static or dynamic. In static obstruction, the dissection flap extends and blocks the branch vessel. In dynamic obstruction, the dissection flap (FL) compresses and true lumen, thereby impairing flow to branch vessels.

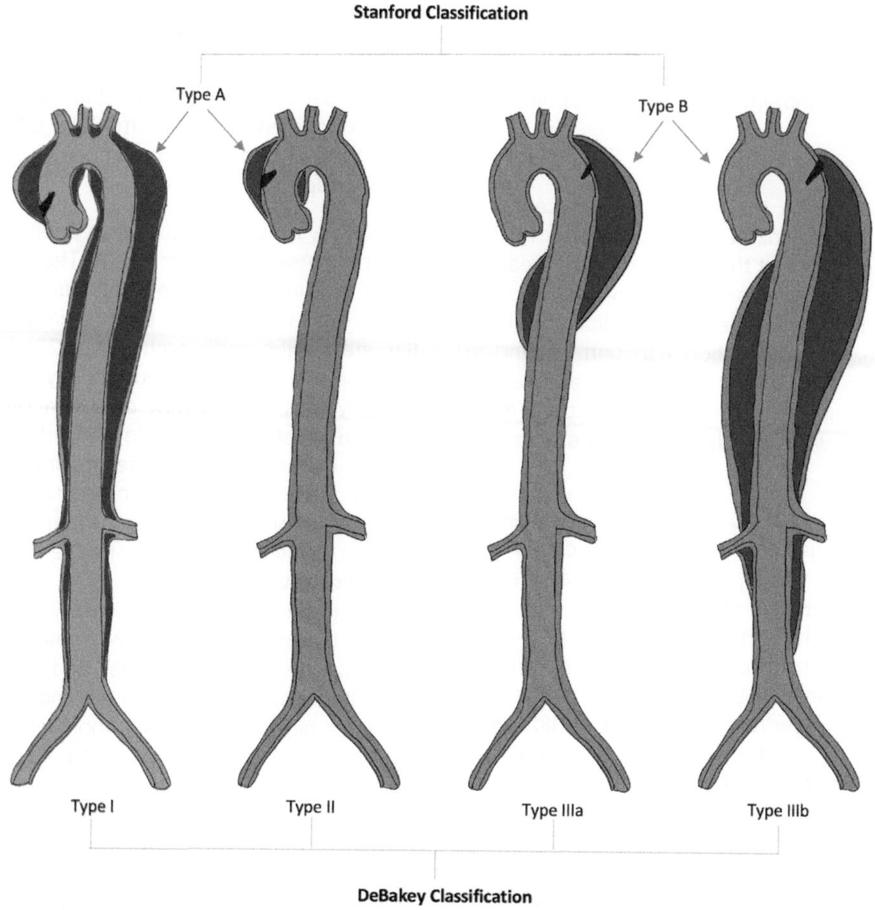


**Fig. 6.** The Stanford and DeBakey classification for aortic dissection and intramural hematoma.

TEE and MRA can help in the early identification of these complications by both direct visualizations of extension of the dissection flap as well as changes in flow pattern (Doppler, 2D or 4D flow map) through the aortic valve (AR) and branch vessels (malperfusion syndrome). It is interesting to note that imaging evidence of malperfusion can be seen in up to 25% of patients with acute aortic dissection on imaging; however, they may not be clinically symptomatic (**Fig. 7**).

**Diagnosis** Imaging is critical to the diagnosis and management of aortic dissection. TEE, CTA, and MRA are all highly accurate for the diagnosis of AAS. One meta-analysis looking at the comparative diagnostic accuracy of different imaging modalities (TEE, CTA, and MRA) showed excellent diagnostic accuracy for all 3 modalities, with sensitivity between 98% and 100% and specificity between 94% and 98%.[40] Clinically CT is the most preferred imaging modality, primarily due to its widespread availability in emergency departments, more user expertise, and rapid image acquisition. However, as discussed previously, better knowledge of MR techniques and use of succinct and focused imaging protocols can bridge the gap.

Imaging of suspected aortic dissection must be able to identify the dissection flap (FL) and its extent, origin, and extent of the aortic wall (intimal) tear, and presence of risk factors (such as a bicuspid aortic valve) and complications. The presence of a dissection flap (FL, channel between the layers of the aortic wall) is pathognomic for aortic dissection. MR imaging has high sensitivity (97%–100%) and specificity (94%–100%) for diagnosing aortic dissection.[62] Black-blood (aortic wall) and 2D or 4D-flow (blood flow patterns) sequences can help distinguish between true and FL (based on flow pattern and anatomic features). It can help identify the origin and extent of aortic dissection. For instance, the presence of bright pericardial effusion on the black-blood sequence may suggest a rupture of ascending aorta rupturing into the pericardial space.[4] Four-dimensional-flow mapping can help quantify the

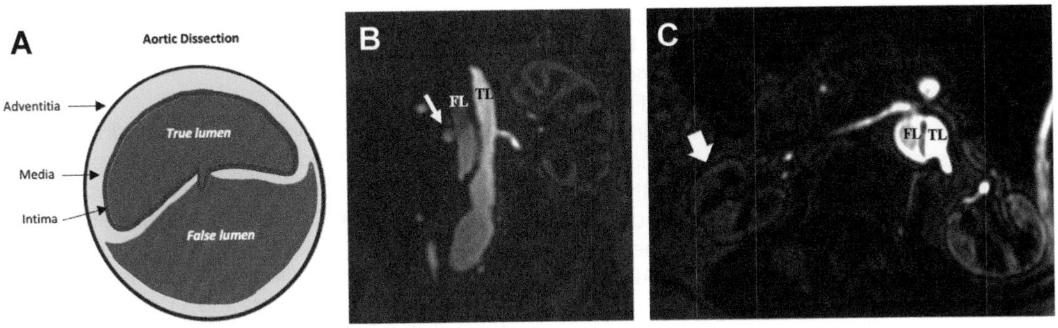


**Fig. 7.** A 63-year-old man with acute aortic dissection. An image (*A*) showing the pathogenesis of aortic dissection. Coronal MRA image (*B*) showing right renal artery (*arrow*) originating from the FL and left renal artery originating from the true lumen (TL). Axial MRA image (*C*) showing differential renal enhancement with decreased right renal perfusion (*block arrow*, C). Although imaging showed malperfusion of the right kidney, the patient was clinically asymptomatic, and the renal function was preserved.

aortic wall stress, flow pattern within the false and true lumen, and presence of thrombus.[63,64] Four-dimensional-flow studies have shown that the technique can detect small flap fenestration in aortic dissection and provide additional information about flow through fenestrations throughout the cardiac cycle, when compared with CTA and conventional MR imaging.[65] In patients with type-B aortic dissection, FL ejection fraction, defined as the ratio of retrograde flow rate at the dominant entry tear during diastole over the antegrade systolic flow rate, is shown to be an independent predictor of aortic growth.[66] Additionally, the presence of high-volume turbulent flow in FL is shown to be associated with higher risk of late complications.[67]

**Management** Early and accurate diagnosis of AAS is important for timely treatment to provide optimum outcomes and prevent acute and chronic complications. Early initiation of medical treatment has been shown to reduce long-term aorta-related adverse events.[68–70] Therefore, it is recommended while undergoing evaluation for definitive treatment (eg, surgical intervention in type-A aortic dissection or endovascular intervention in type-B aortic dissection). Medical management is targeted at aggressive control of blood pressure and heart rate to reduce aortic wall stress, using intravenous beta blockers (or calcium channel blockers if a contraindication to beta blockers) followed by vasodilators adjunctive therapy (ideally started after beta-blockers or calcium channel blockers to avoid compensatory tachycardia).[71,72]

Open surgical or endovascular stent graft repair is the preferred modality for the definitive management of AAS. The type of definitive management is often dictated by the patient's hemodynamic status and complications related to AAS. For instance, type-A aortic dissection, which is associated with potentially life-threatening sequelae, including rupture leading to cardiac tamponade, shock, malperfusion, or the presence of these complications, warrants the earliest surgical intervention is preferred.[73]

Endovascular aortic repair (thoracic endovascular aortic repair [TEVAR]) of type-B aortic dissection is being frequently performed with a goal to place the stent in true lumen and cover the entry and exit tear. Postprocedural imaging is useful for evaluating expansion of stent graft, branch anastomosis, reevaluation for improvement in malperfusion, and detection of endoleaks. A study using 4D flow MR imaging for detecting endoleaks found 4D flow MR imaging to be superior to CTA, allowing the distinction of type II endoleak into subtypes (type IIa and IIb) based on flow patterns of the aortic side branches.[74] It is also worth noting that certain applicability of TEE or intravascular ultrasounds can be limited by the type of stent graft used in the procedure. For instance, stents made of polytetrafluoroethylene or Gore-Tex-based material act as a barrier to ultrasound waves.[8]

Long-term follow-up is crucial for prognostication and early diagnosis of complications. The recommended time frame for follow-up assessment of the aorta is 1, 3, 6, and 12 months after the procedure, followed by yearly examinations.[8] Prognostic factors associated with poor outcomes include an increase in false luminal pressure (seen as compression of the true lumen, thrombosis, and blood flow pattern changes in the FL) and persistence of false patent lumen and aortic diameter. An aortic diameter of more than 45 mm after the acute phase with a false patent lumen or descending thoracic aortic diameter of more than 55 mm or annual growth of more than 5 mm is associated with a high risk of aortic rupture and warrants surgical reintervention.[25]

CT and MR imaging are preferred modalities for a long-term follow-up, given their large field of view and excellent anatomic information, including surrounding structure. MR imaging and MRA offer added advantages, including lack of ionizing radiations and assessment of blood flow using 2D or 4D flow mapping. It has been shown that the combined use of 4D flow MR imaging and computational flow dynamics could predict the post-TEVAR flow dynamics from pre-TEVAR flow data.[75]

### *Penetrating aortic ulcer*

**Etiopathogenesis** A PAU is characterized by an ulceration of an atherosclerotic lesion that disrupts/penetrates the intimal layer. It typically affects elderly patients with severe atherosclerotic disease. It can involve multifocal lesions, as the underlying process of atherosclerosis is generally diffuse.[76] It accounts for 2% to 7% of all AAS.[77] Some isolated PAUs remain asymptomatic and are only incidentally detected on imaging such as CTA or MRA. It is most commonly located in the descending thoracic aorta and is uncommon in the aortic arch and the abdominal aorta. Clinically PAU presents similar to aortic dissection and other AAS.[1]

PAU can progress to IMH (penetrating media), aortic dissection (media with FL), aneurysm, or rupture (penetrating through all the 3 layers of the aortic wall resulting in saccular, fusiform, or pseudoaneurysm, which may ultimately rupture) based on level of penetration. Overall, rupture is uncommon. The presence of progression lesions is a poor prognostic indicator.

**Diagnosis** Diagnosis of PAU and its complications can be evaluated using MR imaging. The commonly seen imaging features include irregular crater-like contrast-filled protrusion/out-pouching from the aortic wall (**Fig. 8**).[17] Calcified atherosclerotic plaques surrounding the ulcer are better seen on CT imaging. Extraluminal outpouchings (saccular, fusiform, or pseudoaneurysm) are well visualized both on CT and MR imaging. A size of more than 13 mm or a neck of more than 10 mm is associated with rapid progression and therefore warrants early definitive treatment.[78] Intramural hematomas are seen as areas of high signal intensity on T-1 weighted images within the aortic wall.[8]

**Management** Current management strategy for PAU treatment even for asymptomatic PAU if they have a diameter of 13 mm or greater to 20 mm or a depth of 10 mm or greater, or if they involve ascending aorta. Any-size symptomatic PAUs are associated with a high risk of early disease progression and treatment through open surgical or endovascular intervention is recommended.[79,80]

### *Intramural hematoma*

**Etiopathogenesis** IMH is characterized by hemorrhage within the media. It has a distinct pathologic condition to aortic dissection or PAU. It typically affects elderly patients with hypertension and severe atherosclerotic disease.[81] It is most commonly located in the descending thoracic aorta (60%), followed by ascending aorta (30%) and aortic arch (10%).[81] It accounts for 6% to 44% (6%–23% in North America and Europe and 26%–44% in Asia) of all AAS.[1] Clinically, it presents with similar symptoms to aortic dissection and other AAS.

IMH can progress to aortic dissection, aneurysm, or rupture or lead to malperfusion (through similar mechanisms seen in aortic dissection). In some cases, the hematoma can also be resorbed. Intramural hematomas use the same classification system as aortic dissection. Type-A IMH is associated with an 18% risk of rupture at presentation and 100% mortality without surgical intervention.[79] Type-B IMH is associated with a lower mortality rate ranging from 4% to 6% with medical management while in-hospital and 9% at 1-year follow-up.[81,82]

**Diagnosis** On MR imaging, the signal intensity of the hematoma varies with the stage or age of the thrombus. Hyperacute intramural hematoma seems isointense on T1-weighted images and hyperintense on T2-weighted while the late subacute stage is characterized by change from oxyhemoglobin to methemoglobin that changes the signal characteristics to bright crescentic appearance on T1-weighted and T2-weighted images (**Fig. 9**). Given the small size of the IMH-associated lesion, MR imaging may offer an advantage by providing better soft-tissue characterization and luminal evaluation, especially compared with CT in situations iodinated contrast use is relatively or absolutely contraindicated (**Fig. 10**).

Imaging can also be used for risk stratification and guiding treatment approaches. High-risk imaging features associated with intramural hematomas include focal intimal disruption (FID), increasing aortic diameter, increasing hematoma thickness, hematoma thickness 10 mm or greater to 13 mm ($\geq$13 in type B and $\geq$10 mm in type A), pericardial effusion, maximum aortic diameter greater than 45 mm to 50 mm ($\geq$47–50 in type B and $\geq$45–50 mm in type A).[83,84] FID is characterized by contrast-filled outpouching 3 mm or greater from the aortic wall (intraluminal), similar to a PAU. However, unlike PAUs, these FID are

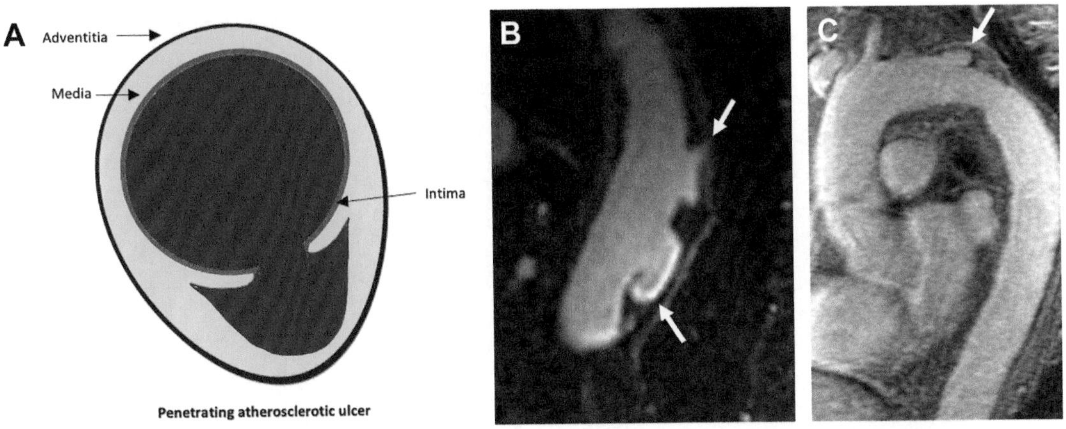


Fig. 8. An image (A) showing pathogenesis of PAU. Coronal (*B*) and Sagittal (*C*) images showing intimal discontinuity with a contained contrast-filled outpouching along the thoracic aorta (*arrows*) consistent with PAUs.

not associated with atherosclerotic plaque. Benign tiny intimal disruptions share a similar physical appearance to FID but are smaller 3 mm or lesser projections.[84] MR imaging may also offer an advantage in serial surveillance imaging for monitoring the dynamic evolution of intramural hematoma, that is, progression to aortic dissection, aneurysm, or rupture.[8]

**Management** Similar to PAU, there is no evidence of directed management guidelines for IMH. For type A IMH, open surgical intervention is recommended. The timing of the procedure remains unclear, with some authors suggesting a delay of 1 to 3 days may offer some advantage by allowing the hematoma to mature.[85] Although in medically unstable patients, urgent intervention is recommended. For the management of type B intramural hematoma, open surgical, TEVAR, and medical management have shown similar results. However, good outcomes were reported with open surgical repair.[86]

### *Traumatic aortic injury*

TAI is often lethal, with more than 80% of patients dying before reaching the hospital.[6,87] TAI can be from sharp (penetrating/direct trauma) or blunt (indirect trauma) force. Penetrating aortic trauma is usually fatal. MR imaging has a limited role in the assessment of acute TAI, given the validated diagnostic accuracy of rapid CTA examinations. However, MR imaging is a great option for serial assessment of chronic aortic trauma because it provides better soft-tissue characterization, assessment of hemorrhagic component of a blunt traumatic thoracic aortic injury, and changes in aorta morphology (sheer wall pressure, blood flow patterns in FL, endoleaks).[4,88]

## *Aortic Aneurysm*

Aneurysm is defined as a permanent localized dilatation of the artery, at least 50% greater than the normal luminal diameter. True aneurysms contain all 3 layers of the vessel wall. Based on

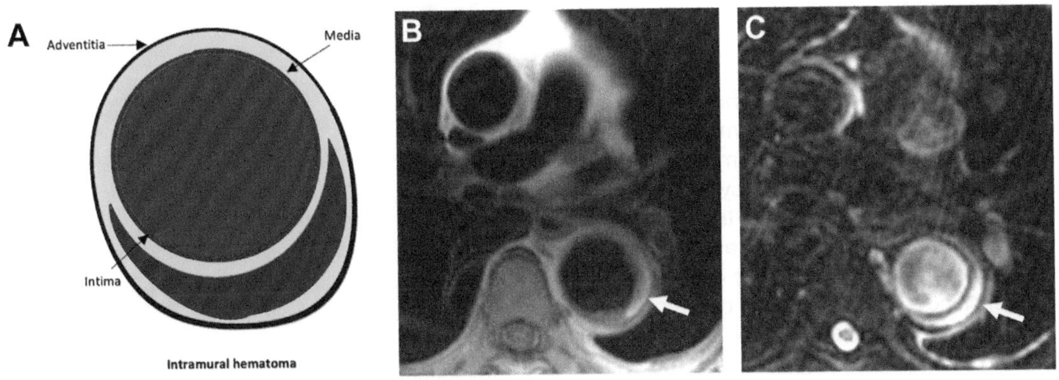


Fig. 9. A diagram (*A*) showing pathogenesis of intramural hematoma. Axial T1-weighted (*B*) and T2-weighted (*C*) images showing subacute stage intramural hematoma with high T1 and T2 signal in the wall of descending thoracic aorta.

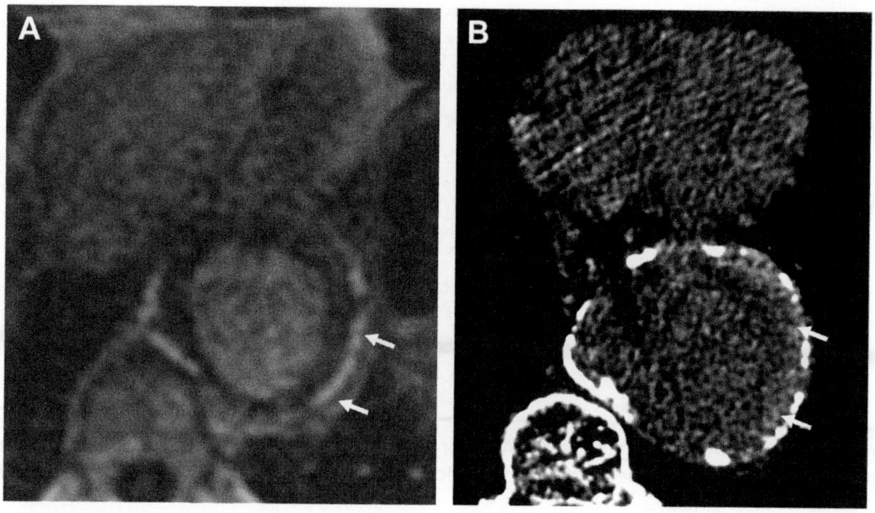


Fig. 10. A 72-year-old woman with history of iodinated contrast severe allergy and known TAA, presenting with acute chest pain. Contrast-enhanced MR angiogram (*A*) showing high signal (*white arrows*) in the periphery of the aneurysm aorta. Although a noncontrast follow-up CT (*B*) also allowed faint delineation of high-density peripheral IMH (*white arrows, B*), MRA, with luminal evaluation, enabled both the diagnosis and presurgical planning.

morphology, the aneurysm can be fusiform (more common) or saccular (less common). Fusiform results from diffuse circumferential weakening of the aortic wall. Saccular aneurysms result from the weakening of the partial segment of the circumferential aortic wall. Usually patients with aortic aneurysm present in their fifth or sixth decades. However, people with connective tissue disorders or congenital aortic diseases may present at a younger age. The incidence of thoracic aortic aneurysm (TAA) ranges from 5 to 10 per 100,000 person-years.[89] The incidence of AAA ranges from 1.3% to 8.9% in men and 1% to 2.2% in women.[90] For TAA, the most common site involved is the aortic root or ascending aorta (60%), followed by descending aorta (30%) and aortic arch (10%). Infrarenal aorta is the most common site for AAA.

### *Etiopathogenesis*

The most common risk factors include hypertension, smoking, hypercholesterolemia, heritable genetic disorders (Marfan syndrome, Loeys-Dietz syndrome, and Ehlers-Danlos syndrome), BAV, history of aortic diseases, and trauma.[91] Aneurysms of the aortic root and ascending aorta tend to be from heritable genetic disorders (fibrillin-1 deficiency being the most common cause) and are often associated with the bicuspid aortic valve.[1] The "tulip bulb" sign refers to the characteristic appearance of annuloaortic ectasia due to symmetric dilatation of the sinuses of Valsalva, with extension into the ascending aorta and effacement of the sinotubular junction (**Fig. 11**). This appearance is typically seen in patients with Marfan syndrome. AAA tends to be from atherosclerosis. It is characterized by cystic medial degeneration of the aortic wall.[1] Although, it is worth remembering that the development of an

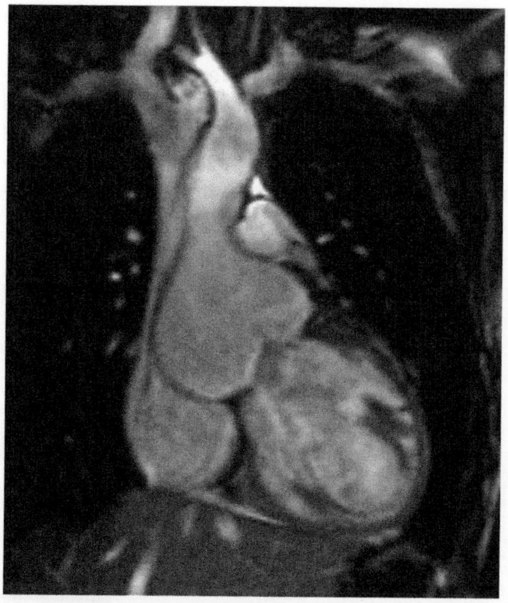

Fig. 11. A 12-year-old girl with Marfan syndrome. Three-dimensional SSFP coronal MRA image showing classical annuloaortic ectasia with sinuses of Valsalva aneurysm and effacement of the sinotubular junction (also known as "Tulip bulb" sign).

aneurysm involves a complex interplay of various hereditary and environmental risk factors.

### *Diagnosis and treatment planning*

Most patients with either TAA or AAA are asymptomatic, and diagnosis is often made on screening or incidentally on imaging. Imaging also plays a key role in risk stratification and treatment planning of aortic aneurysms.

**Role of imaging in screening and diagnosis** Size thresholds are often used for screening, diagnosis, prognostication, or treatment planning. However, single aortic diameter measurements are limited by interindividual variability based on age, sex, height, and body surface area and, therefore, may not be the most accurate assessment of pathologic dilatation. Traditional size thresholds used for diagnosis of TAA and AAA are 4.5 cm and 3 cm, respectively.

Screening of AAA is suggested in patients aged between 65 and 75 years with either a family history of AAA (grade 1 recommendation in men and grade 2a recommendation in women) or has ever smoked (grade 1 recommendation in both men and women), using abdominal ultrasound. Some randomized clinical trials have shown screening associated with significant mortality benefit (Odd ratio, OR: 0.65; 95% confidence interval, CI: 0.57–0.74) and reduction in AAA-related ruptures (OR: 0.62; 95% CI: 0.55–0.70).[1]

TTE and TEE are often limited in their capacity to visualize certain segments of the aorta (distal ascending aorta, aortic arch, and descending aorta) due to normal anatomic structures obscuring the view. MDCT and MR imaging offer excellent alternatives for the assessment of the aorta that cannot be adequately visualized on ultrasound.

**Role of imaging in serial monitoring and risk stratification** The goal of serial monitoring is to prevent complications by providing timely therapeutic interventions. Aortic aneurysm dissection and rupture are 2 of the most dreaded and catastrophic complications of aortic aneurysm. For instance, the mortality rate of ruptured AAA is approximated between 80% and 90%, with many patients dying before even reaching the hospital.[5] Imaging using ultrasound, CT, or MR imaging can provide a simultaneous assessment of aortic diameter, aortic morphology, the extent of involvement of the aorta and its branches, and tools for serial follow-ups.

Aortic diameter is an important prognostic indicator of aortic rupture or dissection.[92] This is based on Laplace's law, meaning that an increase in aortic diameter will lead to a proportional increase in wall stress. Accordingly, a maximum aortic diameter threshold of 5.5 cm is the most used parameter in deciding elective aneurysm repair. However, various studies have shown that as much as 60% of patients with an aortic diameter of less than 5.5 cm can still have aortic dissection or rupture.[93,94] Therefore, it is important to consider additional factors while risk-stratifying aortic aneurysm, including gender (women may have higher rupture risk at smaller diameter compared with men), aneurysm growth of greater than 10 mm/y, severe aortic or mitral regurgitation, uncontrolled hypertension, and inherited or family history of the aortic disease.[1,2,95]

Four-dimensional-flow MR imaging may offer several potential advantages over CT and conventional MR imaging sequences. For instance, 4D-flow MR imaging can be used for accurate assessment (qualitative and quantitative) of the hemodynamic changes (increased turbulence, wall shear stress, pulse wave velocity) that cause aortic wall dysfunction and subsequent aneurysm.[96,97] These metrics may help improve risk stratification and treatment guidelines in aneurysms (particularly ascending aortic aneurysms).

**Role of imaging in treatment planning** Imaging can provide important information on the landing zone (proximal and distal), characteristics of the aneurysm sac (tortuosity and angulation), the relationship of the aneurysm sac with surrounding structures (eg, compression), and assessment of potential vascular access site (patency and lumen size). This information, in turn, helps in deciding between an open surgical versus endovascular approach, vascular access site, and appropriate size (lumen and length) of the stent.

### *Management*

Optimum management of aortic aneurysm requires an appropriate risk stratification based on aortic diameter, site, and extent of involvement of the aneurysm, and existing comorbidities. Based on the risk-stratification, the patient can be managed using the medical and medical plus surgical-endovascular approach.

**Medical management** Asymptomatic patients with aneurysms less than 5.5 cm are often managed using medical treatment strategies. This treatment approach can provide primary (decrease the need for aortic repair by reducing growth rates and rupture or dissection) and secondary (reducing recurrence rate and postintervention complications) preventative strategies for aortic aneurysms. This includes a combination of lifestyle modifications, such as smoking cessation, weight reduction, a well-balanced diet and

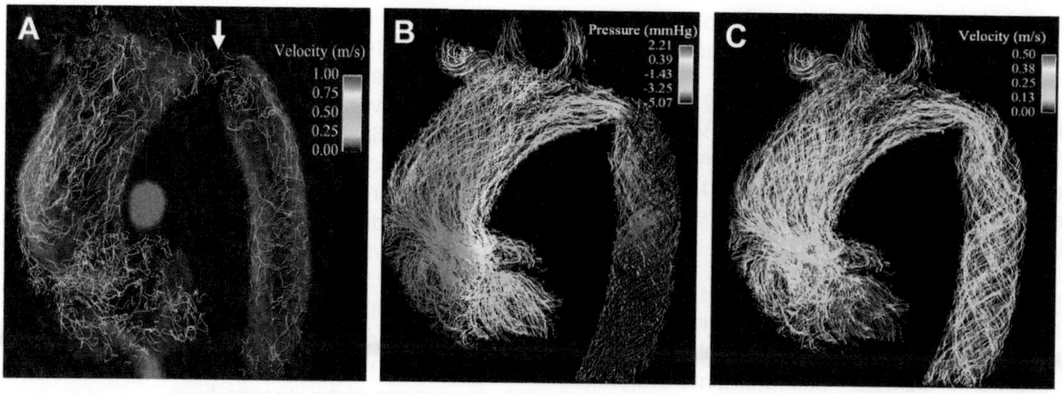


**Fig. 12.** Patient with aortic dissection, status after aortic arch graft repair. Anatomic image from 4D flow data (*A*) showing anatomic narrowing at the graft anastomosis (*white arrow,* A). Pressure (*B*) and velocity (*C*) data showing less than 5 mm Hg drop across the stenosis with no significant flow velocity acceleration suggesting functionally nonsignificant stenosis.

pharmacotherapy with statins (targeting inflammatory and atherosclerotic pathways), antihypertensives (reducing sheer stress on the aortic wall), and antithrombotic therapy (thrombus has been hypothesized to have a role in the pathogenesis of AAA).[1]

**Surgical and endovascular management** In symptomatic patients (resulting from aneurysmal rupture, dissection, or mass effect on surrounding structures), surgical or endovascular interventions are recommended. As most patients are asymptomatic, the need and type of intervention are often dictated by the imaging findings, especially maximal aortic diameter and rate of growth.[1]

An open surgical approach is often associated with higher operative mortality risk as compared with an endovascular approach.[98] Therefore, surgical management is often reserved for patients with unfavorable anatomy for an endovascular intervention.[99]

### *Surveillance after aneurysm repair*

The goal of follow-up examination postintervention is to allow early identification of treatment complications and monitoring of residual disease process. In patients with open repair and anatomic suspicion of anastomotic narrowing, 4D Flow imaging can help measure the pressure gradient and characterize the significance of anastomotic

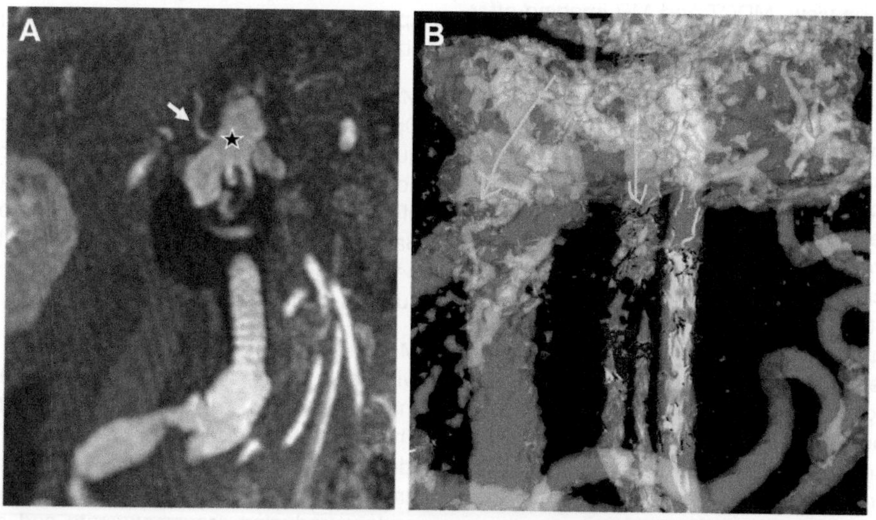


**Fig. 13.** Patient with complex endovascular thoracoabdominal aortic aneurysm repair. Three-dimensional MRA image (*A*) showing endoleak (*star*) with right phrenic artery communicating with the endoleak. It was unclear if the right phrenic artery is being supplied by the endoleak or is the feeding vessel for this endoleak. Four-dimensional Flow (*B*) was performed which showed that the direction of the blood flow in the right phrenic artery is toward the endoleak (*yellow arrows, B*) and confirmed that it is the source of the endoleak for this patient.

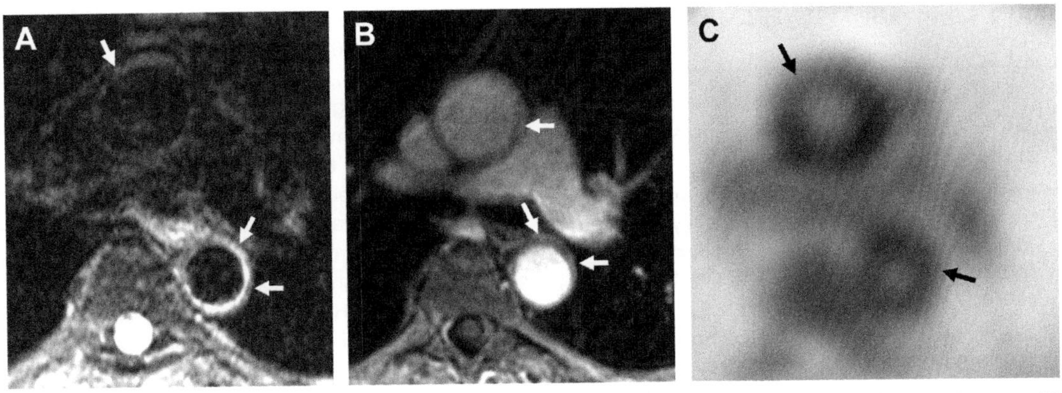


**Fig. 14.** 68-year-old woman with suspected giant cell aortitis. Axial T2 weighted image (*A*) showing increased T2 signal in the ascending and descending aorta (*white arrows, A*). Contrast enhanced MRA (B) showing wall thickening (*white arrows, B*). F18-Deoxy Glucose positron emission tomography (FDG-PET) image (*C*) confirmed high metabolic activity (*black arrows, C*) suggesting active vasculitis.

stenosis (**Fig. 12**). CT is often the preferred modality for post-TEVAR surveillance, which can be helpful in the detection of endoleaks, stent migration, stent-graft fracture or collapse, and aneurysmal dilation of other aortic segments. MR imaging-based follow-up can be limited by metallic artifacts. Although, as discussed previously, MR imaging and flow mapping (2D and 4D) may provide excellent surveillance tools, particularly for the detection of endoleaks and evaluate directionality of blood-flow in suspected type-2 endoleak (**Fig. 13**). MR imaging may also be preferred in younger-middle-aged patients to avoid side effects related to ionizing radiation and iodinated contrast needed in CT-based evaluation.[100]

## *Other Aortic Conditions*

### *Aortitis*

**Infectious aortitis (mycotic aneurysm)** Infectious aortitis is quite rare and often results from septic emboli from endocarditis.[101] It can result in a mushroom-shaped aneurysm, hence the name. It is interesting to note that almost all mycotic aneurysms have a bacterial source, although fungal causes (from *Candida or Aspergillus*) may be seen in immunocompromised patients.[1] Similar to other aortic aneurysms, imaging (CT, MR imaging) can help assess the aneurysm and cardiovascular and valvular function to help formulate a treatment plan.

**Inflammatory aortitis** It is caused by the deposition of inflammatory tissues in the adventitia layer. The 2 most common causes include Takayasu arteritis and giant cell arteritis, primarily affecting the thoracic aorta.[102,103] In comparison, immunoglobulin G4–related diseases primarily affect the abdominal aorta.[102] Takayasu arteritis typically affects young women and is most prevalent in Asia and South America while giant cell arteritis typically presents with new onset headache in patients aged older than 50 years with tenderness of the temporal arteries or decreased pulsation in that region.[104] Imaging can show vascular wall thickening (on CT or MR imaging) and an increase in [$^{18}$F]Fluorodeoxyglucose ($^{18}$F-FDG) uptake on FDG-PET[105] (**Fig. 14**). In chronic stage, areas of stenosis or strictures can be seen.[103] Imaging can help differentiate between infectious and inflammatory aortitis because periaortic fluid and air in periaortic region favor infectious cause.[106] Treatment options include anti-inflammatory therapy and revascularization procedures.

## SUMMARY

MR imaging has an integral role in the screening, diagnosis, management, and posttherapeutic surveillance of aortic pathologic conditions. Advances in imaging that allow improved ECG-gating and techniques such as 4D flow MR imaging, may offer a new paradigm in the management of aortic pathologic conditions by improving the accuracy of anatomic assessment and complementing the anatomic data with physiologic flow disturbances that are involved in the pathogenesis of the aortic disorder, respectively. However, faster and improved 4D flow processing and further systematic evaluation are critical for these advances to integrated into clinical practice guidelines for the management of aortic disorders.

## CLINICS CARE POINTS

- Aortic diseases have diverse presentations and urgent treatment needs.
- Imaging is crucial for early diagnosis and treatment. MRI Imaging is primarily reserved for non-emergent aortic diseases, but is routinely used even for acute cases in many centers.
- Advancements in imaging technology, like 4D-flow MR imaging, and therapeutic interventions offer new possibilities for managing aortic diseases and improving clinical outcomes.
- Use of Gadolinium or Ferumoxytol is an excellent alternative for CT imaging in patients with contraindication to iodinated contrast or when radiation risk needs to be mitigated.

## SUPPLEMENTARY DATA

Supplementary data related to this article can be found online at https://doi.org/10.1016/j.mric.2023.05.002.

## REFERENCES

1. Members WC, Isselbacher EM, Preventza O, et al. 2022 ACC/AHA Guideline for the diagnosis and management of aortic disease: a report of the American Heart Association/American College of Cardiology Joint Committee on Clinical Practice Guidelines. J Am Coll Cardiol 2022;80(24):e223–393.
2. Nagpal P, Khandelwal A, Saboo SS, et al. Modern imaging techniques: applications in the management of acute aortic pathologies. Postgrad Med 2015;91(1078):449–62.
3. Nagpal P, Mullan BF, Sen I, et al. Advances in imaging and management trends of traumatic aortic injuries. Cardiovasc Interv Radiol 2017;40:643–54.
4. Fattori R, Nienaber CA. MRI of acute and chronic aortic pathology: Pre-operative and postoperative evaluation. J Magn Reson Imag 1999;10(5):741–50.
5. Hoornweg L, Storm-Versloot M, Ubbink D, et al. Meta analysis on mortality of ruptured abdominal aortic aneurysms. Eur J Vasc Endovasc Surg 2008;35(5):558–70.
6. Fox N, Schwartz D, Salazar JH, et al. Evaluation and management of blunt traumatic aortic injury. J Trauma Nurs 2015;22(2):99–110.
7. Rodriguez-Palomares JF, Teixido-Tura G, Galuppo V, et al. Multimodality assessment of ascending aortic diameters: comparison of different measurement methods. J Am Soc Echocardiogr 2016;29(9):819–26. e4.
8. Goldstein SA, Evangelista A, Abbara S, et al. Multimodality imaging of diseases of the thoracic aorta in adults: from the American Society of Echocardiography and the European Association of Cardiovascular Imaging: endorsed by the Society of Cardiovascular Computed Tomography and Society for Cardiovascular Magnetic Resonance. J Am Soc Echocardiogr 2015;28(2):119–82.
9. Weinreb JC, Rodby RA, Yee J, et al. Use of intravenous gadolinium-based contrast media in patients with kidney disease: consensus statements from the American College of Radiology and the National Kidney Foundation. Radiology 2021;298(1):28–35.
10. Raman SV, Aneja A, Jarjour WN. CMR in inflammatory vasculitis. J Cardiovasc Magn Reson 2012;14:1–14.
11. Corti R, Fuster V. Imaging of atherosclerosis: magnetic resonance imaging. Eur Heart J 2011;32(14):1709–19.
12. Sakamoto I, Sueyoshi E, Uetani M. MR imaging of the aorta. Radiol Clin 2007;45(3):485–97.
13. Nagpal P, Agrawal MD, Saboo SS, et al. Imaging of the aortic root on high-pitch non-gated and ECG-gated CT: awareness is the key! Insights Imaging 2020;11(1):51.
14. Priya S, Thomas R, Nagpal P, et al. Congenital anomalies of the aortic arch. Cardiovasc Diagn Ther 2018;8(Suppl 1):S26.
15. Davenport MS, Perazella MA, Yee J, et al. Use of intravenous iodinated contrast media in patients with kidney disease: consensus statements from the American College of Radiology and the National Kidney Foundation. Radiology 2020;294(3):660–8.
16. Asch FM, Yuriditsky E, Prakash SK, et al. The need for standardized methods for measuring the aorta: multimodality core lab experience from the GenTAC registry. JACC Cardiovasc Imaging 2016;9(3):219–26.
17. Kpodonu J, Ramaiah VG, Diethrich EB. Intravascular ultrasound imaging as applied to the aorta: a new tool for the cardiovascular surgeon. Ann Thorac Surg 2008;86(4):1391–8.
18. Lortz J, Papathanasiou M, Rammos C, et al. High intimal flap mobility assessed by intravascular ultrasound is associated with better short-term results after TEVAR in chronic aortic dissection. Sci Rep 2019;9(1):7267.
19. Lang RM, Badano LP, Tsang W, et al. EAE/ASE recommendations for image acquisition and display using three-dimensional echocardiography. Eur Heart J Cardiovasc Imaging 2012;13(1):1–46.
20. Abraha I, Luchetta ML, De Florio R, et al. Ultrasonography for endoleak detection after endoluminal abdominal aortic aneurysm repair. Cochrane Database Syst Rev 2017;6.

21. Sebastià C, Pallisa E, Quiroga S, et al. Aortic dissection: diagnosis and follow-up with helical CT. Radiographics 1999;19(1):45–60.
22. Saadi EK. Multidetector computed tomography scanning is still the gold standard for diagnosis of acute aortic syndromes. Interact Cardiovasc Thorac Surg 2010;11(3):359.
23. Roos JE, JrK Willmann, Weishaupt D, et al. Thoracic aorta: motion artifact reduction with retrospective and prospective electrocardiography-assisted multi-detector row CT. Radiology 2002; 222(1):271–7.
24. Wu W, Budovec J, Foley WD. Prospective and retrospective ECG gating for thoracic CT angiography: a comparative study. Am J Roentgenol 2009;193(4):955–63.
25. Erbel R, Aboyans V, Boileau C, et al. 2014 ESC guidelines on the diagnosis and treatment of aortic diseases. Kardiol Pol 2014;72(12):1169–252.
26. Kinno M, Nagpal P, Horgan S, et al. Comparison of Echocardiography, Cardiac Magnetic Resonance, and Computed Tomographic Imaging for the Evaluation of Left Ventricular Myocardial Function: Part 2 (Diastolic and Regional Assessment). Curr Cardiol Rep 2017;19(1):6.
27. Kinno M, Nagpal P, Horgan S, et al. Comparison of Echocardiography, Cardiac Magnetic Resonance, and Computed Tomographic Imaging for the Evaluation of Left Ventricular Myocardial Function: Part 1 (Global Assessment). Curr Cardiol Rep 2017; 19(1):9.
28. Moore AG, Eagle KA, Bruckman D, et al. Choice of computed tomography, transesophageal echocardiography, magnetic resonance imaging, and aortography in acute aortic dissection: International Registry of Acute Aortic Dissection (IRAD). Am J Cardiol 2002;89(10):1235–8.
29. Kuo AH, Nagpal P, Ghoshhajra BB, et al. Vascular magnetic resonance angiography techniques. Cardiovasc Diagn Ther 2019;9(Suppl 1):S28–36.
30. Jalili MH, Yu T, Hassani C, et al. Contrast-enhanced MR Angiography without Gadolinium-based Contrast Material: Clinical Applications Using Ferumoxytol. Radiol Cardiothorac Imaging 2022;4(4): e210323.
31. Bollache E, van Ooij P, Powell A, et al. Comparison of 4D flow and 2D velocity-encoded phase contrast MRI sequences for the evaluation of aortic hemodynamics. Int J Cardiovasc Imag 2016;32: 1529–41.
32. Lotz J, Meier C, Leppert A, et al. Cardiovascular flow measurement with phase-contrast MR imaging: basic facts and implementation. Radiographics 2002;22(3):651–71.
33. Hope MD, Meadows AK, Hope TA, et al. Evaluation of bicuspid aortic valve and aortic coarctation with 4D flow magnetic resonance imaging. Circulation 2008;117(21):2818–9.
34. Töger J, Kanski M, Carlsson M, et al. Vortex ring formation in the left ventricle of the heart: analysis by 4D flow MRI and Lagrangian coherent structures. Ann Biomed Eng 2012;40:2652–62.
35. Goubergrits L, Riesenkampff E, Yevtushenko P, et al. MRI-based computational fluid dynamics for diagnosis and treatment prediction: Clinical validation study in patients with coarctation of aorta. J Magn Reson Imag 2015;41(4):909–16.
36. JU Fluckiger, Goldberger JJ, Lee DC, et al. Left atrial flow velocity distribution and flow coherence using four-dimensional FLOW MRI: A pilot study investigating the impact of age and Pre-and Postintervention atrial fibrillation on atrial hemodynamics. J Magn Reson Imag 2013;38(3):580–7.
37. Odagiri K, Inui N, Miyakawa S, et al. Abnormal hemodynamics in the pulmonary artery seen on time-resolved 3-dimensional phase-contrast magnetic resonance imaging (4D-flow) in a young patient with idiopathic pulmonary arterial hypertension. Circ J 2014;78(7):1770–2.
38. Garcia J, Barker AJ, Markl M. The role of imaging of flow patterns by 4D flow MRI in aortic stenosis. JACC Cardiovasc Imaging 2019;12(2):252–66.
39. Campbell-Washburn AE, Faranesh AZ, Lederman RJ, et al. Magnetic resonance sequences and rapid acquisition for MR-guided interventions. Magnetic Resonance Imaging Clinics 2015;23(4):669–79.
40. Shiga T, Wajima ZI, Apfel CC, et al. Diagnostic accuracy of transesophageal echocardiography, helical computed tomography, and magnetic resonance imaging for suspected thoracic aortic dissection: systematic review and meta-analysis. Arch Intern Med 2006;166(13):1350–6.
41. Bansal RC, Chandrasekaran K, Ayala K, et al. Frequency and explanation of false negative diagnosis of aortic dissection by aortography and transesophageal echocardiography. J Am Coll Cardiol 1995;25(6):1393–401.
42. Vasan RS, Larson MG, Levy D. Determinants of echocardiographic aortic root size: the Framingham Heart Study. Circulation 1995;91(3):734–40.
43. Schulz-Menger J, Bluemke DA, Bremerich J, et al. Standardized image interpretation and post processing in cardiovascular magnetic resonance: Society for Cardiovascular Magnetic Resonance (SCMR) board of trustees task force on standardized post processing. J Cardiovasc Magn Reson 2013;15(1):1–19.
44. Potthast S, Mitsumori L, Stanescu LA, et al. Measuring aortic diameter with different MR techniques: Comparison of three-dimensional (3D) navigated steady-state free-precession (SSFP), 3D contrast-enhanced magnetic resonance

angiography (CE-MRA), 2D T2 black blood, and 2D cine SSFP. J Magn Reson Imag 2010;31(1): 177–84.
45. Beebe HG, Kritpracha B, Serres S, et al. Endograft planning without preoperative arteriography: a clinical feasibility study. J Endovasc Ther 2000;7(1):8–15.
46. Zafar MA, Li Y, Rizzo JA, et al. Height alone, rather than body surface area, suffices for risk estimation in ascending aortic aneurysm. J Thorac Cardiovasc Surg 2018;155(5):1938–50.
47. Vilacosta I, San Román JA. Acute aortic syndrome. Heart; 2001. p. 365–8.
48. Chen C-W, Tseng Y-H, Lin C-C, et al. Aortic dissection assessment by 4D phase-contrast MRI with hemodynamic parameters: The impact of stent type. Quant Imag Med Surg 2021;11(2):490.
49. Ramanath VS, Oh JK, Sundt TM III, et al. Acute aortic syndromes and thoracic aortic aneurysm. Mayo Clin Proc 2009;84(5):465–81.
50. Meszaros I, Morocz J, Szlavi J, et al. Epidemiology and clinicopathology of aortic dissection. Chest 2000;117(5):1271–8.
51. Clouse WD, Hallett JW, Schaff HV, et al. Acute aortic dissection: population-based incidence compared with degenerative aortic aneurysm rupture. Mayo Clin Proc 2004;79(2):176–80.
52. De Bakey ME, Henly WS, Cooley DA, et al. Surgical management of dissecting aneurysms of the aorta. J Thorac Cardiovasc Surg 1965;49(1):130–49.
53. Nienaber CA, Eagle KA. Aortic dissection: new frontiers in diagnosis and management: Part I: from etiology to diagnostic strategies. Circulation 2003;108(5):628–35.
54. Czerny M, Schmidli J, Adler S, et al. Current options and recommendations for the treatment of thoracic aortic pathologies involving the aortic arch: an expert consensus document of the European Association for Cardio-Thoracic surgery (EACTS) and the European Society for Vascular Surgery (ESVS). Eur J Cardio Thorac Surg 2019; 55(1):133–62.
55. Lombardi JV, Hughes GC, Appoo JJ, et al. Society for Vascular Surgery (SVS) and Society of Thoracic Surgeons (STS) reporting standards for type B aortic dissections. Ann Thorac Surg 2020;109(3): 959–81.
56. Booher AM, Isselbacher EM, Nienaber CA, et al. The IRAD classification system for characterizing survival after aortic dissection. Am J Med 2013; 126(8):730.e19-24.
57. Tsai TT, Nienaber CA, Eagle KA. Acute aortic syndromes. Circulation 2005;112(24):3802–13.
58. Movsowitz HD, Levine RA, Hilgenberg AD, et al. Transesophageal echocardiographic description of the mechanisms of aortic regurgitation in acute type A aortic dissection: implications for aortic valve repair. J Am Coll Cardiol 2000;36(3):884–90.
59. La Canna G, Maisano F, De Michele L, et al. Determinants of the degree of functional aortic regurgitation in patients with anatomically normal aortic valve and ascending thoracic aorta aneurysm. Transoesophageal Doppler echocardiography study. Heart 2009;95(2):130–6.
60. Geirsson A, Szeto WY, Pochettino A, et al. Significance of malperfusion syndromes prior to contemporary surgical repair for acute type A dissection: outcomes and need for additional revascularizations. Eur J Cardio Thorac Surg 2007; 32(2):255–62.
61. Berretta P, Trimarchi S, Patel HJ, et al. Malperfusion syndromes in type A aortic dissection: what we have learned from IRAD. J Vis Surg 2018;4.
62. Nienaber C, Spielmann R, Von Kodolitsch Y, et al. Diagnosis of thoracic aortic dissection. Magnetic resonance imaging versus transesophageal echocardiography. Circulation 1992;85(2):434–47.
63. Pitcher A, Cassar TE, Leeson P, et al. Aortic dissection: visualisation of aortic blood flow and quantification of wall shear stress using time-resolved, 3D phase-contrast MRI. J Cardiovasc Magn Reson 2011;13(1):1–2.
64. Clough R, Hussain T, Uribe S, et al. An MRI examination for evaluation of aortic dissection using a blood pool agent. J Cardiovasc Magn Reson 2010;12(1):1–2.
65. Allen BD, Aouad PJ, Burris NS, et al. Detection and Hemodynamic Evaluation of Flap Fenestrations in Type B Aortic Dissection with 4D Flow MRI: Comparison with Conventional MRI and CTA. Radiol Cardiothorac Imaging 2019;1(1). https://doi.org/10.1148/ryct.2019180009.
66. Burris NS, Nordsletten DA, Sotelo JA, et al. False lumen ejection fraction predicts growth in type B aortic dissection: preliminary results. Eur J Cardio Thorac Surg 2020;57(5):896–903.
67. Takahashi K, Sekine T, Miyagi Y, et al. Four-dimensional flow analysis reveals mechanism and impact of turbulent flow in the dissected aorta. Eur J Cardio Thorac Surg 2021;60(5):1064–72.
68. Berretta P, Patel HJ, Gleason TG, et al. IRAD experience on surgical type A acute dissection patients: results and predictors of mortality. Ann Cardiothorac Surg 2016;5(4):346.
69. Umana-Pizano JB, Nissen AP, Sandhu HK, et al. Acute type A dissection repair by high-volume vs low-volume surgeons at a high-volume aortic center. Ann Thorac Surg 2019;108(5):1330–6.
70. Hattori S, Noguchi K, Gunji Y, et al. Acute type A aortic dissection in non-agenarians: to cut or not. Interact Cardiovasc Thorac Surg 2020;31(1): 102–7.
71. Trimarchi S, Nienaber CA, Rampoldi V, et al. Contemporary results of surgery in acute type A aortic dissection: The International Registry of

Acute Aortic Dissection experience. J Thorac Cardiovasc Surg 2005;129(1):112–22.
72. Long SM, Tribble CG, Raymond DP, et al. Preoperative shock determines outcome for acute type A aortic dissection. Ann Thorac Surg 2003;75(2):520–4.
73. Zindovic I, Sjögren J, Bjursten H, et al. Impact of hemodynamic instability and organ malperfusion in elderly surgical patients treated for acute type A aortic dissection. J Cardiovasc Surg 2015;30(11):822–9.
74. Sakata M, Takehara Y, Katahashi K, et al. Hemodynamic analysis of endoleaks after endovascular abdominal aortic aneurysm repair by using 4-dimensional flow-sensitive magnetic resonance imaging. Circ J 2016;80(8):1715–25.
75. Pirola S, Guo B, Menichini C, et al. 4-D Flow MRI-Based Computational Analysis of Blood Flow in Patient-Specific Aortic Dissection. IEEE Trans Biomed Eng 2019;66(12):3411–9.
76. Coady MA, Rizzo JA, Hammond GL, et al. Penetrating ulcer of the thoracic aorta: what is it? How do we recognize it? How do we manage it? J Vasc Surg 1998;27(6):1006–16.
77. Eggebrecht H, Plicht B, Kahlert P, et al. Intramural hematoma and penetrating ulcers: indications to endovascular treatment. Eur J Vasc Endovasc Surg 2009;38(6):659–65.
78. Rocchi G, Lofiego C, Biagini E, et al. Transesophageal echocardiography–guided algorithm for stent-graft implantation in aortic dissection. J Vasc Surg 2004;40(5):880–5.
79. Chou AS, Ziganshin BA, Charilaou P, et al. Long-term behavior of aortic intramural hematomas and penetrating ulcers. J Thorac Cardiovasc Surg 2016;151(2):361–73. e1.
80. Yang L, Zhang QY, Wang XZ, et al. Long-Term Imaging Evolution and Clinical Prognosis Among Patients With Acute Penetrating Aortic Ulcers: A Retrospective Observational Study. J Am Heart Assoc 2020;9(18):e014505.
81. Harris KM, Braverman AC, Eagle KA, et al. Acute aortic intramural hematoma: an analysis from the International Registry of Acute Aortic Dissection. Circulation 2012;126(11_suppl_1):S91–6.
82. Tolenaar JL, Harris KM, Upchurch GR Jr, et al. The differences and similarities between intramural hematoma of the descending aorta and acute type B dissection. J Vasc Surg 2013;58(6):1498–504.
83. Moral S, Ballesteros E, Roque M, et al. Intimal disruption in type B aortic intramural hematoma. Does size matter? A systematic review and meta-analysis. Int J Cardiol 2018;269:298–303.
84. Moral S, Cuéllar H, Avegliano G, et al. Clinical implications of focal intimal disruption in patients with type B intramural hematoma. J Am Coll Cardiol 2017;69(1):28–39.
85. Matsushita A, Fukui T, Tabata M, et al. Preoperative characteristics and surgical outcomes of acute intramural hematoma involving the ascending aorta: A propensity score–matched analysis. J Thorac Cardiovasc Surg 2016;151(2):351–8.
86. Chakos A, Twindyawardhani T, Evangelista A, et al. Endovascular versus medical management of type B intramural hematoma: a meta-analysis. Ann Cardiothorac Surg 2019;8(4):447.
87. Neschis DG, Scalea TM, Flinn WR, et al. Blunt aortic injury. N Engl J Med 2008;359(16):1708–16.
88. Gavelli G, Canini R, Bertaccini P, et al. Traumatic injuries: imaging of thoracic injuries. Eur Radiol 2002;12(6):1273–94.
89. Sampson UK, Norman PE, Fowkes FGR, et al. Global and regional burden of aortic dissection and aneurysms: mortality trends in 21 world regions, 1990 to 2010. Global heart 2014;9(1):171–80. e10.
90. Mathur A, Mohan V, Ameta D, et al. Aortic aneurysm. J Transl Int Med 2016;4(1):35–41.
91. Singh K, Bønaa K, Jacobsen B, et al. Prevalence of and risk factors for abdominal aortic aneurysms in a population-based study: The Tromsø Study. Am J Epidemiol 2001;154(3):236–44.
92. Davies RR, Goldstein LJ, Coady MA, et al. Yearly rupture or dissection rates for thoracic aortic aneurysms: simple prediction based on size. Ann Thorac Surg 2002;73(1):17–28.
93. Rylski B, Blanke P, Beyersdorf F, et al. How does the ascending aorta geometry change when it dissects? J Am Coll Cardiol 2014;63(13):1311–9.
94. Pape LA, Tsai TT, Isselbacher EM, et al. Aortic diameter$\geq$ 5.5 cm is not a good predictor of type A aortic dissection: observations from the International Registry of Acute Aortic Dissection (IRAD). Circulation 2007;116(10):1120–7.
95. Forbes TL, Lawlor DK, DeRose G, et al. Gender differences in relative dilatation of abdominal aortic aneurysms. Ann Vasc Surg 2006;20(5):564–8.
96. Markl M, Wallis W, Harloff A. Reproducibility of flow and wall shear stress analysis using flow-sensitive four-dimensional MRI. J Magn Reson Imag 2011;33(4):988–94.
97. Bürk J, Blanke P, Stankovic Z, et al. Evaluation of 3D blood flow patterns and wall shear stress in the normal and dilated thoracic aorta using flow-sensitive 4D CMR. J Cardiovasc Magn Reson 2012;14(1):1–11.
98. Mori M, Shioda K, Wang X, et al. Perioperative risk profiles and volume-outcome relationships in proximal thoracic aortic surgery. Ann Thorac Surg 2018;106(4):1095–104.
99. Picel AC, Kansal N. Essentials of endovascular abdominal aortic aneurysm repair imaging: preprocedural assessment. Am J Roentgenol 2014;203(4):W347–57.

100. Weigel S, Tombach B, Maintz D, et al. Thoracic aortic stent graft: comparison of contrast-enhanced MR angiography and CT angiography in the follow-up: initial results. Eur Radiol 2003;13:1628–34.
101. Sakalihasan N, Michel J-B, Katsargyris A, et al. Abdominal aortic aneurysms. Nat Rev Dis Prim 2018;4(1):34.
102. Svensson LG, Arafat A, Roselli EE, et al. Inflammatory disease of the aorta: patterns and classification of giant cell aortitis, Takayasu arteritis, and nonsyndromic aortitis. J Thorac Cardiovasc Surg 2015;149(2):S170–5.
103. Rodriguez F, Degnan KO, Nagpal P, et al. Insidious: Takayasu Arteritis. Am J Med 2015;128(12):1288–91.
104. Ghouri MA, Gupta N, Bhat AP, et al. CT and MR imaging of the upper extremity vasculature: pearls, pitfalls, and challenges. Cardiovasc Diagn Ther 2019;9(Suppl 1):S152–73.
105. Veeranna V, Fisher A, Nagpal P, et al. Utility of multimodality imaging in diagnosis and follow-up of aortitis. J Nucl Cardiol 2016;23(3):590–5.
106. Pennell RC, Hollier LH, Lie J, et al. Inflammatory abdominal aortic aneurysms: a thirty-year review. J Vasc Surg 1985;2(6):859–69.

# MR Angiography of Extracranial Carotid Disease

Anthony Peret, MD[a], Griselda Romero-Sanchez, MD[b], Mona Dabiri, MD[c], Joseph Scott McNally, MD, PhD[d], Kevin M. Johnson, PhD[e], Mahmud Mossa-Basha, MD[f], Laura B. Eisenmenger, MD[a,*]

**KEYWORDS**

• Magnetic resonance angiography • MR imaging • Atherosclerosis • Carotid artery • Vessel wall imaging

**KEY POINTS**

- Magnetic resonance angiography (MRA) provides imaging of vascular structures while having capability to concomitantly provide tissue characterization using structural, diffusion, and perfusion contrast in addition to vessel wall imaging (VWI).
- MR imaging VWI is a promising noninvasive method to evaluate vessel wall pathologic condition. It can depict important plaque features such as intraplaque hemorrhage (IPH), lipid-rich necrotic core, and fibrous cap.
- Atherosclerotic plaques with a similar degree of stenosis may vary from a histopathological standpoint with high-risk plaque composition associated with plaque rupture, thrombosis, and cerebral ischemic events.
- IPH is a marker of plaque vulnerability and has been associated with plaque rupture, plaque progression, distal embolization, and cerebrovascular events.
- MRA can also help in the diagnosis and management of nonatherosclerotic conditions of the extracranial carotid artery such as blunt trauma, inflammatory vasculopathies, pseudoaneurysms, and carotid webs.

## INTRODUCTION

A properly functioning central nervous system necessitates a reliable blood supply. Indeed, although the brain merely represents 2% of the total body weight on average, it consumes 20% to 25% of the body's total energy requirement. The carotid-vertebral system is the main route for blood delivery to the encephalon and cerebellum. The extracranial carotid artery is susceptible to primary vascular pathologic conditions such as atherosclerosis, the most frequent extracranial carotid disease, as well as vascular trauma and inflammatory vasculopathies.

Catheter-based, digital subtraction angiography (DSA) has conventionally been the gold standard in carotid imaging since its invention. However, DSA is invasive and requires arterial access,

[a] Department of Radiology, University of Wisconsin-Madison, 600 Highland Avenue, Madison, WI 53705, USA; [b] Department of Radiology, Instituto Nacional de Ciencias Medicas y Nutricion Salvador Zubiran, Avenida Vasco de Quiroga No.15, Colonia Belisario Domínguez Sección XVI, Delegación Tlalpan C.P.14080, Ciudad de México, Mexico City, Mexico; [c] Radiology Department, Children's Medical Center, Tehran University of Medical Science, No 63, Gharib Avenue, Keshavarz Blv, Tehran 1419733151, Iran; [d] Department of Radiology, University of Utah, 50 N Medical Dr, Salt Lake City, UT 84132, USA; [e] Department of Medical Physics, University of Wisconsin-Madison, 600 Highland Avenue, Madison, WI 53705, USA; [f] Department of Radiology, University of Washington School of Medicine, 1959 NE Pacific Street, Seattle, WA 98195, USA

* Corresponding author.
*E-mail address:* LEisenmenger@uwhealth.org

Magn Reson Imaging Clin N Am 31 (2023) 395–411
https://doi.org/10.1016/j.mric.2023.04.003

exposes the patient to ionizing radiation, and uses potentially nephrotoxic iodinated contrast agents.[1] Computed tomography angiography (CTA) is a common noninvasive alternative. However, CTA has similar risks related to radiation dose and iodinated contrast administration. Magnetic resonance angiography (MRA) provides imaging of vascular structures while having capability to concomitantly provide tissue characterization using structural, diffusion, and perfusion contrast in addition to VWI.[2] MRA is a noninvasive method of evaluating the intracranial and extracranial vasculature that provides exceptional anatomic detail without the cost of ionizing radiation and has become the modality of choice in many clinical situations.[3]

Here we aim to review the applications of MRA and MR VWI in extracranial carotid imaging, with an emphasis on atherosclerotic disease and a brief review of other diagnostically relevant carotid pathologic conditions.

## *Normal Anatomy and Imaging Technique*

### *Normal Anatomy*

The extracranial segments of the carotid artery include the common carotid artery (CCA), the cervical internal carotid artery (ICA), and the external carotid artery (ECA). The ICA and ECA provide blood supply to the structures of the brain and the face, respectively, although there are numerous ICA-ECA anastomoses. The left CCA emerges directly from the aortic arch, whereas the right CCA emerges from the brachiocephalic artery. Each CCA divides into ICA and ECA at the carotid bifurcation, approximately at the C4 vertebral level. The carotid bifurcation is a site of predilection for atherosclerotic plaque formation as the blood flow is locally turbulent.[4]

## *Lumen MR Imaging*

MRA sequences such as time-of-flight (TOF) angiography and postgadolinium contrast-enhanced (CE) angiography are dedicated to luminal imaging and to stenosis quantification.[5,6] TOF is a conventional gradient echo sequence that utilizes radiofrequency pulses to saturate the signal from stationary tissues and maximize inflow signal enhancement. It can either be done in two-dimensional (2D) or three-dimensional (3D). 2D-TOF offers high signal and is relatively robust to slow flow. Three-dimensional TOF, however, uses smaller voxels and thus provides weaker signal with slow flow but has the advantage of higher resolution. This limitation is improved by the use of multiple overlapping thin-slab acquisition, a technique that consists of multiple overlapping 3D-TOF slabs to minimize saturation effects for through-plane or in-plane flow.[1] The main advantage of TOF over CE-MRA is that it does not require gadolinium. Therefore, TOF can be used in patients with contraindications to gadolinium such as pregnancy or renal failure, particularly if the glomerular filtration rate is less than 30 mL/min/1.73 $m^2$.[7]

Although used frequently for intracranial imaging, TOF often overestimates moderate carotid bifurcation stenosis.[8] Conversely, CE-MRA is highly accurate for occlusion or high-grade stenosis[8,9] and has therefore largely replaced TOF for cervical carotid evaluation. Current CE-MRA methods provide better definition of vessel contours, increased coverage, shorter acquisition times, robust signal-to-noise ratio, and fewer artifacts. The main CE-MRA limitation is the need for gadolinium-based contrast agents. A recent concern is parenchymal gadolinium deposition in the brain, especially in patients requiring multiple follow-up examinations,[10] although the consequences, if any, of gadolinium deposition are not clearly known to date.

## *Vessel Wall MR Imaging*

MR imaging VWI is a promising noninvasive method to evaluate vessel wall pathologic condition. Most cervical carotid studies focus on a limited field of view (FOV) including the carotid bifurcation and the proximal ICA. At minimum, VWI protocols either include precontrast and postcontrast T1-weighted imaging, for instance "Sampling Perfection with Application optimized Contrast using different flip angle Evolution" (SPACE - Siemens) "Volume ISotropic Turbo spin echo Acquisition" (VISTA - Phillips), or CUBE (GE Healthcare). In addition, protocols can include a sequence focused on IPH such as magnetization-prepared rapid acquisition with gradient echo (MPRAGE) (**Fig. 1**). Some institutions incorporate T2-weighted and proton density-weighted imaging. This multicontrast approach seeks to more comprehensively describe plaque composition, although focusing on IPH can also have value and help in the identification of stroke sources as well as stroke prediction.[11–13] Note that in patients with a contraindication to gadolinium, TOF can provide both luminal imaging, IPH evaluation and calcification detection, although TOF is somewhat limited for calcification assessment.[14] Without gadolinium contraindications, CE-MRA and postcontrast T1-weighted VWI can evaluate plaque features such as fibrous cap and lipid core.[15,16]

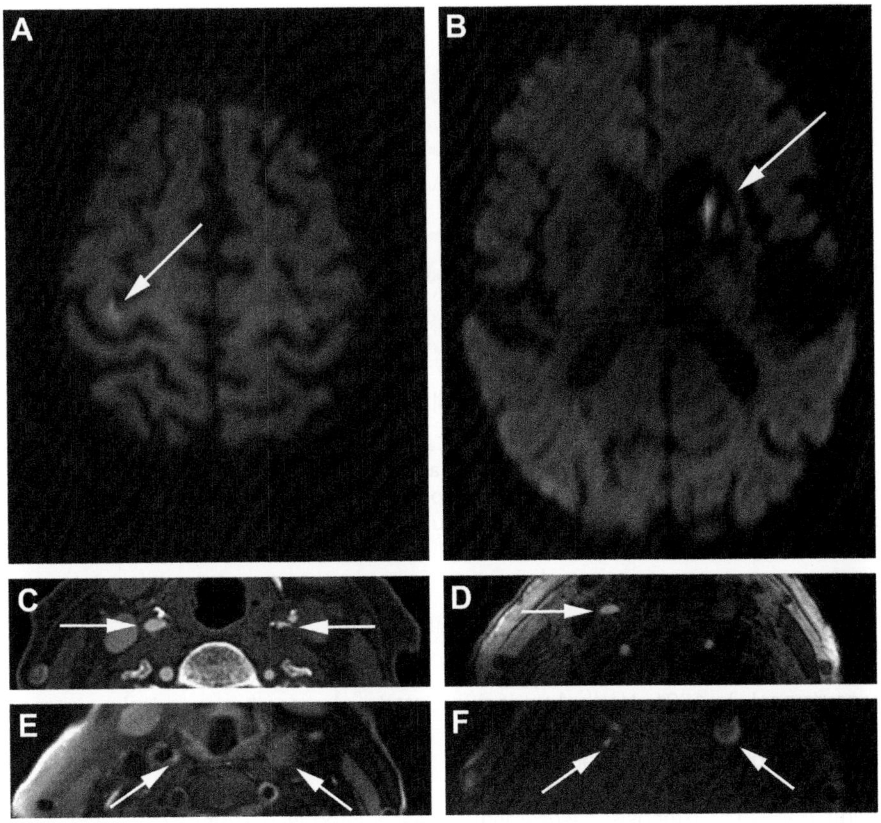


**Fig. 1.** Case of a patient with bilateral internal carotid IPH and bilateral infarcts. On diffusion-weighted imaging, recent infarcts seem as hyperintense, diffusion-restricted areas (*A* and *B*, *arrows*). Computed tomography angiogram shows thick ICA atherosclerotic plaques, predominantly in the left ICA (*C*, *arrows*). Three-dimensional axial TOF (*D*), T1-weighted imaging with fat saturation (*E*), and MPRAGE (*F*) show hyperintense signal within the plaque, corresponding to IPHs (*arrows*).

According to the American Society of Neuroradiology (ASNR), the minimum VWI requirements include[17] the following:

- Field strength = 3T (optimal option) or 1.5 T (acceptable alternative)
- In-plane resolution = 0.6 mm, through-plane resolution = 2 mm
- Longitudinal coverage = 3 to 4 cm centered on the carotid bifurcation (for 2D-VWI)
- Effective blood suppression (for a plaque burden visualization sequence)
- Either 2D or 3D sequences, or a combination of both
- Carotid coils recommended for all protocols

## *Atherosclerotic Disease Imaging Findings/Pathology*

Atherosclerosis is characterized by progressive formation of plaques rich in lipidic aggregates, inflammatory cells, and connective tissue. Its prevalence increases with cardiovascular risk factors such as obesity, age older than 55 years, hyperlipidemia, hypertension, and diabetes.[18] Atherosclerotic carotid artery narrowing is reported in up to 75% of men and 62% of women aged 65 years and older.[19] Atherosclerosis is a major cause of stroke, the second most common cause of mortality worldwide,[20] with 18% to 25% of strokes caused by carotid atherosclerosis.[21]

In routine clinical practice, extracranial carotid atherosclerosis is assessed with ultrasonography (US), DSA, CTA, and MRA.[22,23] The goal of these techniques is to quantify luminal stenosis and evaluate for surface irregularities.[24,25] However, atherosclerotic plaques with a similar degree of stenosis may vary from a histopathological standpoint (**Fig. 2**). Plaque composition is associated with plaque rupture, thrombosis, and ischemic events.[26–28] Advanced imaging techniques such as multicontrast VWI can depict these plaque features (**Table 1**), which can serve to stratify plaque risk based on plaque composition.[29,30]

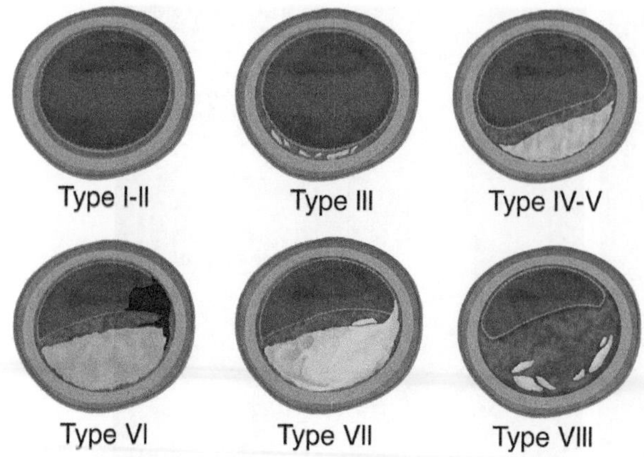

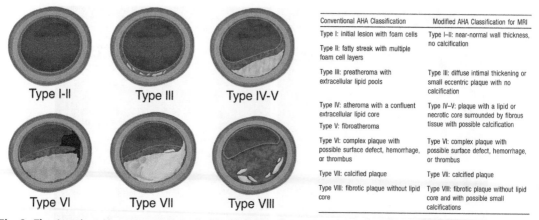

| Conventional AHA Classification | Modified AHA Classification for MRI |
|---|---|
| Type I: initial lesion with foam cells<br>Type II: fatty streak with multiple foam cell layers | Type I–II: near-normal wall thickness, no calcification |
| Type III: preatheroma with extracellular lipid pools | Type III: diffuse intimal thickening or small eccentric plaque with no calcification |
| Type IV: atheroma with a confluent extracellular lipid core<br>Type V: fibroatheroma | Type IV–V: plaque with a lipid or necrotic core surrounded by fibrous tissue with possible calcification |
| Type VI: complex plaque with possible surface defect, hemorrhage, or thrombus | Type VI: complex plaque with possible surface defect, hemorrhage, or thrombus |
| Type VII: calcified plaque | Type VII: calcified plaque |
| Type VIII: fibrotic plaque without lipid core | Type VIII: fibrotic plaque without lipid core and with possible small calcifications |

**Fig. 2.** The American Heart Association classification for atherosclerosis describes the different types of atherosclerotic plaques based on histological findings. Vessel wall MR imaging allows the depiction of plaque features such as hemorrhage and LRNCs, with good correlation to histology. Plaques with similar degree of stenosis but different content present variable risks of rupture and subsequent ischemic events.

## *Stenosis*

DSA is the luminal gold standard,[31,32] although US, CTA, and MRA can also be used for luminal stenosis measurement. In 1991, North American Symptomatic Carotid Endarterectomy Trial (NASCET) cemented the role of carotid stenosis as a stroke predictor, leading to our current approach for intervention (**Fig. 3**).[33] Stenosis assessment alone, however, is inadequate in stroke risk stratification, because stable stenotic plaques will frequently remain asymptomatic, whereas plaques with vulnerable features causing only mild-to-moderate stenosis frequently lead to acute cerebral infarction.[34–41] Similarly, there is a poor correlation between stenosis and plaque burden, which are other known risk factors for stroke.[42–44] Several vulnerable plaque features are good candidates to better stratify stroke risk regardless of the degree of luminal narrowing.[45–48]

## *Plaque Volume*

Increased carotid plaque volume has been shown to be a good marker of plaque vulnerability and correlated with risk of cardiovascular events.[43,49–51] Plaque volume is an indirect indicator of plaque composition, in that an increased proportion of lipid and calcifications is found in larger plaques, with increased likelihood of IPH.[52] VWI is a reproducible technique to evaluate plaque volume, with a interreader variability between 3% and 6%.[53,54] Several VWI studies showed that increasing plaque volume was associated with progression of low-grade asymptomatic lesions into higher grade plaques with increased rupture risk.[44,55,56] VWI assessing plaque volume could be useful in monitoring treatment response.[57]

## *Plaque Surface*

Morphologically, atherosclerotic plaque surface can be classified as smooth, irregular, or ulcerated.[58] A smooth plaque lacks surface ulceration or irregularity. An irregular surface indicates small fissures of the luminal surface of the plaque and is considered a risk factor for embolism and is associated with TIA/stroke.[59] Plaque ulceration is "an intimal defect larger than 1 mm in width, exposing the necrotic core of the atheromatous plaque"[60]; however, other authors suggested alternative (smaller) sizes.[61–63] The NASCET trial demonstrated a significantly increased cerebrovascular risk in ulcerated plaques.[24] MR imaging/MRA detects plaque ulcerations with a sensitivity similar to CT,[64] with VWI directly depicting thinning or disruption of the fibrous cap and exposed lipid core. In addition, CE-MRA improves the sensitivity for ulcerations by 37.5% compared with unenhanced TOF.[64]

## *Intraplaque Hemorrhage*

IPH is the accumulation of blood products within atherosclerotic plaque due to neovessel rupture or plaque rupture itself. This phenomenon is precipitated by inflammation, metabolic disease, elevated blood pressure, and diabetes.[65–67] IPH is a marker of plaque vulnerability[41] and has been associated with plaque rupture, plaque progression, distal embolization, and cerebrovascular events.[26,61,68,69]

VWI is the best technique to detect IPH and numerous authors therefore recommend that it becomes a standard in the identification of carotid artery vulnerable plaques.[41,70–73] Meta-analyses demonstrated that MR imaging-detected carotid

**Table 1**
**Signal intensity changes of the plaque components on different VW-MR imaging sequences**

| Plaque Components | TlWI | TlWI + Gd | T2WI | PD | 3D-TOF |
|---|---|---|---|---|---|
| Lipid core (2) | Iso/high | No | Low | Low | Low |
| Fibrous cap | Iso | Yes: High | Mixed | Mixed | Low |
| Fibrous Tissue (1) | Iso/high | Yes: High | Mixed | Mixed | Iso/Low |
| Calcifications (4) | Low | No | Low | Low | Low |
| Hemorrhage (3) | | | | | |
| Acute (<1 wk) | High | No | Low/Iso | Low/Iso | High |
| Subacute (1–6 wk) | High | No | High | High | High |
| Chronic (>6 wk) | Low | No | Low | Low | Low |
| Scheme of signal intensity changes of the plaque components on MR imaging | 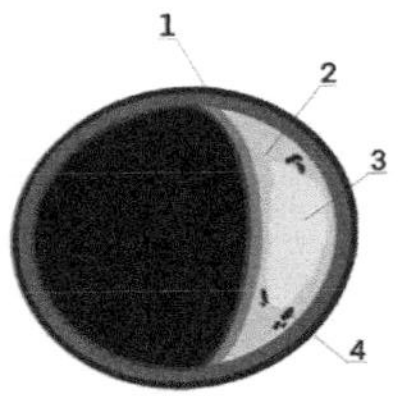  | 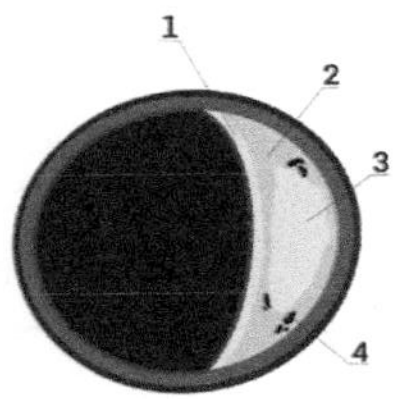  | 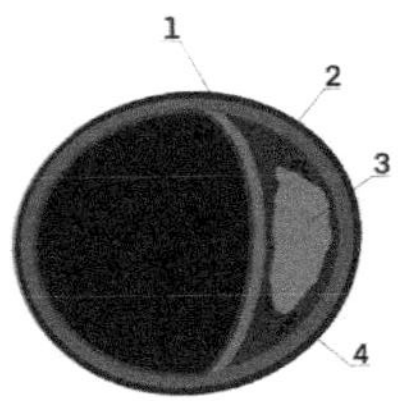  | 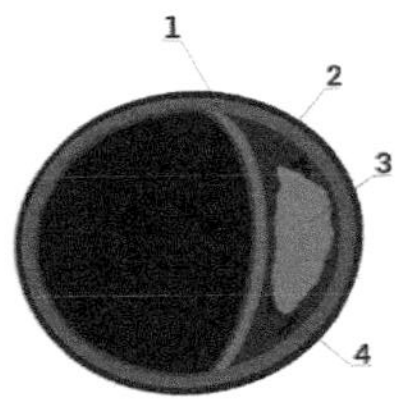  | 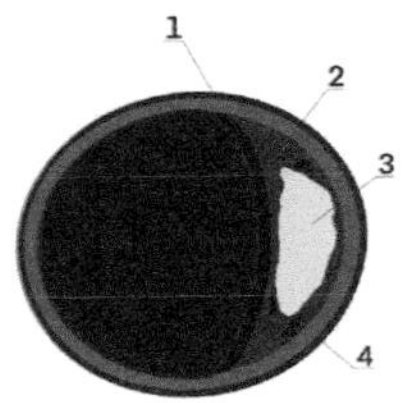  |

Here are shown the signal intensity of different plaque features in multiple MR imaging pulse sequences, including precontrast and postcontrast T1-weighted imaging, T2-weighted imaging, proton density-weighted imaging, and 3D TOF. Note that MPRAGE (frequently used to depict IPH) is a heavily T1-weighted pulse sequence.

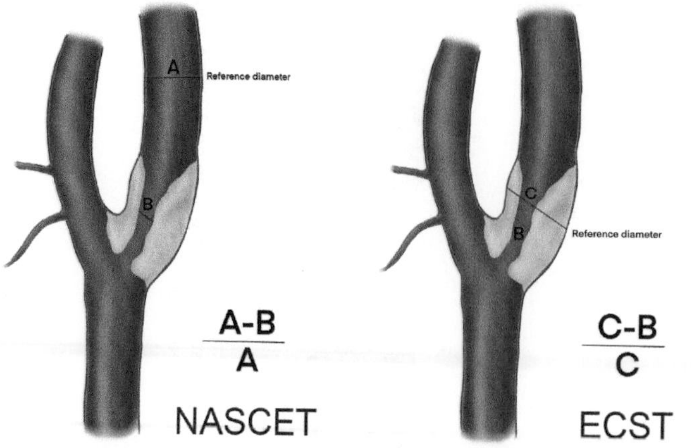


**Fig. 3.** NASCET versus European Carotid Surgery Trial (ECST). Clinical trials, such as the NASCET and the ECST aimed to define the threshold for the degree of stenosis in which surgery was indicated to reduce risk of subsequent stroke. NASCET cemented the role of carotid stenosis as a stroke predictor, leading to our current approach for intervention, and found that surgery outperformed medical therapy with a number needed to treat of 6. The degree of diameter-based luminal narrowing is therefore the quantitative metric used in current guidelines for the selection of patients undergoing carotid endarterectomy.

IPH were associated with increased risk for future ischemic events (HR = 5.69, 95% CI = 2.98–10.87).[74,75] During a median follow-up of 19.6 months, the presence of IPH was associated with a 6-fold higher risk for cerebrovascular events.[75] Conversely, the absence of IPH is a good predictor of plaque stability and low risk for ischemic events, even in the case of symptomatic moderate-to-severe carotid stenosis (50%–99%).[76]

Nonacute IPH seems hyperintense on T1-weighted imaging due to the short T1 of methemoglobin (**Fig. 4**).[77] Heavily T1-weighted sequences, including MPRAGE, are the method of choice for the depiction of IPH. IPH is typically defined as intraplaque signal intensity at least 2-fold higher relative to adjacent sternocleidomastoid muscle.[78] MPRAGE is superior to conventional MR imaging sequences and shows higher sensitivity, specificity, and interreader agreement compared with 3D-TOF and T1-weighted fast spin echo sequences.[14,79,80] Note that acute IPH will look isointense on T1-weighted and T2-weighted sequences.

Other heavily T1-weighted sequences also have the ability to depict IPH. Coregistered multicontrast acquisitions allow visualization of background in other weightings.[81,82] Multicontrast

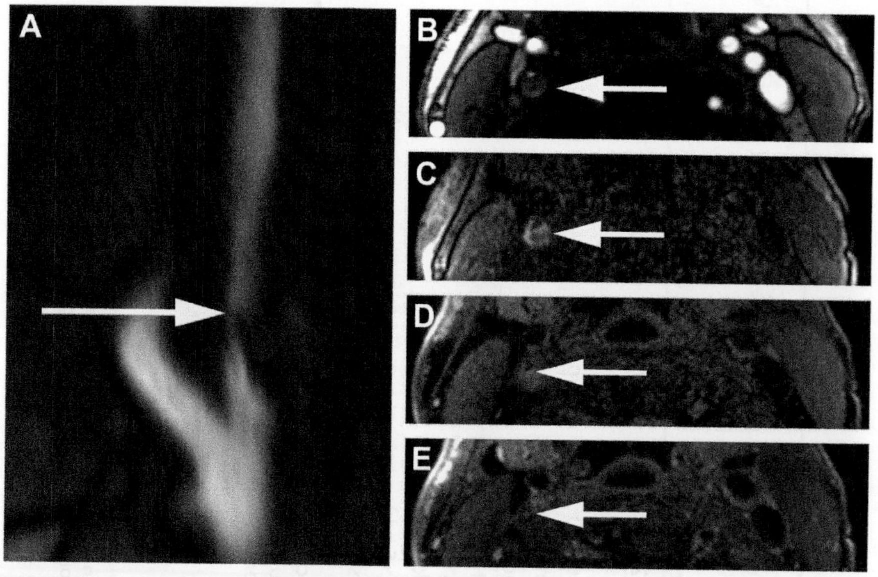


**Fig. 4.** Case of a 70-year-old man with symptomatic right ICA atherosclerotic plaque. Sagittal TOF imaging shows a severe more than 70% stenosis in the right proximal ICA (*arrow* in *A*). IPH was present and depicted as hyperintense signal on both axial TOF (*arrow* in *B*) and MPRAGE imaging (*arrow* in *C*). T1 SPACE before (*D*) and after (*E*) intravenous injection of gadolinium demonstrates some enhancement of collagen rich tissue along the fibrous cap (*arrows*).

atherosclerosis characterization (MATCH) uses inversion preparation to depict IPH with a near-dark background. Simultaneous noncontrast angiography and intraplaque hemorrhage (SNAP) provides bright and black blood reconstructions and has the advantage of delineating the lumen boundary better than MPRAGE.[83,84] Dedicated carotid coils for bifurcation imaging is preferred but IPH can be detected using large-FOV neck coils, at the cost of lower sensitivity and specificity.

### Lipid-Rich Necrotic Core

In atherosclerotic plaques, lipid-rich necrotic core (LRNC) results from the death of macrophages after they phagocytize lipid streaks (then called foam cells).[18] The volume of the LRNC is directly correlated to the development of cerebrovascular events and is a marker of plaque vulnerability.[52] LRNCs are best detected with CE T1-weighted VWI, where they appear as focal nonenhancing regions[15,59] (**Fig. 5**), although they may also be visible as hypointense regions on T2-weighted VWI.[85,86] Again, dedicated carotid coils are the preferred option to depict LRNC because they improve their detection and quantification compared with large-FOV neck coils.

### Fibrous Cap

The fibrous cap is a connective tissue layer rich in macrophages and smooth-muscle cells that separate the LRNC, and in general the internal plaque contents, from the lumen.[87] Its integrity is a marker of stability, whereas vulnerable plaques are characterized by fibrous cap thinning and/or disruption. The size of the LRNC is associated with fibrous cap thinning and disruption.[46,88] Fibrous cap rupture initiates the thromboembolic process from exposure of underlying thrombogenic plaque contents to flowing blood, leading to stroke. Both fibrous cap status and LRNC volume are therefore good indicators of plaque stability.[69,74,89]

Fibrous cap can be assessed with VWI better than with CT and US.[59,90,91] In stable atherosclerotic plaques, a thick fibrous cap can be depicted as a thick and regular juxtaluminal band of low signal intensity on TOF and high signal intensity on CE T1-weighted VWI (**Fig. 6**). The detection of thin fibrous cap is more challenging and often requires the use of a dedicated carotid coil. Fibrous cap thinning can be suggested if the fibrous cap cannot be visualized on TOF or CE T1-weighted VWI. Fibrous cap rupture can also be depicted and is suspected when the fibrous cap is thin or not visible and a focal region of intermediate-to-high signal is present adjacent to the lumen (corresponding to thrombus).[15,92] Both 1.5 T and 3T scanners allow for the assessment of the fibrous cap, though 3T is preferred.[17]

### Neovascularization and Inflammation

Atherosclerotic disease is characterized by inflammatory changes including the recruitment of inflammatory cells and neovascularization. Inflammation is thought to drive plaque growth and contributes to plaque disruption. Inflammatory cells are mostly found in the fibrous cap and aggregate in advanced plaques.[93,94] Among all inflammatory cells in atherosclerotic plaques, macrophages are associated with the highest risk of plaque rupture.[90,95,96] Their identification with ultrasmall superparamagnetic iron oxide (USPIO) imaging has therefore found its place in several

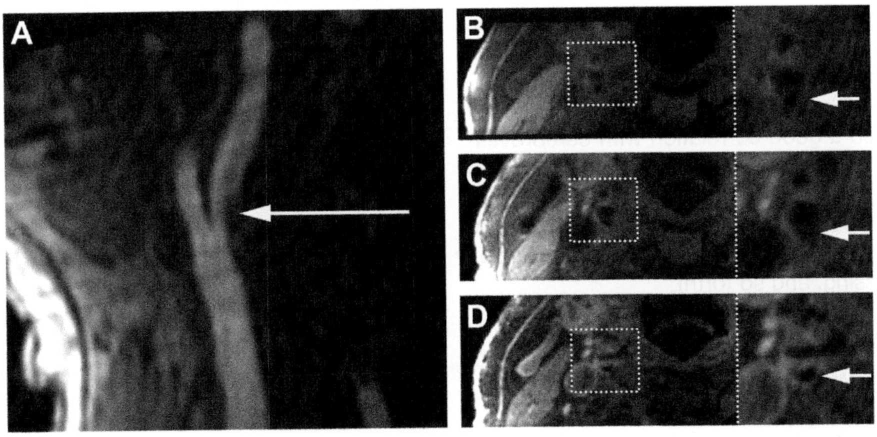


Fig. 5. Lipid rich necrotic core. A 69-year-old man with noncalcified plaque causing moderate right carotid stenosis on TOF MRA (*arrow* in *A*). The right carotid plaque was negative for IPH on MPRAGE (*B*) with central nonenhancing lipid-rich necrotic core comparing pre (*C*) and postcontrast T1 SPACE (*D*). *Square dotted boxes* indicate the zoomed area visible on the right of images *B*, *C* and *D*.

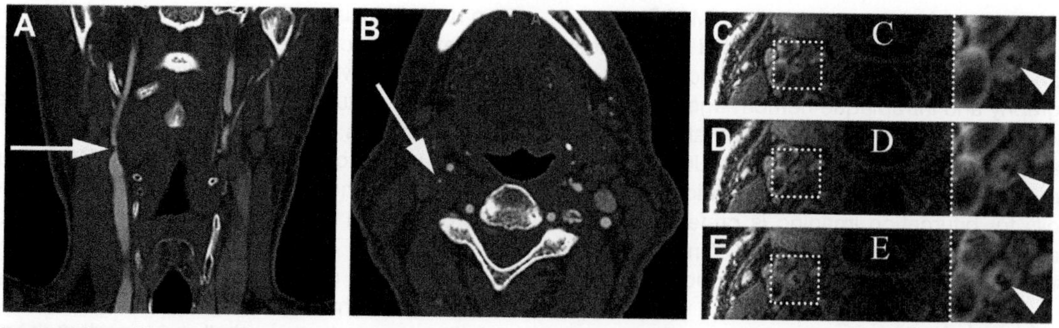


**Fig. 6.** Thinned fibrous cap. A 75-year-old man with noncalcified plaque causing severe right carotid stenosis on CTA, coronal (*arrow* in *A*) and axial (*arrow* in *B*). Axial T1 MERGE postcontrast black blood images from superior to inferior (*C–E*) with thinned fibrous cap as demonstrated by thinned delayed enhancement along the posteromedial intimal margin (inset, *arrowheads*). *Square dotted boxes* indicate the zoomed area visible on the right of images *C, D* and *E*.

studies.[97–101] Intraplaque neovascularization is also associated with plaque inflammation. Neovessels originate from the adventitia and tend to be immature, tortuous, and fragile. As a result, they are particularly prone to rupture with resultant IPH. Neovascularization is a good marker of plaque vulnerability.[102,103]

MR imaging techniques dedicated to the characterization of inflammatory changes within atherosclerotic plaques aim to image macrophage infiltration and/or neovascularization. Imaging macrophages in inflamed vessel wall is achievable thanks to the great avidity of these phagocytic cells to iron oxide particles, specifically USPIO.[102,104] The use of these contrast agents with MR imaging allows for plaque inflammation to be depicted as focal areas of signal loss.[100] Postgadolinium enhancement of carotid plaque is also associated with neovascularization, which has been confirmed histologically.[105] Adventitial neovascularization is a good marker of inflammation as the adventitia is rich in vasa vasorum and is a fundamental source for neovessel formation in both early and advanced plaques.[106] Postgadolinium adventitial enhancement on T1-weighted VWI showed a good correlation with cerebrovascular ischemic events.[107] Dynamic CE perfusion MR imaging showed similar results,[108,109] although this technique is more challenging for routine clinical applications (compliance, complex postprocessing, and so forth).

## *Nonatherosclerotic Disease Imaging Findings/Pathology*

### *Dissection and Blunt Cerebrovascular Injury*

Cervicocranial artery dissection (CCAD) is an important cause of stroke among young and middle-aged patients, representing up to 20% of strokes in this population and an annual incidence rate of 2.6 to 2.9 per 100,000.[110] CCAD is either traumatic or spontaneous in origin. CCAD results from intimal or adventitial side arterial wall tear, or both. Intramural blood may dissect longitudinally, spreading along the vessel proximally and distally.[111,112] Head and neck pain is the most common symptom in CCAD.[110] Ischemic symptoms and cerebral infarction can be caused by either hypoperfusion or thromboembolism.[112,113] Conventional angiography, CTA, MRA, and VWI can be used for diagnostic imaging. The classic angiographic findings include the "pearl and string sign," "string sign," intimal flap with false lumen, luminal dilation, tapered stenosis/occlusion, and irregular stenosis.[114,115]

MRA can be used to assess luminal changes relating to arterial dissection, with a sensitivity of 95% and a specificity of 99%. CE-MRA can provide better results than 3D-TOF MRA.[116]

VWI can well depict dissection findings including double lumen, intimal flap, intramural hematoma, pseudoaneurysm, irregular surface, and intraluminal thrombus (**Table 2**).[117–119] A systematic review and meta-analysis to evaluate patients with acute to subacute CCAD who underwent VWI indicated that wall hematoma and intimal flap are the most common and double lumen the least common direct imaging findings.[120] VWI can serve as a second-line agent to confirm indeterminate and low-grade blunt cerebrovascular injuries detected on CTA.[121] Intraluminal thrombus on VWI is strongly associated with territorial ischemic stroke.[115]

## *Inflammatory Vasculopathies*

### *Takayasu arteritis*

TA is a rare form of chronic inflammatory disorder of unclear cause.[122] Diagnosis is based on American College of Rheumatology guidelines, with presence of at least 3 of the following: (1) age

**Table 2**
**Definition and schemes of the different dissection types**

| Type of Dissection | Double Lumen Sign | Intimal Flap | Intramural Hematoma | Irregular Surface | Intraluminal Thrombus | Pseudoaneurysm |
|---|---|---|---|---|---|---|
| Definition by Wu et al[92] | Blood flow is divided into a true and a false lumen | Curvilinear line crossing the flow void lumen or between a hyperintense hematoma that extended to sidewall | Crescent-shaped thickening of the arterial wall that was iso-high signal on precontrast images | Discontinuity of the juxtaluminal surface of the intraluminal contrast enhancement on postcontrast images | Hyperintense filling within the lumen on precontrast images and an area of intraluminal contrast enhancement on postcontrast images | Diameter of aneurysmal vessels dilated more than 1.5× than the normal distal artery |
| Scheme of dissections | 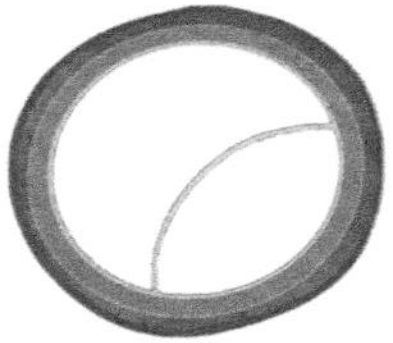 | 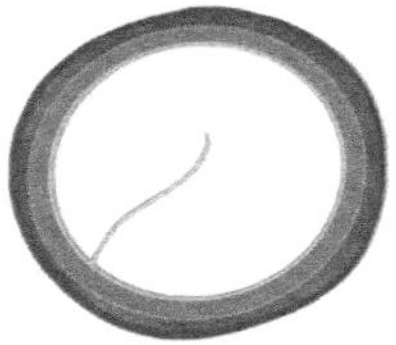 | 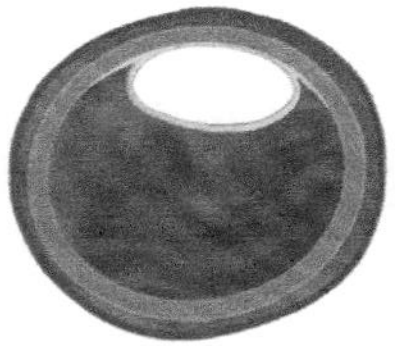 | 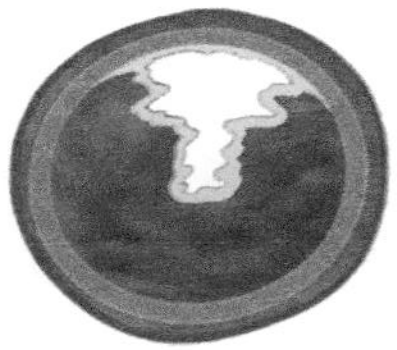 | 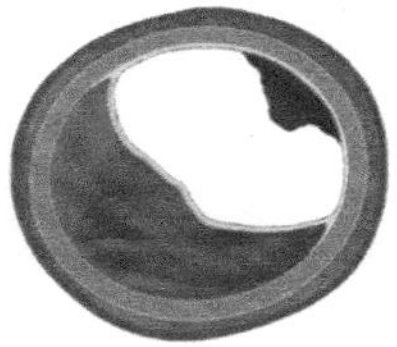 | 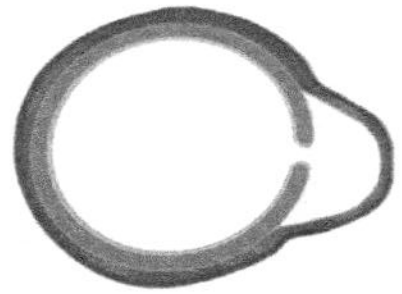 |

MR angiography can be used to assess luminal changes relating to arterial dissection. MR VWI can depict dissection findings with great accuracy, including double lumen, intimal flap, intramural hematoma, pseudoaneurysm, irregular surface, and intraluminal thrombus.

less than 40 years, (2) extremity claudication, (3) decreased brachial artery pulse, (4) arm blood pressure difference greater than 10 mm Hg, (5) bruit over subclavian arteries or aorta, and (6) arteriogram abnormality. These criteria, however, are frequently negative in early TA, before the development of stenosis, and once luminal changes develop they are frequently irreversible due to intimal fibrosis.[123,124] According to the European Alliance of Associations of Rheumatologists guidelines, MR imaging is the imaging test of choice to capture disease extent and activity in TA.[125] Inflammatory changes such as mural edema, wall thickening, and wall enhancement are important for early detection of disease and immunosuppression treatment before the development of permanent stenosis, occlusion, or aneurysms that can lead to downstream ischemia or local hemorrhage.

#### *Giant cell arteritis*

Giant cell arteritis (GCA) is a chronic inflammatory disease that affects medium and large-caliber arteries.[126] MR imaging findings in GCA include smooth, concentric vessel wall enhancement, thickening, and edema of the extracranial and intracranial arteries.[127] There is frequent involvement of the superficial temporal arteries, which can be detected by US or VWI, with characteristics extensive inflammatory changes spilling into the adjacent perivascular soft tissues. Early immunosuppressive treatment is needed to prevent acute complications of untreated GCA, such as vision loss or occasionally stroke, can be devastating.[124]

### *Transient Perivascular Inflammation of the Carotid Artery Syndrome*

Transient perivascular inflammation of the carotid artery (TIPIC), also called carotidynia, is a self-limiting inflammatory disease affecting the extracranial carotid artery. Clinically, it is characterized by self-limiting neck pain and tenderness. On MRA, TIPIC is associated with inflammatory changes in the soft tissue adjacent to the cervical carotid artery, namely contrast-enhancement after intravenous gadolinium injection (**Fig. 7**). The exact mechanism of this pathologic condition remains elusive.[128]

### *Carotid Webs*

Carotid webs (CaWs) are intraluminal shelf-like fibrotic projections into the ICA bulb on CTA, MRA, or US. CaWs are associated with ischemic strokes in young adults without risk factors. Recurrent stroke is very high (25%–35%) with CaWs. Alteration in hemodynamic patterns leading to thrombus formation is the likely pathogenesis of strokes from CaWs.[129,130]

Traditionally, surgery has been used to resect webs. Endovascular treatment with stent replacement is a safe alternative. In a systematic review by Patel and colleagues, in 289 patients with CaW, the group treated invasively had no recurrent stroke, whereas the group treated medically showed recurrent ischemic cerebral events. They concluded that carotid intervention for webs in combination with appropriate medical therapy is the most effective option.[131]

## OTHER DISEASE ENTITIES

### *Fibromuscular Dysplasia*

Fibromuscular dysplasia (FMD) is a vascular disease most commonly seen in women, caused by arterial wall overgrowth, specifically affecting the renal and internal carotid arteries. FMD is associated with serious complications such as dissection, pseudoaneurysm, and stroke from

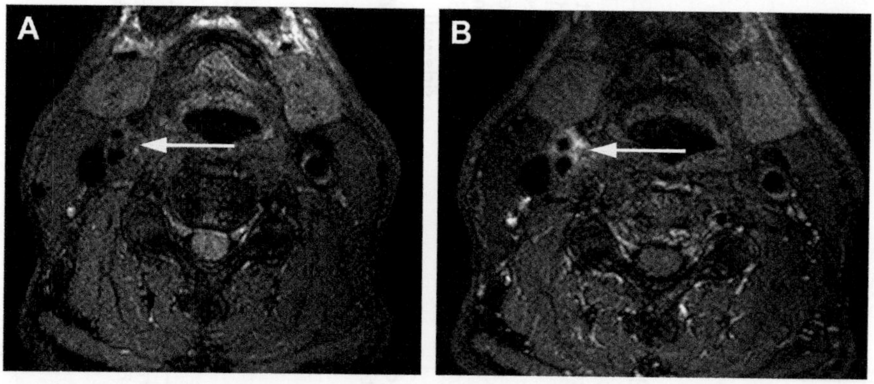


Fig. 7. TIPIC syndrome in a 59-year-old male patient with right-sided carotidynia and no neurological deficit. Pregadolinium (*A*) and post-gadolinium (*B*) T1-weighted imaging (SPACE) with flow suppression shows a thick, enhancing area around the external and internal carotid arteries (*arrows*). This corresponds to a TIPIC. The patient completely recovered after treatment with anti-inflammatories.

concomitant thrombi. Medial FMD is the most common type and affects the middle layer of arteries and has a string of beads appearance. Catheter angiography is the gold standard imaging of FMD. CTA and MRA are also used for FMD but particularly for cerebral arteries. Ultrasound can be used for both diagnosis and follow-up of patients with FMD.[132] There is no role for VWI in routine evaluation, although it may be useful for the detection of complications such as dissection. There is no known cure for FMD but percutaneous balloon angioplasty can help widen narrowed arteries, leading to improved blood flow. In patients with FMD-induced dissection, angioplasty with stenting is recommended.[132]

## *Radiation Vasculopathy and Pseudoaneurysm*

Radiation vasculopathy of the extracranial carotid arteries is typically caused after head and neck radiotherapy for the treatment of squamous cell carcinomas of the aerodigestive system and lymphoma. Acute vascular rupture, macrovascular thrombosis, and atherosclerotic disease can occur in medium arteries (>100 μm). Occlusive vasculopathy and vasa vasorum injury can be seen in large arteries (>500 μm). Vascular anomalies, such as aneurysms, cavernous malformations, and carotid stenosis may be the result of radiation. In a study by Haddy and colleagues,[133] 4227 patients who had undergone head and neck radiation during childhood were examined. They found that nearly 23 deaths were the result of cerebrovascular diseases after 29 years of follow-up. Apart from radiation dose, other factors such as genetic (neurofibromatosis type 1), childhood radiation history, using chemotherapy agents (cisplatin), and radiation fields can be contributed in the risk of cerebrovascular diseases.[134]

Cheng and colleagues[135] found that 3 years after neck radiotherapy, 10% (24/240) of patients had internal carotid stenosis (>70%) and 5% had common carotid stenosis. Due to the fast progression of radiation-induced carotid stenosis, yearly ultrasound screening is recommended 3 years postradiation. Thalhammer and colleagues examined 60 postradiation patients and found 30% to 40% had significant carotid artery changes. In addition, they found complete internal or CCA occlusion in some asymptomatic subjects. Approximately one-third of patients had no plaques.[136] After radiotherapy, in order to decrease inflammation, using neuroprotective agents (erythropoietin), angiogenesis inhibitors (bevacizumab), transplantation of neural stem cells, and renin-angiotensin system blockage is highly recommended.[134]

## *Carotid Blowout Syndrome*

Carotid blowout syndrome (CBS) is a serious fatal postradiation complication associated with weakened arterial wall leading to carotid artery rupture. A meta-analysis of 1554 patients showed nearly 2.6% of reirradiated patients developed CBS, which was fatal in 76%.[137] Endovascular treatment with stents, coils, balloons, and open surgery should be performed emergently.[138]

## *Future Directions*

### *Vessel Wall Imaging Clinical Implementation*

The role of VWI in the clinical diagnostic algorithm for stroke secondary to carotid disease is still undetermined. New randomized control trials will be needed to determine how to translate VWI into clinical decision-making. VWI may, however, be used to better visualize atherosclerotic plaque extent and composition to assist surgical planning. VWI could be useful in stroke etiology assessment in cryptogenic stroke, or for decision-making in moderate stenosis.

## *Atherosclerotic Plaque Segmentation*

Novel techniques have emerged in an effort to assist neuroradiologists in interpreting and quantifying plaque composition. Automated and semiautomated segmentation tools have proven useful in VWI plaque characterization. These tools are able to quantify the different plaque components (calcium, IPH, fibrous cap, LRNC) with similar performance to manual segmentation[139] and with good histological agreement.[140] Recently developed machine learning algorithms demonstrated the ability to distinguish low versus high-risk plaques on VWI.[141]

## *Improvement of MR Techniques*

Several advanced VWI sequences, including SNAP, have been developed and can provide both luminal and vessel wall images for IPH detection.[118,142] Three-dimensional spoiled gradient-recalled echo pulse sequence for hemorrhage assessment using inversion recovery and multiple echoes (3D-SHINE) not only offers detection but also characterizes IPH based on T2* relaxivity.[143] MATCH is a multicontrast sequence that allows comprehensive analysis of plaque content in 5 minutes.[82] Finally, 3D multiple-echo recombined gradient-echo (3D-MERGE)[144] and 3D delay-alternating with nutation for tailored excitation with fast low-angle shot (3D-DASH)[145] provide blood-suppressed, high-resolution, large FOV coverage VWI for plaque burden measurements. Although these VWI techniques are promising, some technical improvements are needed for routine clinical implementation.

In 2018, the ASNR Vessel Wall Imaging Study Group suggested technical improvements for VWI, including higher spatial resolution and improved blood suppression to allow for better depiction of finer structures such as the fibrous cap. The use of dedicated carotid coils and better motion correction methods could also improve image quality. These improvements combined with the continued efforts to develop abbreviated VWI protocols are necessary to incorporate carotid VWI into daily clinical practice. Education and training of technologists and radiologists on VWI applications, sequences and interpretation is also necessary for increased adoption.[146] Finally, it is essential to carry out prospective interventional studies that have the potential to generate new guidelines in carotid atherosclerosis management that correlate better with histopathological findings.

## SUMMARY

Carotid artery atherosclerosis is traditionally assessed by luminal stenosis imaging; however, plaque composition can improve ischemic stroke prediction over stenosis alone. VWI can depict plaque features that correlate with ischemic risk and may be superior to luminal imaging in selecting patients that could benefit most from surgery and in the prediction of future ischemic stroke, as well as assisting in the evaluation of other extracranial carotid diseases.

## DISCLOSURE

This study is supported by the Clinical and Translational Science, United States Award program/ NIH, United States, National Center for Advancing Translational Sciences, United States UL1TR002373 and KL2TR002374 (L.B. Eisenmenger), and Wisconsin Alzheimer's Disease Research Center grant P30-AG062715 (L.B. Eisenmenger).

## CLINICS CARE POINTS

- The NASCET trial demonstrated a significantly increased cerebrovascular risk in ulcerated plaques.
- VWI is the best technique to detect IPH and numerous authors therefore recommend that it becomes a standard in the identification of vulnerable plaques in extracranial carotid artery.
- VWI could be useful in stroke etiology assessment in cryptogenic stroke, or for decision-making in moderate stenosis; new randomized control trials will be needed to determine how to translate VWI into clinical decision-making.

## REFERENCES

1. Morelli JN, Gerdes CM, Schmitt P, et al. Technical considerations in MR angiography: an image-based guide. J Magn Reson Imaging 2013;37(6): 1326–41.
2. Costello J, Alexander MD, McNally JS, et al. MR angiography series: neurovascular MR angiography. Radiographics 2021;41(7):E204–e205.
3. Papke K, Brassel F. Modern cross-sectional imaging in the diagnosis and follow-up of intracranial aneurysms. Eur Radiol 2006;16(9):2051–66.
4. Bradac GB. Cerebral angiography: normal anatomy and vascular pathology. Heidelberg: Springer Berlin; 2011.
5. DeMarco JK, Willinek WA, Finn JP, et al. Current state-of-the-art 1.5 T and 3 T extracranial carotid contrast-enhanced magnetic resonance angiography. Neuroimaging Clin N Am 2012;22(2): 235–57, x.
6. Weber J, Veith P, Jung B, et al. MR angiography at 3 Tesla to assess proximal internal carotid artery stenoses: contrast-enhanced or 3D time-of-flight MR angiography? Clin Neuroradiol 2015;25(1):41–8.
7. Woolen SA, Shankar PR, Gagnier JJ, et al. Risk of nephrogenic systemic fibrosis in patients with stage 4 or 5 chronic kidney disease receiving a group ii gadolinium-based contrast agent: a systematic review and meta-analysis. JAMA Intern Med 2020;180(2):223–30.
8. Willig DS, Turski PA, Frayne R, et al. Contrast-enhanced 3D MR DSA of the carotid artery bifurcation: preliminary study of comparison with unenhanced 2D and 3D time-of-flight MR angiography. Radiology 1998;208(2):447–51.
9. Platzek I, Sieron D, Wiggermann P, et al. Carotid artery stenosis: comparison of 3D time-of-flight MR angiography and contrast-enhanced MR angiography at 3T. Radiol Res Pract 2014;2014:508715.
10. McDonald RJ, McDonald JS, Kallmes DF, et al. Intracranial gadolinium deposition after contrast-enhanced MR imaging. Radiology 2015;275(3): 772–82.
11. Yamada N, Higashi M, Otsubo R, et al. Association between signal hyperintensity on T1-weighted MR imaging of carotid plaques and ipsilateral ischemic events. AJNR Am J Neuroradiol 2007;28(2): 287–92.

12. McNally JS, Kim SE, Mendes J, et al. Magnetic resonance imaging detection of intraplaque hemorrhage. Magn Reson Insights 2017;10:1–8.
13. McNally JS, McLaughlin MS, Hinckley PJ, et al. Intraluminal thrombus, intraplaque hemorrhage, plaque thickness, and current smoking optimally predict carotid stroke. Stroke 2015;46(1):84–90.
14. Ota H, Yarnykh VL, Ferguson MS, et al. Carotid intraplaque hemorrhage imaging at 3.0-T MR imaging: comparison of the diagnostic performance of three T1-weighted sequences. Radiology 2010; 254(2):551–63.
15. Cai J, Hatsukami TS, Ferguson MS, et al. In vivo quantitative measurement of intact fibrous cap and lipid-rich necrotic core size in atherosclerotic carotid plaque: comparison of high-resolution, contrast-enhanced magnetic resonance imaging and histology. Circulation 2005;112(22):3437–44.
16. Takaya N, Cai J, Ferguson MS, et al. Intra- and interreader reproducibility of magnetic resonance imaging for quantifying the lipid-rich necrotic core is improved with gadolinium contrast enhancement. J Magn Reson Imaging 2006;24(1):203–10.
17. Saba L, Yuan C, Hatsukami TS, et al. Carotid artery wall imaging: perspective and guidelines from the ASNR vessel wall imaging study group and expert consensus recommendations of the American society of neuroradiology. AJNR Am J Neuroradiol 2018;39(2):E9–e31.
18. Lusis AJ. Atherosclerosis. Nature 2000;407(6801): 233–41.
19. Yanez ND, Burke GL, Manolio T, et al. Sibling history of myocardial infarction or stroke and risk of cardiovascular disease in the elderly: the Cardiovascular Health Study. Ann Epidemiol 2009; 19(12):858–66.
20. Katan M, Luft A. Global Burden of Stroke. Semin Neurol 2018;38(2):208–11.
21. Ooi YC, Gonzalez NR. Management of extracranial carotid artery disease. Cardiol Clin 2015;33(1): 1–35.
22. von Arbin M, Britton M, De Faire U, et al. Non invasive assessment of the internal carotid artery in stroke patients. Scand J Clin Lab Invest 1983; 43(4):275–83.
23. Weinberger J. Clinical applications of noninvasive carotid artery testing. J Am Coll Cardiol 1985; 5(1):137–48.
24. Barnett HJ, Taylor DW, Eliasziw M, et al. Benefit of carotid endarterectomy in patients with symptomatic moderate or severe stenosis. North American Symptomatic Carotid Endarterectomy Trial Collaborators. N Engl J Med 1998;339(20):1415–25.
25. Howarth JC, Klotz JG. The diagnostic value of carotid arteriography; a preliminary report. Cleve Clin Q 1951;18(3):179–83.
26. Imparato AM, Riles TS, Gorstein F. The carotid bifurcation plaque: pathologic findings associated with cerebral ischemia. Stroke 1979;10(3):238–45.
27. Jeziorska M, Woolley DE. Local neovascularization and cellular composition within vulnerable regions of atherosclerotic plaques of human carotid arteries. J Pathol 1999;188(2):189–96.
28. Redgrave JN, Lovett JK, Gallagher PJ, et al. Histological assessment of 526 symptomatic carotid plaques in relation to the nature and timing of ischemic symptoms: the Oxford plaque study. Circulation 2006;113(19):2320–8.
29. Naghavi M, Libby P, Falk E, et al. From vulnerable plaque to vulnerable patient: a call for new definitions and risk assessment strategies: Part II. Circulation 2003;108(15):1772–8.
30. Naghavi M, Libby P, Falk E, et al. From vulnerable plaque to vulnerable patient: a call for new definitions and risk assessment strategies: Part I. Circulation 2003;108(14):1664–72.
31. Croft RJ, Ellam LD, Harrison MJ. Accuracy of carotid angiography in the assessment of atheroma of the internal carotid artery. Lancet 1980;1(8176): 997–1000.
32. Wardlaw JM, Chappell FM, Best JJ, et al. Non-invasive imaging compared with intra-arterial angiography in the diagnosis of symptomatic carotid stenosis: a meta-analysis. Lancet 2006;367(9521): 1503–12.
33. Barnett HJM, Taylor DW, Haynes RB, et al. Beneficial effect of carotid endarterectomy in symptomatic patients with high-grade carotid stenosis. N Engl J Med 1991;325(7):445–53.
34. Wasserman BA, Wityk RJ, Trout HH 3rd, et al. Low-grade carotid stenosis: looking beyond the lumen with MRI. Stroke 2005;36(11):2504–13.
35. Spagnoli LG, Mauriello A, Sangiorgi G, et al. Extracranial thrombotically active carotid plaque as a risk factor for ischemic stroke. JAMA 2004; 292(15):1845–52.
36. Lovett JK, Gallagher PJ, Hands LJ, et al. Histological correlates of carotid plaque surface morphology on lumen contrast imaging. Circulation 2004;110(15):2190–7.
37. Astor BC, Sharrett AR, Coresh J, et al. Remodeling of carotid arteries detected with MR imaging: atherosclerosis risk in communities carotid MRI study. Radiology 2010;256(3):879–86.
38. Redgrave JN, Lovett JK, Rothwell PM. Histological features of symptomatic carotid plaques in relation to age and smoking: the oxford plaque study. Stroke 2010;41(10):2288–94.
39. Lovett JK, Gallagher PJ, Rothwell PM. Reproducibility of histological assessment of carotid plaque: implications for studies of carotid imaging. Cerebrovasc Dis 2004;18(2):117–23.

40. Freilinger TM, Schindler A, Schmidt C, et al. Prevalence of nonstenosing, complicated atherosclerotic plaques in cryptogenic stroke. JACC Cardiovasc Imaging 2012;5(4):397–405.
41. Altaf N, Daniels L, Morgan PS, et al. Detection of intraplaque hemorrhage by magnetic resonance imaging in symptomatic patients with mild to moderate carotid stenosis predicts recurrent neurological events. J Vasc Surg 2008;47(2):337–42.
42. Mono ML, Karameshev A, Slotboom J, et al. Plaque characteristics of asymptomatic carotid stenosis and risk of stroke. Cerebrovasc Dis 2012;34(5–6):343–50.
43. Rozie S, de Weert TT, de Monyé C, et al. Atherosclerotic plaque volume and composition in symptomatic carotid arteries assessed with multidetector CT angiography; relationship with severity of stenosis and cardiovascular risk factors. Eur Radiol 2009;19(9):2294–301.
44. Saam T, Yuan C, Chu B, et al. Predictors of carotid atherosclerotic plaque progression as measured by noninvasive magnetic resonance imaging. Atherosclerosis 2007;194(2):e34–42.
45. Albuquerque LC, Narvaes LB, Maciel AA, et al. Intraplaque hemorrhage assessed by high-resolution magnetic resonance imaging and C-reactive protein in carotid atherosclerosis. J Vasc Surg 2007;46(6):1130–7.
46. Ota H, Yu W, Underhill HR, et al. Hemorrhage and large lipid-rich necrotic cores are independently associated with thin or ruptured fibrous caps: an in vivo 3T MRI study. Arterioscler Thromb Vasc Biol 2009;29(10):1696–701.
47. Saba L, Montisci R, Sanfilippo R, et al. Multidetector row CT of the brain and carotid artery: a correlative analysis. Clin Radiol 2009;64(8):767–78.
48. Saba L, Tamponi E, Raz E, et al. Correlation between fissured fibrous cap and contrast enhancement: preliminary results with the use of CTA and histologic validation. AJNR Am J Neuroradiol 2014;35(4):754–9.
49. Miura T, Matsukawa N, Sakurai K, et al. Plaque vulnerability in internal carotid arteries with positive remodeling. Cerebrovasc Dis Extra 2011;1(1):54–65.
50. Vukadinovic D, Rozie S, van Gils M, et al. Automated versus manual segmentation of atherosclerotic carotid plaque volume and components in CTA: associations with cardiovascular risk factors. Int J Cardiovasc Imaging 2012;28(4):877–87.
51. Wannarong T, Parraga G, Buchanan D, et al. Progression of carotid plaque volume predicts cardiovascular events. Stroke 2013;44(7):1859–65.
52. Saba L, Sanfilippo R, Sannia S, et al. Association between carotid artery plaque volume, composition, and ulceration: a retrospective assessment with MDCT. AJR Am J Roentgenol 2012;199(1):151–6.
53. Saam T, Kerwin WS, Chu B, et al. Sample size calculation for clinical trials using magnetic resonance imaging for the quantitative assessment of carotid atherosclerosis. J Cardiovasc Magn Reson 2005;7(5):799–808.
54. Saam T, Raya JG, Cyran CC, et al. High resolution carotid black-blood 3T MR with parallel imaging and dedicated 4-channel surface coils. J Cardiovasc Magn Reson 2009;11(1):41.
55. Boussel L, Arora S, Rapp J, et al. Atherosclerotic plaque progression in carotid arteries: monitoring with high-spatial-resolution MR imaging–multicenter trial. Radiology 2009;252(3):789–96.
56. Corti R, Fayad ZA, Fuster V, et al. Effects of lipid-lowering by simvastatin on human atherosclerotic lesions: a longitudinal study by high-resolution, noninvasive magnetic resonance imaging. Circulation 2001;104(3):249–52.
57. Zhao XQ, Dong L, Hatsukami T, et al. MR imaging of carotid plaque composition during lipid-lowering therapy a prospective assessment of effect and time course. JACC Cardiovasc Imaging 2011;4(9):977–86.
58. Saba L, Anzidei M, Marincola BC, et al. Imaging of the carotid artery vulnerable plaque. Cardiovasc Intervent Radiol 2014;37(3):572–85.
59. Wasserman BA, Smith WI, Trout HH 3rd, et al. Carotid artery atherosclerosis: in vivo morphologic characterization with gadolinium-enhanced double-oblique MR imaging initial results. Radiology 2002;223(2):566–73.
60. Sitzer M, Müller W, Siebler M, et al. Plaque ulceration and lumen thrombus are the main sources of cerebral microemboli in high-grade internal carotid artery stenosis. Stroke 1995;26(7):1231–3.
61. Anderson GB, Ashforth R, Steinke DE, et al. CT angiography for the detection and characterization of carotid artery bifurcation disease. Stroke 2000;31(9):2168–74.
62. Polak JF, O'Leary DH, Kronmal RA, et al. Sonographic evaluation of carotid artery atherosclerosis in the elderly: relationship of disease severity to stroke and transient ischemic attack. Radiology 1993;188(2):363–70.
63. Troyer A, Saloner D, Pan XM, et al. Major carotid plaque surface irregularities correlate with neurologic symptoms. J Vasc Surg 2002;35(4):741–7.
64. Etesami M, Hoi Y, Steinman DA, et al. Comparison of carotid plaque ulcer detection using contrast-enhanced and time-of-flight MRA techniques. AJNR Am J Neuroradiol 2013;34(1):177–84.
65. Sun J, Canton G, Balu N, et al. Blood pressure is a major modifiable risk factor implicated in pathogenesis of intraplaque hemorrhage: an in vivo magnetic resonance imaging study. Arterioscler Thromb Vasc Biol 2016;36(4):743–9.

66. Selwaness M, van den Bouwhuijsen QJ, Verwoert GC, et al. Blood pressure parameters and carotid intraplaque hemorrhage as measured by magnetic resonance imaging: the rotterdam study. Hypertension 2013;61(1):76–81.
67. Pasterkamp G, van der Steen AF. Intraplaque hemorrhage: an imaging marker for atherosclerotic plaque destabilization? Arterioscler Thromb Vasc Biol 2012;32(2):167–8.
68. Takaya N, Yuan C, Chu B, et al. Presence of intraplaque hemorrhage stimulates progression of carotid atherosclerotic plaques: a high-resolution magnetic resonance imaging study. Circulation 2005;111(21):2768–75.
69. Takaya N, Yuan C, Chu B, et al. Association between carotid plaque characteristics and subsequent ischemic cerebrovascular events: a prospective assessment with MRI–initial results. Stroke 2006;37(3):818–23.
70. Bitar R, Moody AR, Leung G, et al. In vivo 3D high-spatial-resolution MR imaging of intraplaque hemorrhage. Radiology 2008;249(1):259–67.
71. Moody AR. Magnetic resonance direct thrombus imaging. J Thromb Haemost 2003;1(7):1403–9.
72. Moody AR, Allder S, Lennox G, et al. Direct magnetic resonance imaging of carotid artery thrombus in acute stroke. Lancet 1999;353(9147):122–3.
73. Qiao Y, Etesami M, Malhotra S, et al. Identification of intraplaque hemorrhage on MR angiography images: a comparison of contrast-enhanced mask and time-of-flight techniques. AJNR Am J Neuroradiol 2011;32(3):454–9.
74. Gupta A, Baradaran H, Schweitzer AD, et al. Carotid plaque MRI and stroke risk: a systematic review and meta-analysis. Stroke 2013;44(11):3071–7.
75. Saam T, Hetterich H, Hoffmann V, et al. Meta-analysis and systematic review of the predictive value of carotid plaque hemorrhage on cerebrovascular events by magnetic resonance imaging. J Am Coll Cardiol 2013;62(12):1081–91.
76. Hosseini AA, Kandiyil N, Macsweeney ST, et al. Carotid plaque hemorrhage on magnetic resonance imaging strongly predicts recurrent ischemia and stroke. Ann Neurol 2013;73(6):774–84.
77. Rudnick MR, Kesselheim A, Goldfarb S. Contrast-induced nephropathy: how it develops, how to prevent it. Cleve Clin J Med 2006;73(1):75–80, 83-77.
78. Scott McNally J, Yoon HC, Kim SE, et al. Carotid MRI Detection of Intraplaque Hemorrhage at 3T and 1.5T. J Neuroimaging 2015;25(3):390–6.
79. Inoue K, Nakayama R, Isoshima S, et al. Semiautomated segmentation and volume measurements of cervical carotid high-signal plaques using 3D turbo spin-echo T1-weighted black-blood vessel wall imaging: a preliminary study. Diagnostics 2022;12(4):1014.
80. Mura M, Della Schiava N, Long A, et al. Carotid intraplaque haemorrhage: pathogenesis, histological classification, imaging methods and clinical value. Ann Transl Med 2020;8(19):1273.
81. Dai Y, Lv P, Lin J, et al. Comparison study between multicontrast atherosclerosis characterization (MATCH) and conventional multicontrast MRI of carotid plaque with histology validation. J Magn Reson Imaging 2017;45(3):764–70.
82. Fan Z, Yu W, Xie Y, et al. Multi-contrast atherosclerosis characterization (MATCH) of carotid plaque with a single 5-min scan: technical development and clinical feasibility. J Cardiovasc Magn Reson 2014;16(1):53.
83. Chen S, Zhao H, Li J, et al. Evaluation of carotid atherosclerotic plaque surface characteristics utilizing simultaneous noncontrast angiography and intraplaque hemorrhage (SNAP) technique. J Magn Reson Imaging 2018;47(3):634–9.
84. Wang J, Börnert P, Zhao H, et al. Simultaneous noncontrast angiography and intraplaque hemorrhage (SNAP) imaging for carotid atherosclerotic disease evaluation. Magn Reson Med 2013;69(2):337–45.
85. Toussaint JF, LaMuraglia GM, Southern JF, et al. Magnetic resonance images lipid, fibrous, calcified, hemorrhagic, and thrombotic components of human atherosclerosis in vivo. Circulation 1996;94(5):932–8.
86. Trivedi RA, U-King-Im JM, Graves MJ, et al. MRI-derived measurements of fibrous-cap and lipid-core thickness: the potential for identifying vulnerable carotid plaques in vivo. Neuroradiology 2004;46(9):738–43.
87. Cury RC, Houser SL, Furie KL, et al. Vulnerable plaque detection by 3.0 tesla magnetic resonance imaging. Invest Radiol 2006;41(2):112–5.
88. Xu D, Hippe DS, Underhill HR, et al. Prediction of high-risk plaque development and plaque progression with the carotid atherosclerosis score. JACC Cardiovasc Imaging 2014;7(4):366–73.
89. Kwee RM, van Oostenbrugge RJ, Mess WH, et al. MRI of carotid atherosclerosis to identify TIA and stroke patients who are at risk of a recurrence. J Magn Reson Imaging 2013;37(5):1189–94.
90. Hatsukami TS, Ross R, Polissar NL, et al. Visualization of fibrous cap thickness and rupture in human atherosclerotic carotid plaque in vivo with high-resolution magnetic resonance imaging. Circulation 2000;102(9):959–64.
91. Saba L, Potters F, van der Lugt A, et al. Imaging of the fibrous cap in atherosclerotic carotid plaque. Cardiovasc Intervent Radiol 2010;33(4):681–9.
92. Yuan C, Zhang SX, Polissar NL, et al. Identification of fibrous cap rupture with magnetic resonance imaging is highly associated with recent transient

ischemic attack or stroke. Circulation 2002;105(2):181–5.
93. de Boer OJ, van der Wal AC, Teeling P, et al. Leucocyte recruitment in rupture prone regions of lipid-rich plaques: a prominent role for neovascularization? Cardiovasc Res 1999;41(2):443–9.
94. van der Wal AC, Becker AE, van der Loos CM, et al. Site of intimal rupture or erosion of thrombosed coronary atherosclerotic plaques is characterized by an inflammatory process irrespective of the dominant plaque morphology. Circulation 1994;89(1):36–44.
95. Lennartz MR, Aggarwal A, Michaud TM, et al. Ligation of macrophage Fcγ receptors recapitulates the gene expression pattern of vulnerable human carotid plaques. PLoS One 2011;6(7):e21803.
96. Moulton KS, Vakili K, Zurakowski D, et al. Inhibition of plaque neovascularization reduces macrophage accumulation and progression of advanced atherosclerosis. Proc Natl Acad Sci U S A 2003;100(8):4736–41.
97. Howarth SP, Tang TY, Trivedi R, et al. Utility of USPIO-enhanced MR imaging to identify inflammation and the fibrous cap: a comparison of symptomatic and asymptomatic individuals. Eur J Radiol 2009;70(3):555–60.
98. Tang TY, Howarth SP, Miller SR, et al. Correlation of carotid atheromatous plaque inflammation using USPIO-enhanced MR imaging with degree of luminal stenosis. Stroke 2008;39(7):2144–7.
99. Annovazzi A, Bonanno E, Arca M, et al. 99mTc-interleukin-2 scintigraphy for the in vivo imaging of vulnerable atherosclerotic plaques. Eur J Nucl Med Mol Imaging 2006;33(2):117–26.
100. Trivedi RA, Mallawarachi C, U-King-Im JM, et al. Identifying inflamed carotid plaques using in vivo USPIO-enhanced MR imaging to label plaque macrophages. Arterioscler Thromb Vasc Biol 2006;26(7):1601–6.
101. Ruehm SG, Corot C, Vogt P, et al. Ultrasmall superparamagnetic iron oxide-enhanced MR imaging of atherosclerotic plaque in hyperlipidemic rabbits. Acad Radiol 2002;9(Suppl 1):S143–4.
102. McCarthy MJ, Loftus IM, Thompson MM, et al. Angiogenesis and the atherosclerotic carotid plaque: an association between symptomatology and plaque morphology. J Vasc Surg 1999;30(2):261–8.
103. Virmani R, Kolodgie FD, Burke AP, et al. Atherosclerotic plaque progression and vulnerability to rupture: angiogenesis as a source of intraplaque hemorrhage. Arterioscler Thromb Vasc Biol 2005;25(10):2054–61.
104. Ouimet T, Lancelot E, Hyafil F, et al. Molecular and cellular targets of the MRI contrast agent P947 for atherosclerosis imaging. Mol Pharm 2012;9(4):850–61.
105. Millon A, Boussel L, Brevet M, et al. Clinical and histological significance of gadolinium enhancement in carotid atherosclerotic plaque. Stroke 2012;43(11):3023–8.
106. Virmani R, Burke AP, Farb A, et al. Pathology of the vulnerable plaque. J Am Coll Cardiol 2006;47(8 Suppl):C13–8.
107. Qiao Y, Etesami M, Astor BC, et al. Carotid plaque neovascularization and hemorrhage detected by MR imaging are associated with recent cerebrovascular ischemic events. AJNR Am J Neuroradiol 2012;33(4):755–60.
108. Chen H, Sun J, Kerwin WS, et al. Scan-rescan reproducibility of quantitative assessment of inflammatory carotid atherosclerotic plaque using dynamic contrast-enhanced 3T CMR in a multi-center study. J Cardiovasc Magn Reson 2014;16(1):51.
109. Gaens ME, Backes WH, Rozel S, et al. Dynamic contrast-enhanced MR imaging of carotid atherosclerotic plaque: model selection, reproducibility, and validation. Radiology 2013;266(1):271–9.
110. Kwak JH, Choi JW, Park HJ, et al. Cerebral artery dissection: spectrum of clinical presentations related to angiographic findings. Neurointervention 2011;6(2):78–83.
111. Blum CA, Yaghi S. Cervical artery dissection: a review of the epidemiology, pathophysiology, treatment, and outcome. Arch Neurosci 2015;2(4):e26670.
112. Caplan LR. Dissections of brain-supplying arteries. Nat Clin Pract Neurol 2008;4(1):34–42.
113. Houser OW, Mokri B, Sundt TM Jr, et al. Spontaneous cervical cephalic arterial dissection and its residuum: angiographic spectrum. AJNR Am J Neuroradiol 1984;5(1):27–34.
114. Benson JC, Lehman VT, Carr CM, et al. Beyond plaque: a pictorial review of non-atherosclerotic abnormalities of extracranial carotid arteries. J Neuroradiol 2021;48(1):51–60.
115. Liu Y, Li S, Wu Y, et al. The added value of vessel wall mri in the detection of intraluminal thrombus in patients suspected of craniocervical artery dissection. Aging Dis 2021;12(8):2140–50.
116. Mehdi E, Aralasmak A, Toprak H, et al. Craniocervical dissections: radiologic findings, pitfalls, mimicking diseases: a pictorial review. Curr Med Imaging Rev 2018;14(2):207–22.
117. Uemura M, Terajima K, Suzuki Y, et al. Visualization of the intimal flap in intracranial arterial dissection using high-resolution 3T MRI. J Neuroimaging 2017;27(1):29–32.
118. Wang Y, Lou X, Li Y, et al. Imaging investigation of intracranial arterial dissecting aneurysms by using 3 T high-resolution MRI and DSA: from the interventional neuroradiologists' view. Acta Neurochir 2014;156(3):515–25.

119. Wu Y, Wu F, Liu Y, et al. High-resolution magnetic resonance imaging of cervicocranial artery dissection: imaging features associated with stroke. Stroke 2019;50(11):3101–7.
120. Cho SJ, Choi BS, Bae YJ, et al. Image findings of acute to subacute craniocervical arterial dissection on magnetic resonance vessel wall imaging: a systematic review and proportion meta-analysis. Front Neurol 2021;12:586735.
121. Vranic JE, Huynh TJ, Fata P, et al. The ability of magnetic resonance black blood vessel wall imaging to evaluate blunt cerebrovascular injury following acute trauma. J Neuroradiol 2020;47(3):210–5.
122. Bond KM, Nasr D, Lehman V, et al. Intracranial and extracranial neurovascular manifestations of takayasu arteritis. AJNR Am J Neuroradiol 2017;38(4):766–72.
123. Gaballah M, Goldfisher R, Amodio JB. The utility of MRI in the diagnosis of takayasu arteritis. Case Rep Pediatr 2017;2017:7976165.
124. Ninan JV, Lester S, Hill CL. Giant cell arteritis: beyond temporal artery biopsy and steroids. Intern Med J 2017;47(11):1228–40.
125. Guggenberger KV, Bley TA. Imaging in vasculitis. Curr Rheumatol Rep 2020;22(8):34.
126. Hoffman GS. Giant cell arteritis. Ann Intern Med 2016;165(9):Itc65–itc80.
127. D'Souza NM, Morgan ML, Almarzouqi SJ, et al. Magnetic resonance imaging findings in giant cell arteritis. Eye (Lond) 2016;30(5):758–62.
128. Micieli E, Voci D, Mumoli N, et al. Transient perivascular inflammation of the carotid artery (TIPIC) syndrome. Vasa 2022;51(2):71–7.
129. Brinjikji W, Agid R, Pereira VM. Carotid stenting for treatment of symptomatic carotid webs: a single-center case series. Interv Neurol 2018;7(5):233–40.
130. Park CC, El Sayed R, Risk BB, et al. Carotid webs produce greater hemodynamic disturbances than atherosclerotic disease: a DSA time-density curve study. J Neurointerventional Surg 2022;14(7):729–33.
131. Patel SD, Otite FO, Topiwala K, et al. Interventional compared with medical management of symptomatic carotid web: a systematic review. J Stroke Cerebrovasc Dis 2022;31(10):106682.
132. Poloskey SL, Olin JW, Mace P, et al. Fibromuscular dysplasia. Circulation 2012;125(18):e636–9.
133. Haddy N, Mousannif A, Tukenova M, et al. Relationship between the brain radiation dose for the treatment of childhood cancer and the risk of long-term cerebrovascular mortality. Brain 2011;134(5):1362–72.
134. Twitchell S, Karsy M, Guan J, et al. Sequelae and management of radiation vasculopathy in neurosurgical patients. J Neurosurg 2018;130(6):1–9.
135. Cheng SW, Wu LL, Ting AC, et al. Irradiation-induced extracranial carotid stenosis in patients with head and neck malignancies. Am J Surg 1999;178(4):323–8.
136. Thalhammer C, Husmann M, Glanzmann C, et al. Carotid artery disease after head and neck radiotherapy. Vasa 2015;44(1):23–30.
137. McDonald MW, Moore MG, Johnstone PA. Risk of carotid blowout after reirradiation of the head and neck: a systematic review. Int J Radiat Oncol Biol Phys 2012;82(3):1083–9.
138. Boesen ME, Eswaradass PV, Singh D, et al. MR imaging of carotid webs. Neuroradiology 2017;59(4):361–5.
139. Xu W, Yang X, Li Y, et al. Deep learning-based automated detection of arterial vessel wall and plaque on magnetic resonance vessel wall images. Front Neurosci 2022;16:888814.
140. Lopez Gonzalez MR, Foo SY, Holmes WM, et al. Atherosclerotic carotid plaque composition: A 3T and 7T MRI-histology correlation study. J Neuroimaging 2016;26(4):406–13.
141. Zhang R, Zhang Q, Ji A, et al. Identification of high-risk carotid plaque with MRI-based radiomics and machine learning. Eur Radiol 2021;31(5):3116–26.
142. Shu H, Sun J, Hatsukami TS, et al. Simultaneous noncontrast angiography and intraplaque hemorrhage (SNAP) imaging: Comparison with contrast-enhanced MR angiography for measuring carotid stenosis. J Magn Reson Imaging 2017;46(4):1045–52.
143. Zhu DC, Vu AT, Ota H, et al. An optimized 3D spoiled gradient recalled echo pulse sequence for hemorrhage assessment using inversion recovery and multiple echoes (3D SHINE) for carotid plaque imaging. Magn Reson Med 2010;64(5):1341–51.
144. Balu N, Yarnykh VL, Chu B, et al. Carotid plaque assessment using fast 3D isotropic resolution black-blood MRI. Magn Reson Med 2011;65(3):627–37.
145. Li L, Chai JT, Biasiolli L, et al. Black-blood multicontrast imaging of carotid arteries with DANTE-prepared 2D and 3D MR imaging. Radiology 2014;273(2):560–9.
146. Mossa-Basha M, Yuan C, Wasserman BA, et al. Survey of the American society of neuroradiology membership on the use and value of extracranial carotid vessel wall MRI. AJNR Am J Neuroradiol 2022;43(12):1756–61.

# Body and Extremity MR Venography: Technique, Clinical Applications, and Advances

Rory L. Cochran, MD, PhD, Brian B. Ghoshhajra, MD, MBA,
Sandeep S. Hedgire, MD*

**KEYWORDS**

- Deep venous thrombosis • Nonocclusive iliocaval venous lesion (NIVL) • May–Thurner syndrome
- Nutcracker syndrome • Paget–Schroetter syndrome • Superior vena cava syndrome
- Pelvic venous congestion syndrome • Tumor thrombus

**KEY POINTS**

- Familiarity with normal and variant venous anatomy is essential for accurate MR venography diagnosis of venous thrombosis, venous compression, and insufficiency syndromes.
- Distinguishing bland thrombus from tumor thrombus at MR venography is a common challenge and critically important for accurate staging of patients with malignancies prone to venous invasion.
- Lack of ionizing radiation, improvements in non-contrast techniques, faster acquisition times, and recent developments in superparamagnetic iron oxide-based contrast agents have fostered increased MR venography utilization for various forms of venous pathology.

## INTRODUCTION

Magnetic resonance venography (MRV) represents a distinct imaging approach that may be used to evaluate a wide spectrum of venous pathology. Despite duplex ultrasound (US) and computed tomography venography representing the dominant imaging modalities in investigating suspected venous disease, MRV is increasingly used due to its lack of ionizing radiation, unique ability to be performed without administration of intravenous contrast, and recent technical improvements resulting in improved sensitivity, image quality, and faster acquisition times. In this review, the authors discuss commonly used body and extremity MRV techniques, different clinical applications, and future directions.

## MR VENOGRAPHY TECHNIQUES

Conventional vascular MR techniques may be categorized as bright-blood or dark-blood sequences with the respective names intuitively describing the appearance of the intravascular constituents on acquired images. Venous patency and direction of flow are best evaluated with bright-blood sequences, whereas dark-blood sequences provide helpful information about the surrounding soft tissue and vessel wall. **Table 1** lists the major bright-blood sequences currently used for various urgent and routine clinical applications. Although many of the different techniques listed present unique advantages for specific applications, the following discussion focuses primarily on the most commonly used clinical approaches for body and extremity venous MR imaging (**Fig. 1**).

### *Venography Without Intravenous Contrast*

Time-of-flight (TOF) imaging has represented the predominant non-contrast, bright-blood technique used in MRV applications for the last 2 decades. Bright-blood TOF imaging relies on the phenomena of flow-related enhancement where blood

Division of Cardiovascular Imaging, Department of Radiology, Massachusetts General Hospital, 55 Fruit Street, Boston, MA 02114, USA
* Corresponding author. Harvard Medical School.
*E-mail address:* hedgire.sandeep@mgh.harvard.edu

Magn Reson Imaging Clin N Am 31 (2023) 413–431
https://doi.org/10.1016/j.mric.2023.04.004

**Table 1**
**Bright-blood MRA/MR venography techniques**

| Non-Contrast | | Contrast-Enhanced |
|---|---|---|
| Time-of-flight (TOF) | 2D<br>3D<br>Cardiac gated | Single phase<br>Time-resolved |
| Steady-state free precession (SSFP) | | |
| Fast spin echo (FSE) | | |
| Phase contrast (PC) | | |
| Arterial spin labeling (ASL) | | |
| Flow sensitive dephasing (FSD) | | |
| Quiescent interval single shot (QISS) | | |

flowing into or out of an imaging volume seems bright relative to suppressed or saturated background soft tissue. Background soft tissue signal saturation is achieved following multiple radiofrequency pulses. Protons within slowly flowing blood, or at an occlusion, will become saturated and seem hypointense similar to background soft tissue. Flow-related signal intensity is highest when the flow is orthogonal to the image slice; conversely, flow parallel to the image plane becomes saturated similar to the background and gives rise to the in-plane artifacts commonly seen with tortuous vessels. Gradient-echo-based sequences, as opposed to spin-echo-based sequences, are preferred to minimize flow-related signal losses. Moderate to high flip angles (eg, 60°) and short time-to-echo (TE) values (<7 msec) are used to maximize contrast and minimize T2*-related signal losses, respectively. Short time-to-repeat (TR) values (<30 msec) are used to maintain background soft tissue suppression and thin slices (1–3 mm) should be used to maximize flow-related enhancement. Given the slower flow of venous blood relative to arterial, larger saturation bands are needed to saturate the higher velocity arterial blood at the opposite end of the imaging volume.

Both two-dimensional (2D) and three-dimensional (3D) TOF image acquisition modes may be performed with the decision to use one over the other reliant on the trade-offs between acquisition time and image resolution. Two-dimensional TOF acquisition is faster than 3D TOF

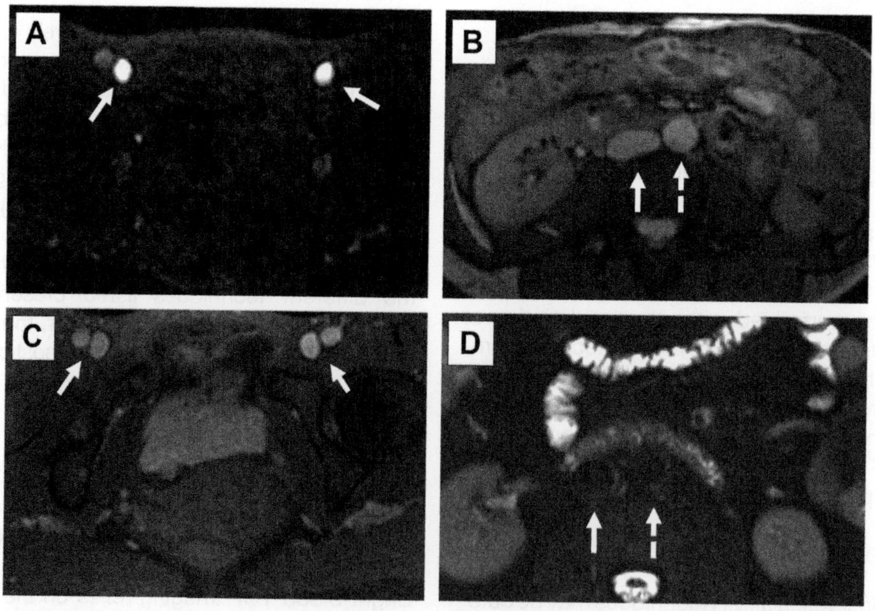


Fig. 1. MR venography techniques. (*A*) Axial gradient-echo-based two-dimensional time-of-flight (2D TOF) image showing hyperintense blood within the bilateral common femoral veins (*solid white arrows*). Note the absence of background soft tissue signal, characteristic of this technique. (*B*) Axial gradient-echo based, steady-state free precession (SSFP) image showing hyperintense signal within the inferior vena cava (*solid white arrow*) and aorta (*dashed white arrow*), and visualization of the surrounding soft tissues. (*C*) Axial T1-weighted fat-suppressed contrast-enhanced image showing excellent visualization of the bilateral common femoral vessels (*solid white arrow*) but also surrounding soft tissue. (*D*) Axial fat-suppressed, fast spin-echo dark blood technique, note the flow void in the aorta and IVC (dashed and solid *white arrows*, respectively).

but has poorer spatial resolution. Therefore, 2D TOF imaging is more commonly used in scenarios where larger anatomic coverage is needed (eg, combined ilio-caval imaging). Three-dimensional TOF imaging is often reserved for cases where anatomy is smaller or where delineating fine detail is necessary (eg, head and neck imaging). Several artifacts are commonly seen with TOF imaging, some of the most commonly encountered in body and extremity imaging include the stair-step (**Fig. 2**) and in-plane artifacts. The stair-step artifacts arise from the relatively thick slab slices that are used and may be reduced by obtaining overlapping slices or reducing slice thickness. As expected, these solutions result in increased scan time. A 2D variant is the "gated TOF"technique, whereby cardiac gating is used to time acquisition to improve image quality through reduction of physical motion artifacts.

Steady-state free precession (SSFP) is a fast bright-blood gradient echo imaging technique that relies on the intrinsic differences in T1 and T2 relaxation times of blood relative to other tissues, specifically the ratio of T2:T1. A major advantage of this approach, aside from the fast acquisition, is that the signal intensity in SSFP imaging predominately relies on the relaxation characteristics of blood and is minimally influenced by flow dynamics (eg, rate or direction of flow). Disadvantages of the SSFP technique include its vulnerability to image degradation from magnetic field inhomogeneities, which is most pronounced at air–tissue interfaces or near the edges of the field of view. The zebra stripe artifact arises from aliasing effects and field inhomogeneities[1] (see **Fig. 2**). Also, as fat and fluid demonstrate a high T2:T1 ratio such as blood, the SSFP technique is less useful for evaluation of smaller vessels, such as in the brain, especially as they are very close to fat/fluid interfaces.

## *Contrast-Enhanced MR Venography*

Despite routine use of multiple non-contrast techniques, contrast-enhanced MRV (CE-MR) remains an invaluable approach, particularly because it is less prone to the artifacts observed with some of the other approaches. CE-MR provides high vessel-to-tissue contrast via gadolinium-mediated T1 relaxation time shortening of adjacent intravascular blood. Most applications use upper extremity (UE) peripheral venous access for administration. However, note should be made of the indication before establishing venous access to minimize potential artifacts in the anatomic area(s) of interest. For single-phase or static imaging, a timed or triggered acquisition should be used according to examination indication. Fat-suppression may be used to increase signal-to-noise ratio. Similar to non-contrast techniques, gradient echo sequences are used to avoid flow-related signal losses.

In contrast to single-phase CE-MR, the newer technique of time-resolved MR provides high temporal resolution through rapid sequential imaging. Time-resolved MR relies both on view sharing and under-sampling of the periphery of k-space. In order to provide high temporal resolution, the technique uses a full-resolution non-contrast as the first image followed by multiple sequential incomplete acquisitions focusing on the center of k-space. As the center of k-space contains information pertaining to image contrast, while the periphery harbors spatial information, the technique represents a trade-off between image contrast and spatial resolution. Time-resolved MRV relies

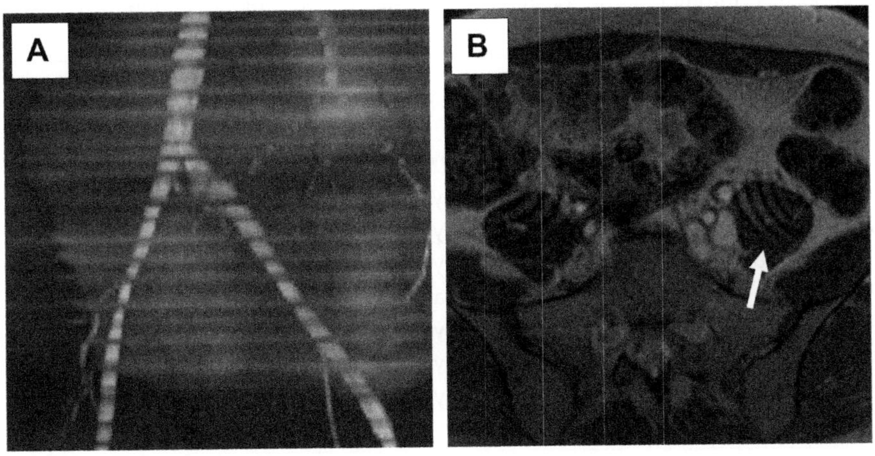


**Fig. 2.** Routinely encountered MRV artifacts. (*A*) TOF stair-step artifact and (*B*) Zebra stripe (Moiré fringes) artifact (*solid white arrow*).

on 3D spoiled gradient-echo sequences using short TR and TE using thin slices.

### Imaging Protocols

At our institution, we prefer to perform all MRV studies with intravenous contrast when feasible. Most protocols use a combination of non-contrast and contrast-enhanced techniques. Gadobutrol (Gadavist; Bayer Healthcare Pharmaceuticals Inc, Wayne, NJ), a class 2 nonionic macrocyclic agent, is the intravenous gadolinium contrast medium used at our institution for most MR venography studies with the administered dose based on body weight (0.1 mL/kg or 0.1 mmol/kg) given at a rate approximately 2 mL/s for adults and 1 to 2 mL for pediatric patients. **Table 2** provides an example MRV protocol for the pelvis.

## MRV CLINICAL APPLICATIONS

### Deep Venous Thrombosis

Venous thromboembolism (VTE) refers to a spectrum of conditions including superficial and deep venous thrombosis (DVT) and pulmonary embolism (PE). Although VTE incidence estimates vary, it is thought to afflict approximately 1 to 2 per 1000 of the US population.[2] Left unrecognized and/or untreated, VTE has the potential for considerable morbidity and mortality owing in large part to the sequela of PE. DVT of the lower extremities (**Box 1**) comprises the majority of new cases of VTE, occurring with a slight left-sided predominance.[3] The most common risk factors for lower extremity DVT include a history of prior DVT, immobility, cancer, and recent surgery.[4] Anticoagulation is the standard mode of treatment for both upper and lower extremity DVT with more invasive management strategies (eg, catheter-directed thrombolysis, thrombectomy, or inferior vena cava (IVC) filter placement) reserved for select cases.[5]

Most lower extremity DVT is believed to arise below the knee (below the popliteal vein), is asymptomatic, and resolves spontaneously.[6] In a subset of cases, however, thrombus can extend above the knee involving the popliteal and more proximal where symptoms become more likely and the risk of subsequent PE increases. According to the ACR Appropriateness Criteria, duplex US is considered the preferred initial imaging approach due to its accessibility, reliability, low cost, and noninvasiveness.[7] Nonetheless, MRV represents a useful, noninvasive complementary imaging tool that harbors certain advantages over US. MRV provides superior soft tissue evaluation, which can aid in diagnosing the underlying thrombosis provocation, such as in cases of congenital or acquired extrinsic venous compression, or provide an alternate explanation for lower extremity swelling (eg, venous insufficiency). Further, MRV permits evaluation of the IVC and pelvic veins, where US has a poorer performance, and enables qualitative and quantitative thrombus evaluation. MRV boasts an estimated sensitivity and specificity of 91.5% and 94.5%, respectively, for diagnosing DVT.[8] Although not routinely performed, prior work has studied the utility of MRV as a quantitative tool to determine the extent of venous thrombosis through volume estimation which may be helpful in determining efficacy of certain anticoagulant management strategies in the future.[9]

Acute thrombus on TOF images and CE-MRV appears as occlusive or partially occlusive hypointense signal (similar to background soft tissue) within the affected vein lumen. In the case of acute occlusive thrombus, the involved vein(s) appear enlarged and perivascular fat stranding may be present. Dark-blood sequences usually portray

**Table 2**
**Protocol overview for infrarenal inferior vena cava and iliac vessel MR venography**

| Sequence and Planes | Anatomic Coverage | Slice Thickness (mm) |
|---|---|---|
| Sagittal, axial SSFSE localizer | Top of kidneys to mid-thighs | 8 |
| Coronal SGR | Top of kidneys to mid-thighs | 5 |
| Axial, coronal, sagittal SSFP BH | Top of kidneys to femoral heads | 5 |
| Axial TOF | Aortic bifurcation to femoral head | 4 |
| Axial T2 FS RT | Top of kidneys to femoral heads | 5 |
| Coronal T1W pre dynamic | Top of kidneys to femoral heads | 1–2 |
| Coronal T1W post dynamic | Top of kidneys to femoral heads | 1–2 |
| Axial SGR FS | Top of kidneys to femoral heads | 1–2 |

*Abbreviations:* 3D, three-dimensional; BH, breath-hold; FS, fat-saturation; PG, peripherally gated; RT, respiratory triggered; SGR, spoiled gradient-echo; SSFP, steady-state free precession; SSFSE, single-shot fast-spin echo; TOF, time-of-flight.

**Box 1**
**Named deep veins of the lower extremities**

Common femoral
Femoral
Deep femoral (profunda femoris)
Popliteal
Posterior tibial
Anterior tibial
Fibular
Soleus and Gastrocnemius

acute thrombus as a luminal filling defect with increased signal intensity (**Fig. 3**). The appearance in the chronic phase depends on the extent of prior thrombosis. With veno-occlusion, there is often evidence of altered flow dynamics with the development of venous collaterals bypassing the site(s) of occlusion. On CE-MRV, chronic thrombosis often manifests as a shrunken, atretic vein with wall irregularity and coexistent venous collaterals. In the setting of nonocclusive thrombosis, there may wall irregularities and with intraluminal fibrous cords (**Fig. 4**; **Table 3**). Dark-blood sequences are usually not helpful for thrombus evaluation in the chronic phase as the thrombus becomes less hyperintense. Notable mimics of DVT include slow flow and in-plane artifacts, as the blood volume signal will become hypointense in these two settings.

UE DVT (**Box 2**), often confined to the axillary and/or subclavian veins, is much less common than lower extremity DVT, comprising approximately 10% of total cases of DVT.[10] Distinct from the lower extremities, UE DVT is often associated with an inciting cause (eg, indwelling venous catheter), which is why UE DVT is routinely dichotomized as primary or secondary. Primary UE DVT is relatively rare and describes cases of DVT that are idiopathic or arise in the setting of venous thoracic outlet obstruction or effort thrombosis, also known as Paget–Schroetter syndrome (PTS) (discussed later). Secondary UE DVT includes cases caused by the presence of an indwelling foreign body, such as a central venous catheter (CVC) or pacemaker leads, cancer-related thrombosis, postsurgical, or following trauma.[10,11] Similar to lower extremity DVT evaluation, the preferred first-line diagnostic test for UE DVT is US. However, as in cases for lower extremity DVT, MRV is particularly useful in soft tissue

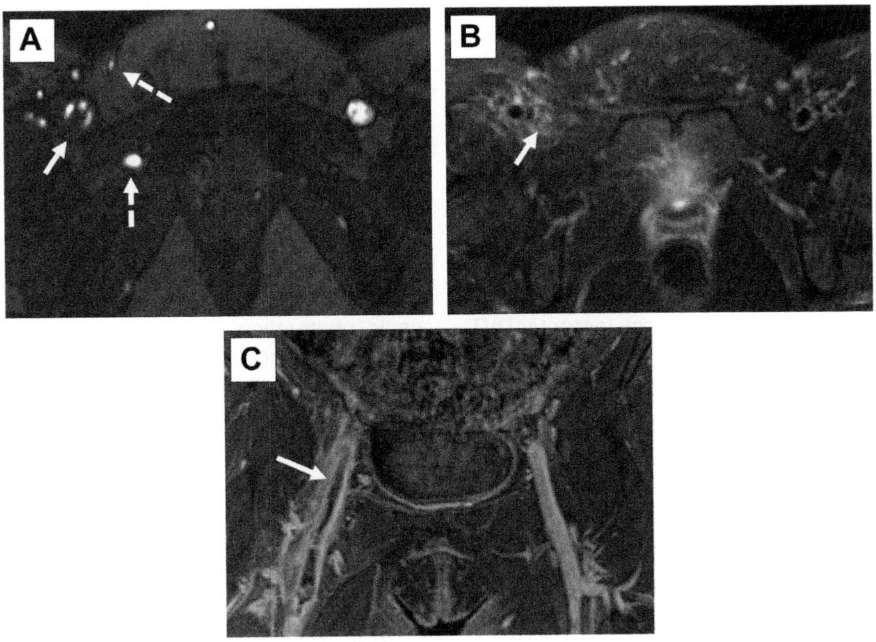


Fig. 3. Acute deep venous thrombosis (DVT). (*A*) Axial TOF image showing acute near occlusive right common femoral vein DVT. Note the mild venous enlargement (*solid white arrow*) and the shunting/engorgement of blood through collateral pathways (*dashed white arrows*). (*B*) Axial fat-saturated fast spin-echo image showing the same patient as in (*A*). Note the hyperintense signal of thrombus (*solid white arrow*) and surrounding fat stranding. (*C*) Coronal fat-suppressed T1-weighted contrast-enhanced image showing hypointense thrombus (*sold white arrow*) within the right common femoral vein extending inferiorly.

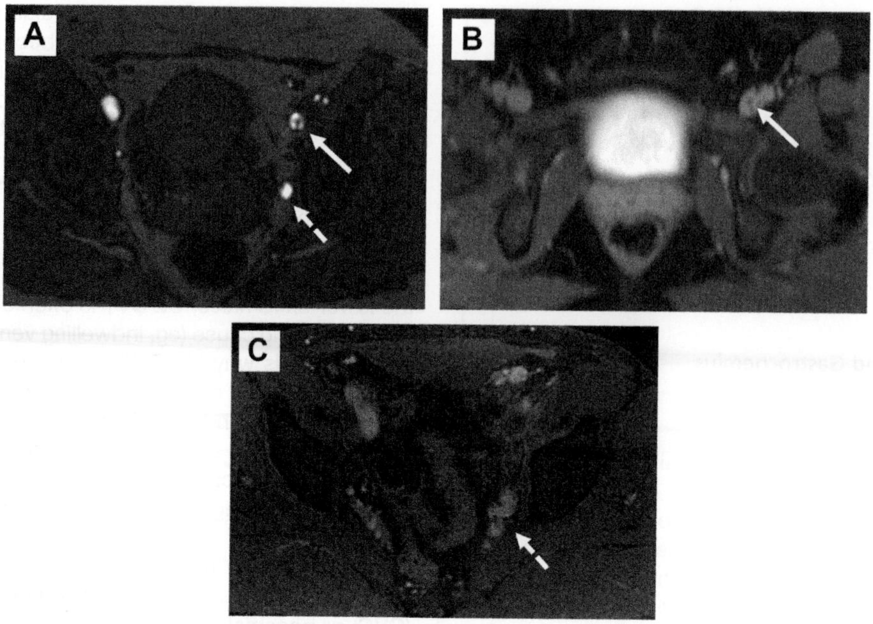


**Fig. 4.** Chronic deep venous thrombosis (DVT). (*A*) Axial TOF image showing atretic left external iliac with nonocclusive chronic thrombus (*solid white arrow*) and development of an enlarged left internal iliac vein (*dashed white arrow*) due to collateralization. (*B*) Axial fat-suppressed T1-weighted image showing same patient from *A* with chronic nonocclusive left common femoral vein thrombosis (*solid white arrow*). (*C*) Axial fat-suppressed contrast-enhanced image of another patient with a chronic left common femoral venous thrombosis with prominent ipsilateral collateral veins (*dashed white arrows*).

characterization, determining extent, potential etiologies for the venous thrombosis, and inspection of the central venous structures where US is unable.[12] MRV imaging features of UE DVT follow the same patterns described seen in lower extremity DVT (**Fig. 5**).

Superficial venous thrombosis (SVT) alone has long been considered a relatively benign, self-limiting entity, diagnosed with compression US. Despite its typically mild clinical course, SVT should not be immediately dismissed before ruling out concurrent DVT, as SVT is a risk factor for DVT and PE.[13] MRV is not routinely used for SVT clinical evaluation.

***Venous Compression Syndromes: May–Thurner***

May–Thurner syndrome (MTS) is the eponymous condition historically describing venous compression of the left common iliac vein (CIV) between the right common iliac artery (CIA) and the anterior aspect of the fifth lumbar vertebral body resulting in ipsilateral DVT[14] (**Fig. 6**). Although May–Thurner "anatomy," which is considered as $\geq$50% narrowing of the left CIV where the right CIA crosses, is commonly seen in normal patients, true MTS is thought to represent a distinct uncommon clinical entity. However, in the absence of consensus diagnostic criteria, the actual prevalence of MTS remains difficult to determine. In addition to conventional MTS, other anatomic variants (so-called variant MTS) giving rise to right CIV or bilateral CIV compression via iliac arterial compression have been described (**Fig. 7**; **Table 4**).[15] From a pathogenesis standpoint, venous endothelial damage arises from chronic compression and pulsation leading to luminal abnormalities, sometimes referred to as webs or spurs, and altered flow dynamics. The acquired luminal irregularities and abnormal flow may result in stenosis, obstruction, and DVT.[16]

MRV is a particularly useful imaging modality for patients with suspected MTS, as MRV enables not

**Table 3**
**Summary of MR venography findings for deep venous thrombosis on bright-blood imaging**

| Acute | Chronic |
|---|---|
| Loss of luminal hyperintense signal | Loss of luminal hyperintense signal |
| Focal venous enlargement | Atretic vein |
| Perivascular fat stranding | Irregular wall thickening |
| | Presence of venous collaterals |

**Box 2**
**Named deep veins of the upper extremities**

Subclavian
Axillary
Brachial
Interosseous
Radial
Ulnar

only evaluation of vessel patency but may be used to evaluate severity and altered flow dynamics. The routine imaging of suspected MTS commonly involves TOF and contrast-enhanced sequences. MRV findings of MTS include focal narrowing of the left CIV in the affected segment, reversal of flow on TOF images, and the presence of ipsilateral pelvic venous collaterals (see **Fig. 6**). A notable pitfall to diagnosing MTS, as well other venous compression syndromes, is in the setting of patient dehydration, which can lead to overestimation of extrinsic venous compression simply due to low intravascular volume.

In pregnant patients, the gravid uterus can lead to mechanical compression of the pelvic vasculature. Pregnant women, and women in the postpartum period, are at an increased risk of thromboembolism secondary to anatomic and physiologic changes promoting venous stasis and hypercoagulability.[17] Thus, the evaluation of MTS in pregnant patient presents a unique clinical and diagnostic challenge. Conventional MR imaging examinations at both 1.5 and 3 T are considered safe in pregnant patients as no known harmful effects have been reported to date.[18] However, pregnancy is considered a relative contraindication to the administration of intravenous gadolinium contrast medium due to concerns for an elevated risk of stillbirth and other adverse fetal effects.[19] The administration of gadolinium contrast media to pregnant patients should only be performed after careful considerations of the risks and benefits, and informed consent is strongly advised. Thus, non-contrast MRV evaluation of suspected MTS in pregnant patients is the most commonly performed approach. Management of MTS usually involves anticoagulation and venous stenting.

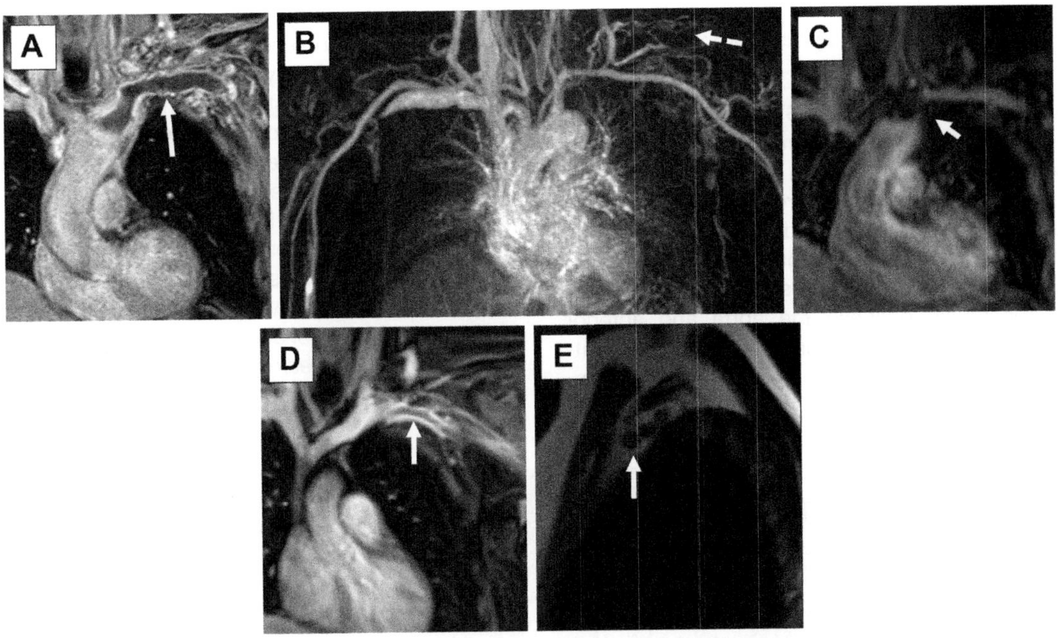


Fig. 5. Upper extremity deep venous thrombosis. (*A*) Coronal T1-weighted contrast-enhanced image demonstrating a left axillosubclavian DVT (*solid white arrow*). (*B*) Coronal maximum intensity projection (MIP) for the same patient in (*A*) illustrating absence of the left brachiocephalic, subclavian and axillary veins with mild ipsilateral engorgement of the collateral pathways (*dashed white arrow*). (*C*) Coronal T1-weighted contrast-enhanced image showing the patient from (*A, B*) following catheter thrombectomy/thrombolysis treatment with stent placement. The apparent absence of flow within the left brachiocephalic vein (*solid white arrow*) is secondary to artifact from the patient's stent. (*D*) Coronal T1-weighted contrast-enhanced image showing another patient with a left axillary DVT (*solid white arrow*). (*E*) Sagittal fast spin-echo image of patient from *D* showing subtle loss of the left axillary vein flow void (*solid white arrow*) and mild vessel enlargement.

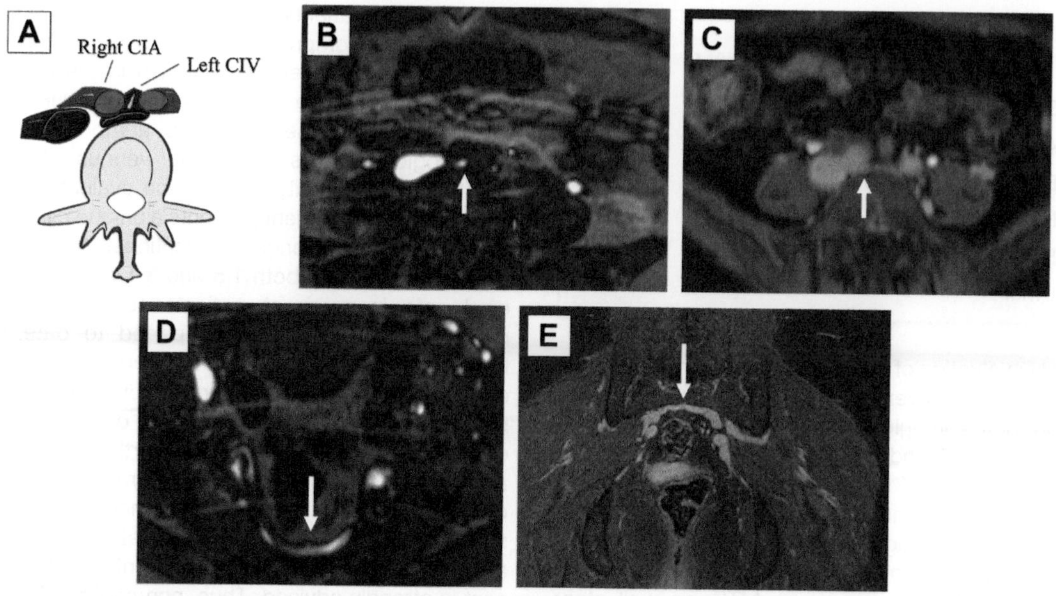


Fig. 6. May–Thurner syndrome. (*A*) Illustration of May–Thurner anatomy with right common iliac artery (CIA) compression of the left common iliac vein (CIV). (*B*) Axial TOF image of a patient with May–Thurner syndrome. Note the near absence of signal in the left CIV (*solid white arrow*). (*C*) Axial fat-suppressed T1-weighted contrast-enhanced image showing hemodynamically significant compression of the left CIV. (*D*) Axial TOF image and (*E*) fat-suppressed coronal T1-weighted contrast-enhanced image showing cross pelvic collateral veins (*solid white arrow*) shunting blood to the contralateral side.

## *Venous Compression Syndromes: Nutcracker Syndrome*

Nutcracker syndrome (NCS) describes left renal vein compression of the left renal vein as it crosses the aorta prior to joining with the IVC (**Fig. 8**). Anterior NCS is defined as compression of the left renal vein between the aorta and superior mesenteric artery (aortomesenteric portion), and posterior NCS is defined by compression of a retroaortic left renal vein between the aorta and anterior aspect of the spine.[20] Similar to MTS, NCS anatomy is often seen in normal patients. The distinguishing feature of NCS from simply variant anatomy is the presence of characteristic signs and symptoms, typically flank pain and hematuria. In males, ipsilateral testicular vein reflux can lead to scrotal swelling, varicocele, and infertility. In females, ipsilateral ovarian vein reflux can lead to pelvic and vulvar varices and symptoms of pelvic venous congestion.[21] NCS clinical features are due to elevated venous pressures. As would be expected, MRV findings of NCS include focal narrowing of the left renal vein as it crosses the aorta similar to the shape of a bird's beak (see **Fig. 8**). In fact, the so-called *beak-sign* has been reported to have a diagnostic sensitivity and specificity of

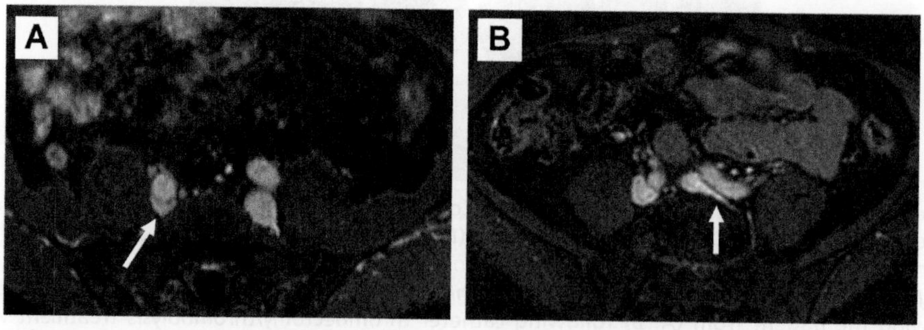


Fig. 7. May–Thurner syndrome variants. (*A*) Axial fat-suppressed T1-weighted contrast-enhanced image showing right common iliac artery compression of the right common iliac vein (*solid white arrow*). (*B*) Axial fat-suppressed T1-weighted contrast-enhanced image showing compression of the left common iliac vein by the left common iliac artery (*solid white arrow*).

Table 4
Reported May–Thurner variants

| Compressed Vein | Artery |
|---|---|
| Right common iliac | Right internal iliac |
| Left common iliac | Left internal iliac |
| Inferior vena cava | Right common iliac |

91.7% and 88.9%, respectively, for diagnosing anterior NCS.[22] Similarly, increasing angle acuity between the SMA and the aorta has also been reported as a useful metric in NCS diagnostic imaging evaluation. Specifically, an angle of less than 41° (normal being ~90°) reportedly has a diagnostic sensitivity and specificity of 100% and 55.6%, respectively.[22,23] Although these findings were described for CT, MRV provides adequate spatial resolution for detection of the same diagnostic findings. MRV can offer better contrast-to-noise ratios as CTV offers only an indirect enhancement when performed via venous access.

Other findings of NCS at MRV include ipsilateral retrograde gonadal vein flow on TOF images and the presences of pelvic varicosities and cross-pelvic collaterals on CE-MRV. Sonography studies have found that left renal vein peak systolic velocities are elevated at the narrowed segment in NCS patients. Given this observation, the investigators have described phase-contrast MR to estimate the left renal vein peak systolic velocity for a patient with NCS,[24] although this is not routinely used in clinical practice. Management of NCS remains patient specific due to the heterogeneity of the condition, strongly influenced by patient age, and includes conservative, surgical, and endovascular treatments (stenting).[25]

### *Venous Compression Syndromes: Paget–Schroetter*

Paget-Schroetter syndrome (PSS), also referred to as effort thrombosis, describes the venous form of thoracic outlet syndrome (vTOS) in individuals developing DVT of the axillary and subclavian veins. vTOS represents the second most common type of TOS behind the neurogenic variant.[26] PSS is rare with an estimated incidence of 1 to 2 per 100,000 population and affects men twice as often as women.[27] PSS arises from dynamic compression of the subclavian vein as it exits the thoracic outlet through the costoclavicular space (**Fig. 9**). The subclavian vein courses anterior to the anterior scalene muscle through the costoclavicular space bordered by the first rib, clavicle, and subclavius muscle. The subclavian vein's path is separate from the subclavian artery and brachial plexus, which exist the thoracic outlet through the scalene triangle.[28] The contemporary

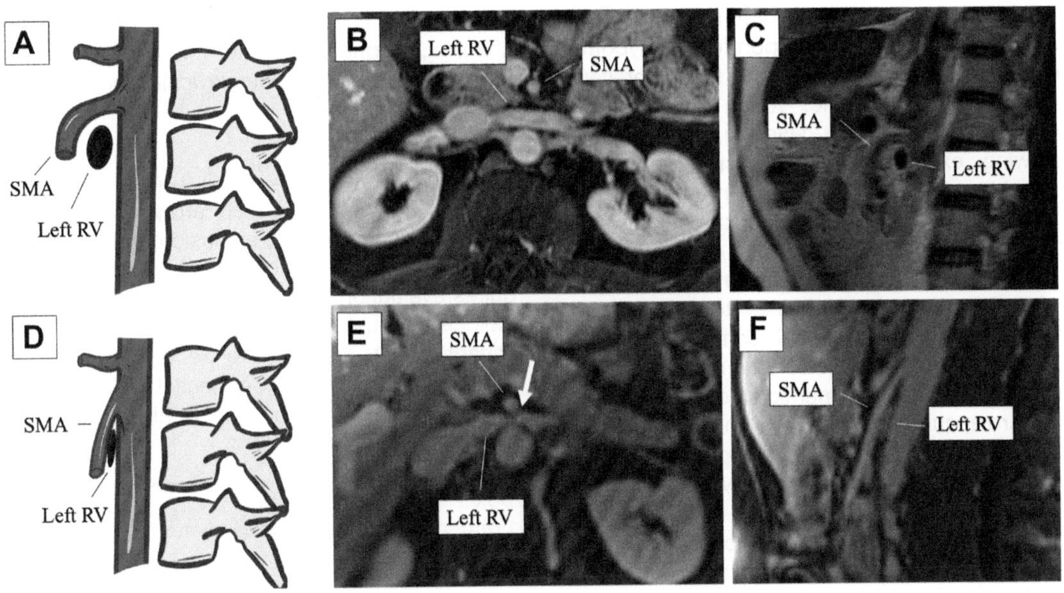


Fig. 8. Nutcracker syndrome. (*A*) Illustration of normal anterior, left renal vein (RV) anatomy in relation to the superior mesenteric artery (SMA). (*B*) Axial fat-suppressed T1-weighted contrast-enhanced and (*C*) sagittal fast spin-echo images showing normal anterior left renal venous anatomy. (*D*) Illustration of anterior Nutcracker syndrome anatomy. (*E*) Axial and sagittal (*F*) T1-weighted contrast-enhanced images showing a patient with Nutcracker syndrome. Note the beak sign on (*E*) at the aortomesenteric interval (*solid white arrow*) and the acute angle of the SMA in (*F*).

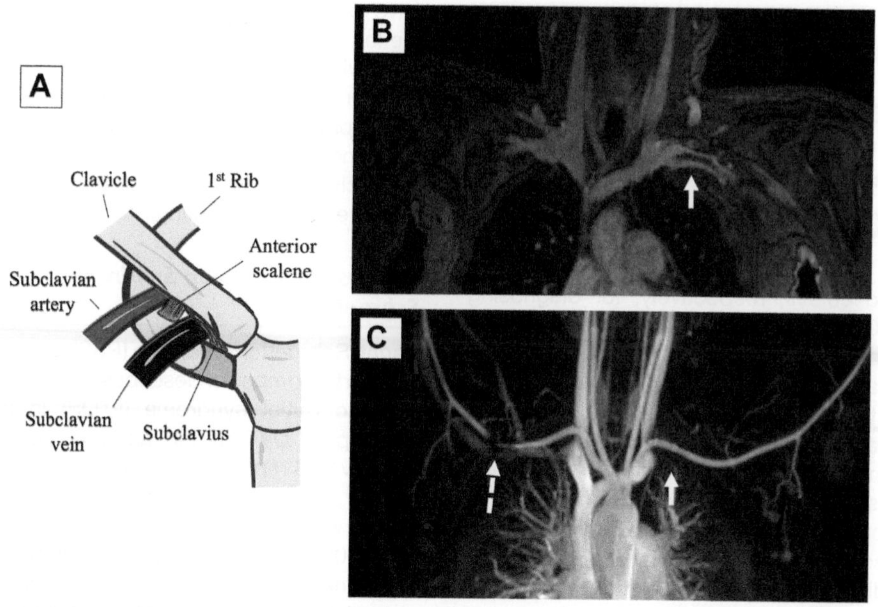


Fig. 9. Paget–Schroetter (PS) syndrome. (*A*) Illustration of the subclavian artery and vein at the cervical inlet. Note the subclavian vein exits through the costoclavicular junction, distinct from the subclavian artery. (*B*) Coronal T1-weighted contrast-enhanced image for a patient with PS-related thrombosis of the left axillosubclavian veins (*solid white arrow*). Note the arms down positioning. (*C*) Coronal maximum intensity projection (MIP) image for the same patient in (*B*) with arms up position. Note the right upper extremity compression without thrombosis in the arms up position (*dashed white arrow*).

pathophysiologic theory posits individuals who perform repetitive UE maneuvers develop locoregional musculature hypertrophy resulting in a predisposition to venous thrombosis at the costoclavicular junction. Support for this hypothesis stems from observations of the unique presenting patient demographic: young athletic males with unilateral UE pain, swelling, and cyanosis following exercise (hence, effort thrombosis). Intermittent subclavian vein compression with symptoms but without thrombosis is known as McCleery syndrome.[16]

MRV is very useful in the imaging evaluation of vTOS. CE-MRV is routinely used to evaluate subclavian vein patency, focal compression, surrounding soft tissue, and venous anatomy. Many institutions perform a dynamic study, whereby images are acquired with arms up and arms down.[29] MRV findings of vTOS include the presence of a dynamic subclavian vein narrowing with arm abduction, a fixed stenosis at the site of dynamic narrowing, venous collaterals bypassing the stenotic segment, the presence of an axillosubclavian vein thrombosis and aberrant osseous, and/or soft tissue anatomy[26] (see **Fig. 9**). It is important to note, however, that like the other venous compression syndromes previously discussed, venous compression alone at the costoclavicular space is not diagnostic of vTOS as many patients without the condition demonstrate focal compression. The mainstay of treatment of patients presenting with acute thrombosis is thrombolytic therapy, mechanical, or pharmacologic, followed by surgery to decompress the costoclavicular junction and prevent recurrence.[27]

## Inferior Vena Cava Imaging

The IVC is involved in an array of disorders, including occlusion (eg, extrinsic compression or thrombosis), malignancy, and infection that requires evaluation by cross-sectional imaging. Radiologists must be familiar with normal and variant caval anatomy to recognize clinically important anomalies. Congenital IVC variants (**Box 3**) result from abnormal embryologic

**Box 3**
**Congenital inferior vena cava anomalies**

- Duplication
- Left-sided IVC
- Azygos/hemiazygos continuation of IVC
- Agenesis
- IVC web

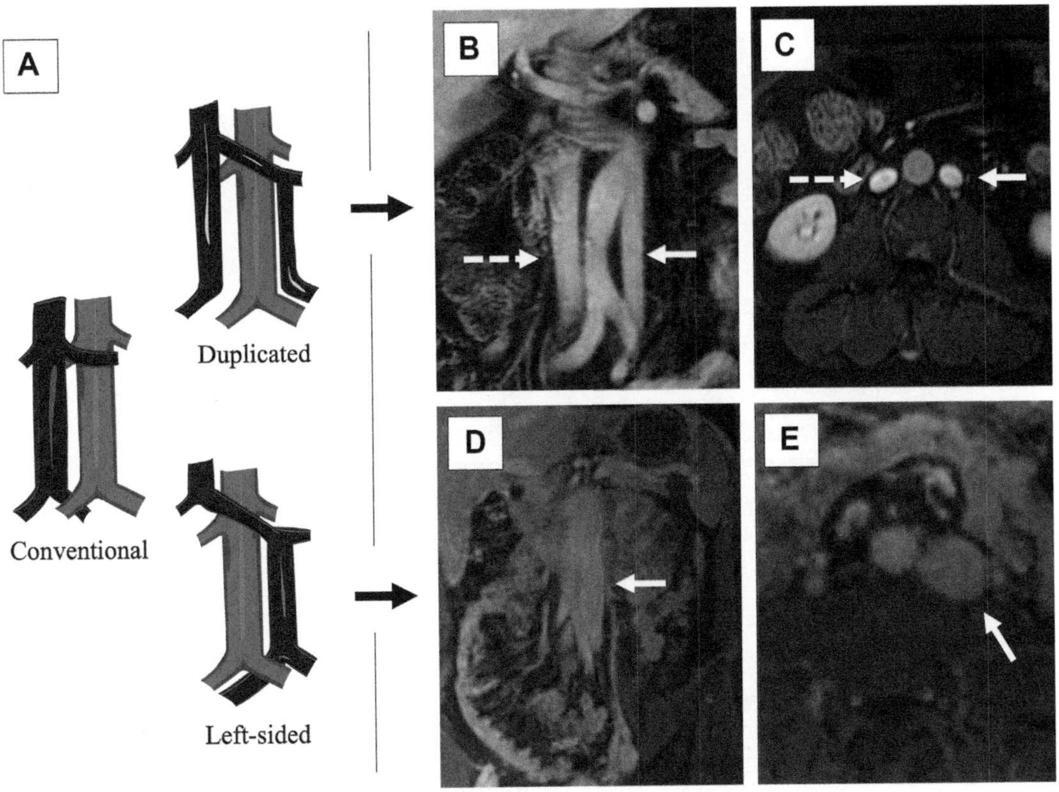


Fig. 10. Inferior vena cava (IVC) anomalies. (*A*) Illustration showing conventional, duplication, and left-sided IVC anatomy. (*B*) Coronal and (*C*) axial fat-suppressed T1-weighted contrast-enhanced images showing a patient with a right-sided (*dashed white arrow*) and left-sided IVC (*solid white arrow*). (*D*) Coronal and (*E*) axial fat-suppressed T1-weighted contrast-enhanced images showing a patient with a left-sided IVC (*solid white arrow*).

development, have a prevalence of approximately 4%,[30] and increase the risk of IVC thrombosis[31,32] (**Fig. 10**). The most commonly encountered anomalies include duplication, persistent left IVC with absent right, and anomalous continuation of the IVC via the azygous/hemi-azygous system. Other variants include mega cava, defined as an IVC diameter greater than 28 mm and IVC agenesis.

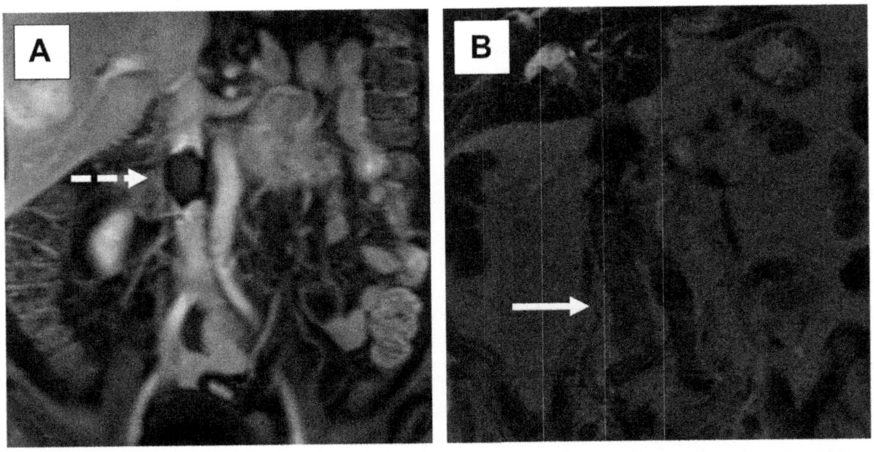


Fig. 11. IVC filter and thrombosis. (*A*) Coronal fat-suppressed T1-weighted contrast-enhanced image of a patient with an indwelling IVC filter (*dashed white arrow*). (*B*) Coronal steady-state free precession image showing a patient with an indwelling IVC filter and extensive thrombosis of the IVC below the level of the filter (*solid white arrow*). Note the mild enlargement of the IVC and mild heterogenous intraluminal signal.

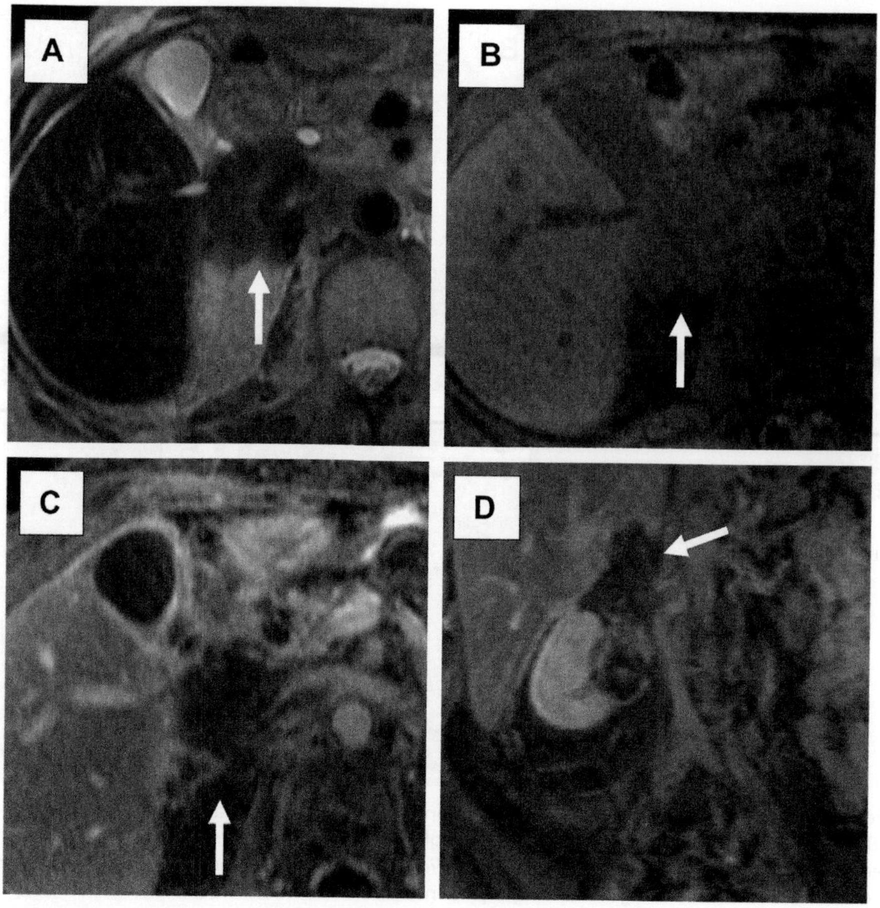


Fig. 12. Primary inferior vena cava (IVC) leiomyosarcoma. (*A*) Axial T2-weighted image and (*B*) axial fat-suppressed T1-weighted image showing a primarily extraluminal suprarenal primary IVC leiomyosarcoma (*solid white arrow*). (*C*) Axial and (*D*) coronal fat-suppressed T1-weighted contrast-enhanced images of the tumor.

CE-MRV and TOF sequences are commonly used to characterize caval anatomy and patency. An important pitfall to avoid on TOF images is mixing artifacts mimicking filling defects at the juxtarenal level.

De novo IVC thrombosis is a relatively rare phenomenon in patients with conventional anatomy but is more common in individuals with anomalous IVC anatomy or who have an indwelling IVC filter. Nonanatomic risk factors for IVC thrombosis include inherited or acquired thrombophilia, malignancy, surgery, trauma, obesity, pregnancy, oral contraceptives, and smoking.[33] Treatment most commonly involves anticoagulation with or without more invasive interventions (eg, thrombectomy/thrombolysis) on a case-by-case basis.[34]

In select patients at risk for life-threatening PE, an IVC filter may be placed.[35] Defining IVC anatomy before placement is essential as aberrant anatomy can influence the procedure. For example, patients with IVC duplication undergoing filter placement must be treated uniquely, often with either two infrarenal filters or a single suprarenal filter, in order for the device to function as intended preventing thrombus from migrating to the heart and lungs. Similarly, patients with mega cava require a special filter (Bird's Nest filter, Cook Medical) that can accommodate the abnormally large luminal diameter.[36] Last, left renal vein anatomy should be defined, as patients with circumaortic left renal vein anatomy require

**Box 4**
**Congenital superior vena cava anomalies**

- Duplication
- Persistent left-sided SVC without right
- Partial anomalous pulmonary venous return (PAPVR)
- SVC aneurysm

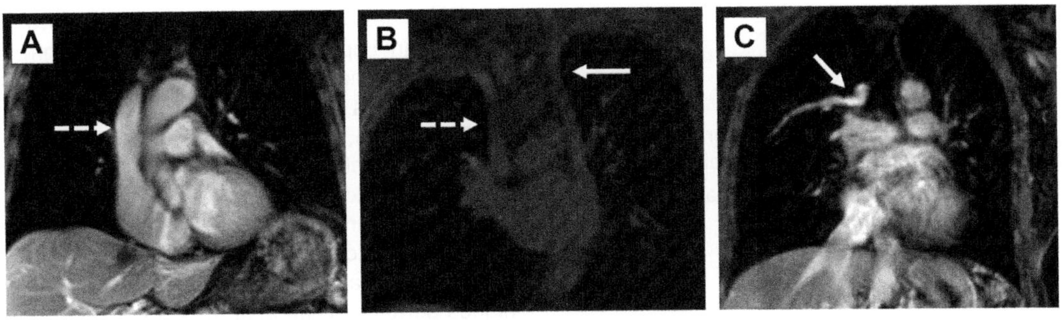


Fig. 13. Superior vena cava (SVC) anomalies. (*A*) Coronal fat-suppressed T1-weighted contrast-enhanced image of conventional, right-sided SVC (*dashed white arrow*) anatomy. (*B*) Coronal fat-suppressed T1-weighted contrast-enhanced images of a patient with a normal right (*dashed white arrow*) and persistent left SVC (*solid white arrow*), duplicated anatomy. (*C*) Coronal fat-suppressed T1-weighted contrast-enhanced image showing a patient with right upper lobe partial anomalous venous return into the SVC (*solid white arrow*).

special procedural planning. Owing to the tendency for the retroaortic limb to lie more inferior relative to the anterior limb, filter placement may need to be placed in the suprarenal position to avoid failure.[37] Most modern permanent and temporary/optional IVC filters are MR compatible made of titanium or non-ferromagnetic alloy. In patients with an indwelling filter, note should be made of infra-filter caval patency, given the increased risk of thrombosis (**Fig. 11**).

Primary tumors of the IVC are rare with leiomyosarcoma being the most common histologic type. IVC leiomyosarcomas are mesenchymal tumors arising from the venous tunica media smooth muscle cells.[38] Interestingly, they are more common in females (~74%) of middle age (median age of 52). Early during tumorigenesis, the cells grow in an intramural fashion before growing extending outward into the retroperitoneum and inward causing caval luminal narrowing with extramural growth more common than intramural growth.[38] At MR, IVC leiomyosarcomas often seem iso-hypointense (to muscle) on T1-weighted images, demonstrate areas of hyperintense signal on T2-weighted images, and may heterogeneously enhance[39,40] (**Fig. 12**). Tumor location predicts outcomes with suprarenal/juxtarenal tumors having the most favorable outcome and intrahepatic IVC tumors having the worst outcomes. Complete en bloc surgical resection is curative.[30] Secondary tumors involving the IVC are much more common than primary IVC tumors and are discussed later.

## *Superior Vena Cava Syndrome and Central Venous Stenosis*

Similar to the IVC, MRV permits characterization of normal superior vena cava (SVC) anatomy and anomalies arising from errors during embryogenesis. It is important to recognize common variants, their associations, and clinical implications. Conventionally, the SVC arises within the visceral mediastinum from the confluence of the left and right brachiocephalic veins and extends inferiorly draining blood into the right atrium. The most commonly encountered congenital SVC variant is a persistent left SVC with or without a coexistent right SVC (**Box 4**; **Fig. 13**). The left-sided SVC arises from the confluence of the left subclavian and jugular veins draining into the coronary sinus, which is often dilated. The estimated prevalence of persistent left SVC is less than 0.5% in the general population but up to 10% in patients with congenital heart disease. Recognition of these anomalies is important in an array of clinical scenarios, including but not limited to accurate CVC placement, pacemaker lead placement, and thromboembolism risk (eg, left SVC with unroofed coronary sinus). Further, in patients with a persistent left and absent right SVC, careful inspection for associated cardiovascular anomalies should be sought (**Box 5**).[41]

SVC syndrome denotes the constellation of signs and symptoms occurring with severe stenosis or complete SVC obstruction, which can include upper body edema, cyanosis, and engorged head and neck veins. The condition afflicts more than 15,000 individuals in the United

**Box 5**
**Left superior vena cava associations**

- Bicuspid aortic valve
- Aortic coarctation
- Septal defects (atrial and ventricular)
- Tetralogy of Fallot
- Mitral atresia
- Cor atriatum

**Table 5**
**Anatomic superior vena cava obstruction classification system**

| | |
|---|---|
| Type 1 | Supra-azygos: bilateral brachiocephalic vein occlusion |
| Type 2 | Supra-azygos: no brachiocephalic vein involvement |
| Type 3 | Azygos SVC |
| Type 4 | Infra-azygos SVC |

States annually.[42] The most common cause of SVC syndrome is malignancy, followed by benign causes from indwelling CVCs and pacemakers. Before the development of antibiotics, however, infectious causes were the dominant etiology of SVC syndrome.[42] The most common malignant cause of SVC syndrome is non-small cell lung cancer.

Imaging findings of SVC syndrome exist along a spectrum depending on the location and degree of obstruction. Using venographic imaging data from affected patients, the Stanford classification was developed, describing four categories based on the degree and level of SVC obstruction relative to the azygos vein. The Stanford classification was proposed as a system that could identify patients at risk for airway and cerebral compromise who would benefit from surgical bypass (types 3 and 4).[43] Given the variability in syndrome severity and newer treatment approaches, Azizi and colleagues proposed a revised classification scheme based on lesion location and severity toward creating an improved management algorithm.[44] **Table 5** lists the types based on lesion location. Severity grades include A, B, and C corresponding to 50% to 90%, greater than 90%, and 100% occlusion, respectively. Although the classification schema may not necessarily be used in imaging reports, the framework can be helpful during image interpretation.

Both static and time-resolved CE-MRV techniques permit evaluation of the central veins[45] toward detecting acute and chronic SVC obstruction. Acute occlusion will result in the absence of signal within the SVC without the development of venous collaterals. In contrast, chronic occlusions will result in collaterals with the degree of collateral formation directly proportional to the hemodynamic severity of occlusion[46](**Fig. 14**). Based on the etiology, severity and patient factors, SVC syndrome may be managed with endovascular therapy (eg, angioplasty and stenting), radiation therapy, or surgery.

Central venous stenosis (CVS) describes venous narrowing of one or more of the large intrathoracic veins in hemodialysis patients, including the internal jugular, subclavian and brachiocephalic veins, and the superior vena cava (**Fig. 15**). CVS occurs in hemodialysis patients with a history of prior CVC access and patients without prior interventions.[47,48] CVS is believed to be the end result of the compensatory responses of venous endothelial injury stimulating smooth muscle proliferation and collagen deposition resulting in wall thickening and luminal

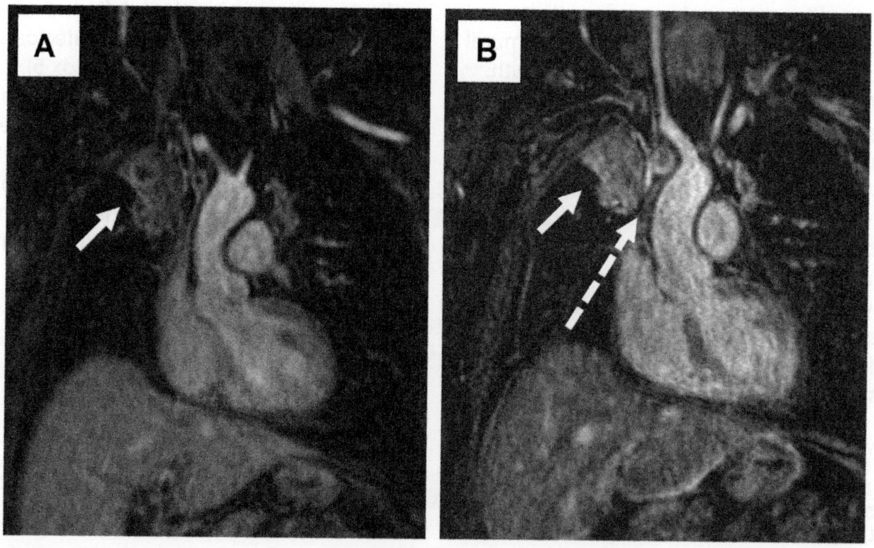


**Fig. 14.** Superior vena cava (SVC) syndrome. (*A*) and (*B*) Coronal fat-suppressed T1-weighted contrast-enhanced images of a patient with a right upper lobe mass (*solid white arrow*) causing extrinsic compression on the SVC (*dashed white arrow*) leading to SVC syndrome.

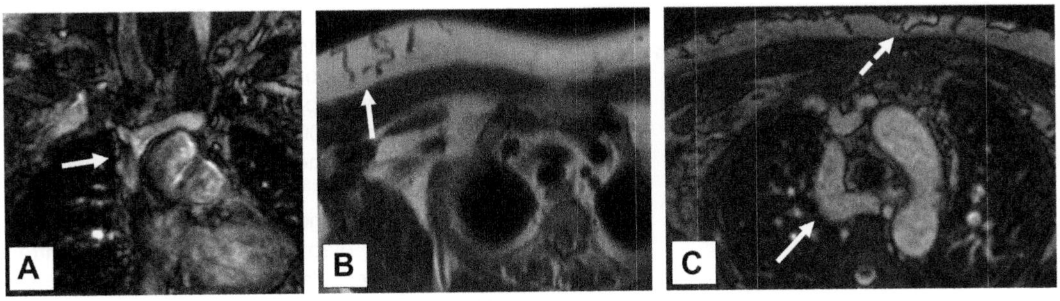


Fig. 15. Central venous stenosis. (*A*) Coronal steady-state free precession (SSFP) image of a patient with superior vena cava (SVC) stenosis (*solid white arrow*) in the setting of an indwelling dialysis catheter. (*B*) Axial T2-weighted image showing developed right chest wall venous collaterals for patient in exhibit A. (*C*) Axial SSFP image for another patient with severe SVC stenosis/occlusion, developed chest wall collaterals and an enlarged azygos vein (*solid white arrow*).

narrowing.[49] Both direct injury from an indwelling line, lead, or catheter and turbulent blood flow can stimulate the response leading to CVS. Various endovascular techniques, including angioplasty and stenting, are commonly used to manage CVS.[50] Although venography has been the historic gold standard for CVS evaluation due to its sensitivity, dynamic nature enabling concurrent same-session intervention, MRV is also routinely used due to its accuracy and noninvasiveness.

## *Venous Insufficiency: Pelvic Venous Congestion*

Venous insufficiency broadly describes the abnormal functional state of veins resulting from valvular incompetence leading to elevated venous pressures and subsequent venous dilatation. The two most commonly described disorders of venous incompetence include pelvic venous insufficiency (PVI) and chronic venous insufficiency of the lower extremities or varicose veins.[51,52] PVI arises from gonadal vein incompetence, which can lead to pelvic venous congestion syndrome (PVCS). Although PVCS can be seen in the setting of PVI with some of the previously discussed compression syndromes (eg, Nutcracker or May–Thurner), it can also be seen with PVI in the absence of a structural abnormality. MRV findings of PVI include dilated parauterine varices, retrograde gonadal venous flow on time-resolved images, loss of the normal flow void within pelvic veins from slow flow, and superficial varices, including vulvar and upper thigh (**Fig. 16**).[53]

## *Oncology: Differentiating Tumor Versus Bland Venous Thrombus*

An incredibly useful application of MRV is in helping distinguish bland from tumor thrombus in oncologic imaging. Several tumor types are well known to invade venous structures (**Box 6**), perhaps most notably renal cell carcinoma (RCC) and hepatocellular carcinoma (HCC). Indeed, the presence of tumor in the vein influences both staging and management strategies for RCC and HCC. Features favoring tumor in vein versus bland thrombus include venous expansion and enhancement of the venous filling defect. The vessel expansion observed with tumor in vein is more prominent than what is observed with an acute bland thrombus. Other features that are characteristic of tumor in vein include enhancement features resembling the primary tumor and malignant

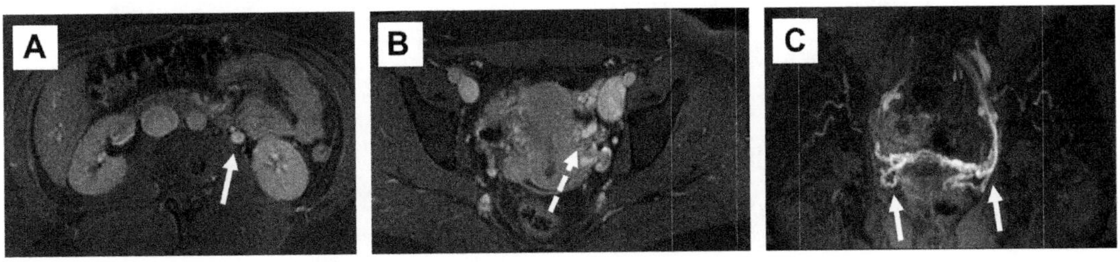


Fig. 16. Pelvic venous congestion syndrome (PVCS). (*A*) and (*B*) Axial fat-suppressed T1-weighted contrast-enhanced images of a patient with an enlarged left ovarian vein (*solid white arrow*) and parauterine varices (*dashed white arrow*) in the setting of PVCS. (*C*) Coronal maximum intensity projection of another patient with PVCS and prominent pelvic venous varicosities (*solid white arrow*).

**Box 6**
**Malignancies commonly demonstrating venous invasion**

Renal cell carcinoma

Hepatocellular carcinoma

Adrenal cortical carcinoma

Wilms tumor

Leiomyosarcoma

thrombus that seems contiguous with the primary tumor (**Fig. 17**).[54] Although diffusion sequences are not routinely performed in routine MRV evaluations, when obtained, tumor thrombus will often restrict diffusion, whereas bland thrombus usually does not (**Box 7**).

## RECENT ADVANCES AND FUTURE DIRECTIONS

### *Ferumoxytol*

Although gadolinium-based compounds have dominated the MR imaging contrast agent space sincenearly their inception, renewed interest and recent clinical studies of iron oxide nanoparticle formulations as contrast agents have emerged in recent years in part due to reports of the drawbacks of gadolinium, namely nephrogenic systemic fibrosis and central nervous system gadolinium retention.[55–57] Iron oxide nanoparticles are superparamagnetic compounds of varying sizes demonstrating utility for both diagnostic and therapeutic applications, including as an MR blood pool contrast agent due to the high longitudinal relaxivity of iron oxide implying T1-shortening effects. Iron oxide-based contrast agents are biodegradable and avoid the potential toxicities associated with gadolinium administration. Among the currently available intravenous preparations, ferumoxytol (Feraheme, AMAG Pharmaceuticals), an ultrasmall dextran-coated formulation, has been studied the most extensively for MR imaging. Ferumoxytol was approved by the Food and Drug Administration in 2009 for intravenous administration in chronic kidney disease patients with iron deficiency anemia.[58] Despite ferumoxytol's therapeutic approval indication, it has been used off-label as a diagnostic MR imaging contrast agent with recent data demonstrating a sufficient safety profile.[59] Compared with gadolinium-based agents, ferumoxytol has a much longer dose-dependent plasma half-life (approximately 14 hours) permitting both immediate and delayed interval imaging, which is particularly advantageous when imaging the body and peripheral vasculature. The notable downside associated with ferumoxytol is the risk of acute hypersensitivity reactions.[59]

Ferumoxytol has been evaluated for various magnetic resonance angiography and venography applications. As a blood pool agent, ferumoxytol harbors great potential for MRV. In a recent report evaluating the now unavailable blood-pool gadolinium agent, gadofosveset, and ferumoxytol, the investigators reported higher ferumoxytol signal-to-noise and contrast-to-noise ratios over a longer period of time in pediatric patients.[60] Stoumpos and colleagues recently reported their findings comparing duplex US and ferumoxytol MRA in chronic kidney disease adult patients undergoing vascular mapping for arteriovenous fistula (AVF) creation. They found that ferumoxytol MR was particularly advantageous enabling both identification of central venous pathology as well as revealing US occult peripheral arterial disease. Indeed, ferumoxytol MRA also independently predicted AVF success.[61] Others have estimated the sensitivity and specificity of ferumoxytol MRV (with invasive venography as the gold standard) for detecting CVS or occlusion to be 99% and 98%,

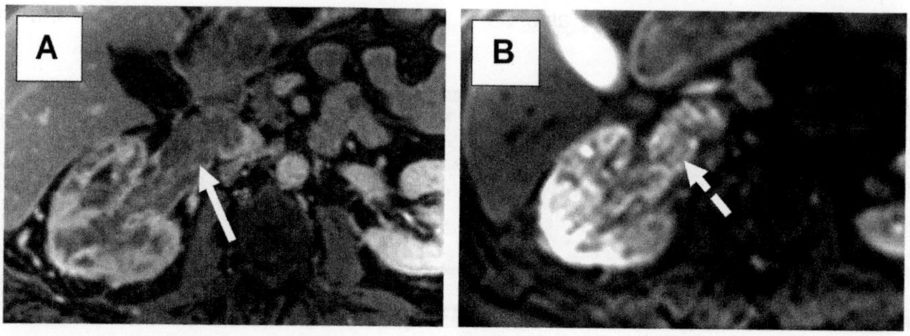


Fig. 17. Tumor thrombus. (*A*) Axial T1-weighted contrast-enhanced image showing renal cell carcinoma tumor thrombus. Note the heterogenous enhancement and right renal vein enlargement, consistent with tumor thrombus (*solid white arrow*). (*B*) Axial diffusion-weighted image showing restricted diffusion of the thrombus (*dashed white arrow*), compatible with tumor thrombus.

**Box 7**
**MR venography features suggesting tumor thrombus**

Enhancing thrombus

Enhancement/characteristics of thrombus are similar to index tumor

Thrombus appears contiguous with index tumor

Diffusion restricting

*Venous enlargement*[a]

[a]This finding can be observed with bland occlusive thrombosis in the acute setting.

respectively.[62] Owing to concerns over ionizing radiation exposure and potential gadolinium toxicities, the investigators have studied ferumoxytol MR as an alternative contrast-enhanced imaging modality in pediatric patients with chronic kidney disease. Prior work has demonstrated both satisfactory tolerability and high concordance between ferumoxytol MRV and invasive venography findings.[63,64]

## SUMMARY

The lack of ionizing radiation and flexible interrogation methods, with or without contrast, positions MRV uniquely among the armamentarium of venous imaging approaches for body and extremity studies. The recognition of variant vascular anatomy, familiarity with various forms of venous pathology, and disease mimics is important for accurate, timely diagnosis.

## DISCLOSURE

The authors have nothing to disclose.

## REFERENCES


1. Stadler A, Schima W, Ba-Ssalamah A, et al. Artifacts in body MR imaging: their appearance and how to eliminate them. Eur Radiol 2007;17(5):1242–55.
2. Beckman MG, Hooper WC, Critchley SE, et al. Venous Thromboembolism. Am J Prev Med 2010; 38(4):S495–501.
3. Thijs W, Rabe KF, Rosendaal FR, et al. Predominance of left-sided deep vein thrombosis and body weight: Letters to the Editor. J Thromb Haemostasis 2010;8(9):2083–4.
4. Goldhaber SZ, Tapson VF. A prospective registry of 5,451 patients with ultrasound-confirmed deep vein thrombosis. Am J Cardiol 2004;93(2):259–62.
5. Wells PS, Forgie MA, Rodger MA. Treatment of Venous Thromboembolism. JAMA 2014;311(7):717.
6. Kearon C. Natural History of Venous Thromboembolism. Circulation 2003;107(23_suppl_1). https://doi.org/10.1161/01.CIR.0000078464.82671.78.
7. Hanley M, Steigner ML, Ahmed O, et al. ACR Appropriateness Criteria® Suspected Lower Extremity Deep Vein Thrombosis. J Am Coll Radiol 2018;15(11):S413–7.
8. Sampson FC, Goodacre SW, Thomas SM, et al. The accuracy of MRI in diagnosis of suspected deep vein thrombosis: systematic review and meta-analysis. Eur Radiol 2007;17(1):175–81.
9. Tamura K, Nakahara H. MR Venography for the Assessment of Deep Vein Thrombosis in Lower Extremities with Varicose Veins. Annals of Vascular Diseases 2014;7(4):399–403.
10. Kucher N. Deep-Vein Thrombosis of the Upper Extremities. N Engl J Med 2011;364(9):861–9.
11. Joffe HV, Goldhaber SZ. Upper-Extremity Deep Vein Thrombosis. Circulation 2002;106(14):1874–80.
12. Desjardins B, Hanley M, Steigner ML, et al. ACR Appropriateness Criteria® Suspected Upper Extremity Deep Vein Thrombosis. J Am Coll Radiol 2020;17(5):S315–22.
13. Scott G, Mahdi AJ, Alikhan R. Superficial vein thrombosis: a current approach to management. Br J Haematol 2015;168(5):639–45.
14. Eliahou R, Sosna J, Bloom AI. Between a Rock and a Hard Place: Clinical and Imaging Features of Vascular Compression Syndromes. Radiographics 2012;32(1):E33–49.
15. Kaltenmeier CT, Erben Y, Indes J, et al. Systematic review of May-Thurner syndrome with emphasis on gender differences. J Vasc Surg: Venous and Lymphatic Disorders 2018;6(3):399–407.e4.
16. Zucker EJ, Ganguli S, Ghoshhajra BB, et al. Imaging of venous compression syndromes. Cardiovasc Diagn Ther 2016;6(6):519–32.
17. ACOG Practice Bulletin No. Thromboembolism in Pregnancy. Obstet Gynecol 2018;132(1):e1–17, 196.
18. ACR manual on MR safety. Version 1.0. American College of Radiology; 2020.
19. ACR manual on contrast media. Version 10.1. American College of Radiology; 2022.
20. Leckie A, Tao MJ, Narayanasamy S, et al. The Renal Vasculature: What the Radiologist Needs to Know. Radiographics 2021;41(5):1531–48.
21. Lamba R, Tanner DT, Sekhon S, et al. Multidetector CT of Vascular Compression Syndromes in the Abdomen and Pelvis. Radiographics 2014;34(1): 93–115.
22. Kim KW, Cho JY, Kim SH, et al. Diagnostic value of computed tomographic findings of nutcracker syndrome: Correlation with renal venography and renocaval pressure gradients. Eur J Radiol 2011;80(3): 648–54.

23. Fong JKK, Poh ACC, Tan AGS, et al. Imaging Findings and Clinical Features of Abdominal Vascular Compression Syndromes. Am J Roentgenol 2014; 203(1):29–36.
24. Goldberg A, Halandras PM, Shea S, et al. Utility of magnetic resonance imaging in establishing a venous pressure gradient in a patient with possible nutcracker syndrome. Journal of Vascular Surgery Cases, Innovations and Techniques 2016;2(3):80–3.
25. Ananthan K, Onida S, Davies AH. Nutcracker Syndrome: An Update on Current Diagnostic Criteria and Management Guidelines. Eur J Vasc Endovasc Surg 2017;53(6):886–94.
26. Raptis CA, Sridhar S, Thompson RW, et al. Imaging of the Patient with Thoracic Outlet Syndrome. Radiographics 2016;36(4):984–1000.
27. Illig KA, Doyle AJ. A comprehensive review of Paget-Schroetter syndrome. J Vasc Surg 2010; 51(6):1538–47.
28. Klaassen Z, Sorenson E, Tubbs RS, et al. Thoracic outlet syndrome: A neurological and vascular disorder: Thoracic Outlet Syndrome. Clin Anat 2014; 27(5):724–32.
29. Ersoy H, Steigner ML, Coyner KB, et al. Vascular Thoracic Outlet Syndrome: Protocol Design and Diagnostic Value of Contrast-Enhanced 3D MR Angiography and Equilibrium Phase Imaging on 1.5- and 3-T MRI Scanners. Am J Roentgenol 2012;198(5):1180–7.
30. Smillie RP, Shetty M, Boyer AC, et al. Imaging Evaluation of the Inferior Vena Cava. Radiographics 2015;35(2):578–92.
31. Gayer G, Luboshitz J, Hertz M, et al. Congenital Anomalies of the Inferior Vena Cava Revealed on CT in Patients with Deep Vein Thrombosis. Am J Roentgenol 2003;180(3):729–32.
32. Chee YL, Culligan DJ, Watson HG. Inferior vena cava malformation as a risk factor for deep venous thrombosis in the young: Short Report. Br J Haematol 2001;114(4):878–80.
33. McAree B, O'Donnell M, Fitzmaurice G, et al. Inferior vena cava thrombosis: A review of current practice. Vasc Med 2013;18(1):32–43.
34. Alkhouli M, Morad M, Narins CR, et al. Inferior Vena Cava Thrombosis. JACC Cardiovasc Interv 2016; 9(7):629–43.
35. Kaufman JA, Barnes GD, Chaer RA, et al. Society of Interventional Radiology Clinical Practice Guideline for Inferior Vena Cava Filters in the Treatment of Patients with Venous Thromboembolic Disease. J Vasc Intervent Radiol 2020;31(10):1529–44.
36. Hicks ME, Malden ES, Vesely TM, et al. Prospective Anatomic Study of the Inferior Vena Cava and Renal Veins: Comparison of Selective Renal Venography with Cavography and Relevance in Filter Placement. J Vasc Intervent Radiol 1995;6(5):721–9.
37. Kalva SP, Chlapoutaki C, Wicky S, et al. Suprarenal Inferior Vena Cava Filters: A 20-Year Single-Center Experience. J Vasc Intervent Radiol 2008;19(7): 1041–7.
38. Hilliard NJ, Heslin MJ, Castro CY. Leiomyosarcoma of the inferior vena cava. Ann Diagn Pathol 2005; 9(5):259–66.
39. Ganeshalingam S, Rajeswaran G, Jones RL, et al. Leiomyosarcomas of the inferior vena cava: diagnostic features on cross-sectional imaging. Clin Radiol 2011;66(1):50–6.
40. Sessa B, Iannicelli E, Caterino S, et al. Imaging of leiomyosarcoma of the inferior vena cava: comparison of 2 cases and review of the literature. Cancer Imag 2010; 10(1). https://doi.org/10.1102/1470-7330.2010.0009.
41. Sonavane SK, Milner DM, Singh SP, et al. Comprehensive Imaging Review of the Superior Vena Cava. Radiographics 2015;35(7):1873–92.
42. Wilson LD, Deterbeck FC, Yahalom J. Superior Vena Cava Syndrome with Malignant Causes. N Engl J Med 2007;356:1862–9.
43. Stanford W, Jolles H, Ell S, et al. Superior vena cava obstruction: a venographic classification. Am J Roentgenol 1987;148(2):259–62.
44. Azizi AH, Shafi I, Shah N, et al. Superior Vena Cava Syndrome. JACC Cardiovasc Interv 2020;13(24): 2896–910.
45. Shinde TS, Lee VS, Rofsky NM, et al. Three-dimensional Gadolinium-enhanced MR Venographic Evaluation of Patency of Central Veins in the Thorax: Initial Experience. Radiology 1999;213(2):555–60.
46. Kim CY, Merkle EM. Time-Resolved MR Angiography of the Central Veins of the Chest. Am J Roentgenol 2008;191(5):1581–8.
47. Oguzkurt L, Tercan F, Yıldırım S, et al. Central venous stenosis in haemodialysis patients without a previous history of catheter placement. Eur J Radiol 2005;55(2):237–42.
48. Hernandez D, Diaz F, Rufino M, et al. Subclavian Vascular Access Stenosis in Dialysis Patients: Natural History and Risk Factors. Journal of American Society of Nephrology 1998;9(8):1507–10.
49. Forauer AR, Theoharis C. Histologic Changes in the Human Vein Wall Adjacent to Indwelling Central Venous Catheters. J Vasc Intervent Radiol 2003; 14(9):1163–8.
50. Tabriz DM, Arslan B. Management of Central Venous Stenosis and Occlusion in Dialysis Patients. Semin Intervent Radiol 2022;39(01):051–5.
51. Knuttinen MG, Xie K, Jani A, et al. Pelvic Venous Insufficiency: Imaging Diagnosis, Treatment Approaches, and Therapeutic Issues. Am J Roentgenol 2015;204(2):448–58.
52. Eberhardt RT, Raffetto JD. Chronic Venous Insufficiency. Circulation 2014;130(4):333–46.
53. Bookwalter CA, VanBuren WM, Neisen MJ, et al. Imaging Appearance and Nonsurgical Management of Pelvic Venous Congestion Syndrome. Radiographics 2019;39(2):596–608.

54. LeGout JD, Bailey RE, Bolan CW, et al. Multimodality Imaging of Abdominopelvic Tumors with Venous Invasion. Radiographics 2020;40(7):2098–116.
55. Mathur M, Jones JR, Weinreb JC. Gadolinium Deposition and Nephrogenic Systemic Fibrosis: A Radiologist's Primer. Radiographics 2020;40(1):153–62.
56. Cowper SE, Robin HS, Steinberg SM, et al. Scleromyxoedema-like cutaneous diseases in renal-dialysis patients. Lancet 2000;356(9234):1000–1.
57. McDonald RJ, McDonald JS, Kallmes DF, et al. Intracranial Gadolinium Deposition after Contrast-enhanced MR Imaging. Radiology 2015;275(3):772–82.
58. Lu M, Cohen MH, Rieves D, et al. FDA report: Ferumoxytol for intravenous iron therapy in adult patients with chronic kidney disease. Am J Hematol 2010. https://doi.org/10.1002/ajh.21656.
59. Nguyen KL, Yoshida T, Kathuria-Prakash N, et al. Multicenter Safety and Practice for Off-Label Diagnostic Use of Ferumoxytol in MRI. Radiology 2019;293(3):554–64.
60. Shahrouki P, Khan SN, Yoshida T, et al. High-resolution three-dimensional contrast-enhanced magnetic resonance venography in children: comparison of gadofosveset trisodium with ferumoxytol. Pediatr Radiol 2022;52(3):501–12.
61. Stoumpos S, Tan A, Hall Barrientos P, et al. Ferumoxytol MR Angiography versus Duplex US for Vascular Mapping before Arteriovenous Fistula Surgery for Hemodialysis. Radiology 2020;297(1):214–22.
62. Gallo CJR, Mammarappallil JG, Johnson DY, et al. Ferumoxytol-enhanced MR Venography of the Central Veins of the Thorax for the Evaluation of Stenosis and Occlusion in Patients with Renal Impairment. Radiology: Cardiothoracic Imaging 2020;2(6):e200339.
63. Luhar A, Khan S, Finn JP, et al. Contrast-enhanced magnetic resonance venography in pediatric patients with chronic kidney disease: initial experience with ferumoxytol. Pediatr Radiol 2016;46(9):1332–40.
64. Nayak AB, Luhar A, Hanudel M, et al. High-resolution, whole-body vascular imaging with ferumoxytol as an alternative to gadolinium agents in a pediatric chronic kidney disease cohort. Pediatr Nephrol 2015;30(3):515–21.

# Four-Dimensional Flow MR Imaging
## Technique and Advances

Oliver Wieben, PhD[a,b,*], Grant S. Roberts, PhD[c], Philip A. Corrado, PhD[d,1], Kevin M. Johnson, PhD[e,f], Alejandro Roldán-Alzate, PhD[g,h]

**KEYWORDS**

• Phase-contrast MR imaging • Flow quantification • 4D flow MR imaging • Hemodynamic analysis • Cine MR imaging • Accelerated imaging • Hemodynamic validation

**KEY POINTS**

- Four-dimensional (4D) flow MR imaging provides comprehensive noninvasive, in vivo assessment of blood flow dynamics in the cardiovascular system.
- 4D flow MR imaging can quantify velocities, flow, and additional hemodynamic parameters such as pulse wave velocity, kinetic energy, and wall shear stress.
- Advances in MR imaging hardware and reconstruction algorithms have greatly reduced scan time for 4D flow MR imaging.
- The availability of rapid 4D flow imaging sequences and established 4D flow processing tools makes this approach readily accessible for research and clinical applications.
- Coupling 4D flow MR imaging with computational fluid dynamics enhances the ability to derive clinically relevant quantitative metrics of blood flow dynamics.

## INTRODUCTION

MR imaging is rich in methodologies to exploit contrast mechanisms for the noninvasive assessment of anatomy and function in the human body. Flow-sensitive MR imaging is based on the phase-contrast (PC) principle for motion encoding[1] and has been adopted for quantifying blood velocities and flow since the early days of MR imaging.[2–4]

PC-MR imaging is available in various modes that include acquisitions with velocity encoding in 1, 2, or 3 spatial directions, 2-dimensional (2D) or 3-dimensional (3D) spatial coverage, and those that are temporally resolved across the cardiac cycle (cine) acquisitions. 2D cine PC-MR imaging with 1-directional velocity encoding is widely used in clinical practice and can be acquired in short scans in a single breath-hold for most patients.[5] PC-MR

[a] Department of Medical Physics, University of Wisconsin-Madison, Wisconsin Institutes for Medical Research, 1111 Highland Avenue, Suite 1127, Madison, WI 53705-2275, USA; [b] Department of Radiology, University of Wisconsin-Madison, Wisconsin Institutes for Medical Research, 1111 Highland Avenue, Suite 1127, Madison, WI 53705-2275, USA; [c] Department of Medical Physics, University of Wisconsin-Madison, Wisconsin Institutes for Medical Research, 1111 Highland Avenue, Madison, WI 53705-2275, USA; [d] Accuray Incorporated, 1414 Raleigh Road, Suite 330, DurhamChapel Hill, NC 27517, USA; [e] Department of Medical Physics, University of Wisconsin-Madison, Wisconsin Institutes for Medical Research, 1111 Highland Avenue, Room 1133, Madison, WI 53705-2275, USA; [f] Department of Radiology, University of Wisconsin-Madison, Wisconsin Institutes for Medical Research, 1111 Highland Avenue, Room 1133, Madison, WI 53705-2275, USA; [g] Department of Mechanical Engineering, University of Wisconsin-Madison, Room: 3035, 1513 University Avenue, Madison, WI 53706, USA; [h] Department of Radiology, University of Wisconsin-Madison, Madison, WI, USA
[1] Present address: 1414 Raleigh Road, Suite 330, Chapel Hill, NC 27517.
* Corresponding author. Department of Medical Physics, University of Wisconsin-Madison, Wisconsin Institutes for Medical Research, Suite L1127, 1111 Highland Avenue, Madison, WI 53705.Department of Medical PhysicsUniversity of Wisconsin-MadisonWisconsin Institutes for Medical ResearchSuite L1127, 1111 Highland AvenueMadisonWI53705
*E-mail address:* owieben@wisc.edu

Magn Reson Imaging Clin N Am 31 (2023) 433–449
https://doi.org/10.1016/j.mric.2023.05.003

imaging with 3-directional velocity encoding, 3D coverage, and acquired for multiple cardiac phases (commonly referred to as 4D flow MR imaging) has recently become viable for clinical use.[6–13] 4D flow captures data sets of inherently coregistered anatomy and the simultaneously acquired dynamic velocity vector field of blood in the vessels and cardiac chambers, providing qualitative and quantitative hemodynamic data not currently available by other means.

Here the authors review the underlying principles of 4D flow MR imaging; technical details on the implementation and scan time reductions; preprocessing steps for data corrections, postprocessing approaches to visualize and measure velocities and flow and derive additional hemodynamic parameters such as pulse wave velocity (PWV), wall shear stress, kinetic energy (KE), vorticity, and flow compartments; and methods for the validation of flow measures. Recent advances including the use of artificial intelligence and respiratory-resolved "5D flow MR imaging" are also briefly discussed.

## FLOW ENCODING

### *Phase in MR Imaging*

Clinical MR imaging uses the principles of frequency and phase encoding to efficiently acquire data in Fourier space, often also referred to as "k-space." Image reconstruction then requires the transform of the acquired data via a Fourier transform. This process generates complex-valued data for each imaging voxel, which are mathematically described by 2 components, either its real and imaginary component or its magnitude and phase (**Fig. 1**).

Most clinical MR imaging scans simply discard the phase information, and only the magnitude data are displayed and stored for diagnosis. However, several MR imaging acquisition schemes are designed to generate image contrast or encode quantitative information into the image phase, for example, MR spectroscopy, temperature mapping, susceptibility weighted imaging, and PC-MR imaging.

### *Velocity Encoding with Bipolar Gradients*

PC-MR imaging uses bipolar velocity-encoding gradients to encode the velocity of moving spins (a hydrogen nucleus's magnetic dipole moment) in the magnetic field. A velocity-encoding gradient takes advantage of the linear relationship between magnetic field and the precessional frequency of spins and encodes spin velocity information into the phase of the MR signal. A bipolar velocity-encoding gradient (**Fig. 2**) produces no net phase accumulation for stationary spins but induces a phase accumulation in moving spins that is linearly proportional to their velocity in the spatial direction of the gradient.[5,14,15] By subtracting the phase of one image taken with a bipolar gradient from one without, phase shifts from other sources such as susceptibility and coil phase are eliminated, yielding a velocity map of the moving blood. The axis on which the gradient is applied determines the direction of flow sensitivity. The sensitivity of the sequence to motion is set by the amplitude and duration of the bipolar gradient and leads to a velocity encoding (Venc) setting. The Venc is the highest measurable velocity that can be uniquely resolved without a phase wrap, $\pm 180°$ or $\pm$ p, respectively, in the cyclic entity of phase. In practice, the operator chooses the Venc such that it slightly exceeds the maximum expected velocity as a balance between high velocity-to-noise performance and the potential for errors from phase wrap. If the velocity is greater than the Venc, the velocity will erroneously wrap, also called velocity aliasing, to appear to be within $\pm$Venc. In practice, gradient echo sequences as shown in **Fig. 2** are used to reduce imaging times.

### *Cine MR Imaging*

Because of the pulsatile nature of blood flow, particularly arterial blood flow, it is often required to measure blood flow at multiple time points across the cardiac cycle. However, MR imaging is an inherently slow imaging modality and not adapted for real-time imaging such as ultrasound and digital subtraction angiography. PC-MR imaging is further slowed due to (1) the need for at least 2 acquisitions for background phase subtraction and (2) longer repetition times because of the addition of the bipolar gradients. In practice, PC-MR imaging is acquired with a "cine" acquisition typical for dynamic cardiac imaging, which resolved the dynamics of the cardiac cycle by repeated acquisition of k-space data over multiple heart beats (**Fig. 3**). The data are sorted with a synchronously acquired electrocardiogram signal to generate a dynamic display of a single heartbeat, even though the data were acquired over a much longer window. Most commonly, 2D cine PC-MR imaging is used with through-plane velocity encoding, where a 2D scan plane is placed orthogonal to the vessel of interest and the through-plane velocity component is measured, enabling quantification of velocities and flow in that vessel.

### *Multidirectional Flow Encoding and 4-Dimensional Flow MR Imaging*

Flow-encoding gradients can also be played on more than one gradient axis. By successively acquiring data with flow-encoding gradients in each of the 3 spatial directions, velocity can be

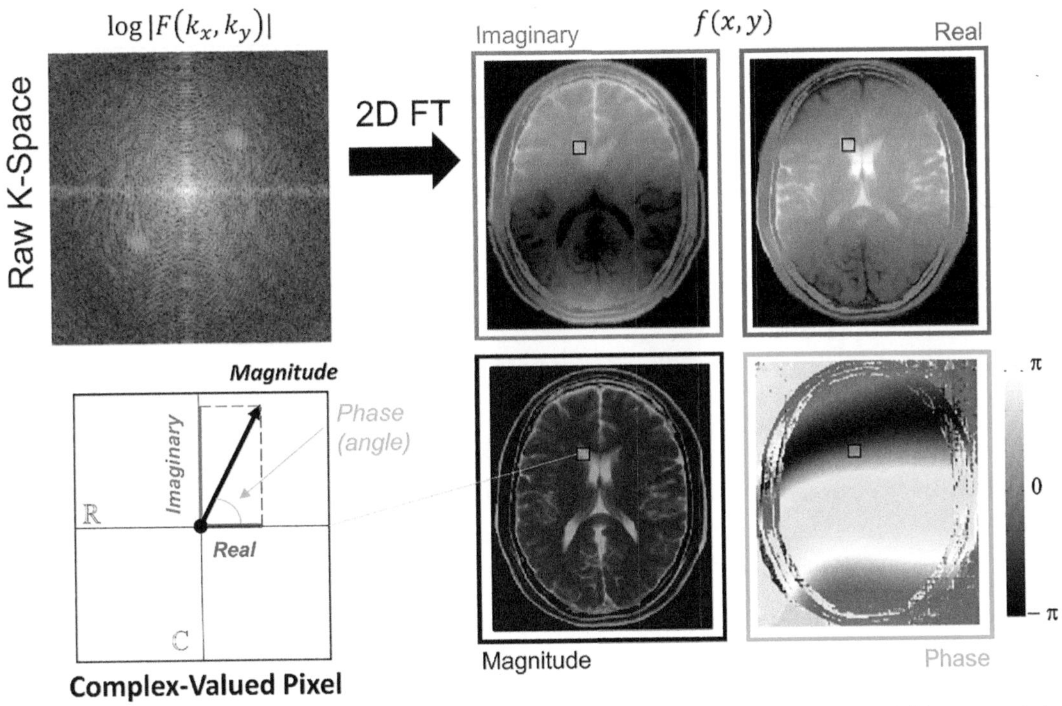


**Fig. 1.** MR image reconstruction and phase in MR imaging. During image reconstruction, spatial frequency information (k-space) is transformed into image using the 2-dimensional Fourier transform (2D FT). Because the raw data are acquired with quadrature coils, both k-space and image space data are complex valued, meaning that each voxel is characterized by a real and imaginary component representing the projection of the net magnetization vector onto the transverse plane. Alternatively, this measure can be represented by magnitude and phase, which corresponds to the length and the angle of the magnetization vector within the coordinate system in the transverse plane.

encoded in all 3 directions, thereby capturing velocity as a vector quantity; this requires at least 4 acquisitions: velocity encodings in x, y, and z and a reference scan to separate the unknown background phase. Several variations of this principle, including simple 4-point, balanced 4-point, and Hadamard encoding, exist with advantages and disadvantages to each approach.[16,17]

Similar to other MR imaging sequences, PC-MR imaging can be acquired as a 3D imaging volume rather than a single 2D slice. PC-MR imaging with 3D cine coverage and 3-directional velocity encoding is often referred to as "4D flow MR imaging" (**Fig. 4**), where the fourth dimension refers to time within the cardiac cycle. 4D flow MR imaging requires a considerably longer acquisition than traditional 2D PC-MR imaging but offers advantages in its ability to comprehensively capture complex blood flow dynamics in multiple vessels or in a complex region of interest such as the heart.

## *Use of Contrast Agents*

In many clinical 4D flow scans, patients are imaged after injection of an MR vascular contrast agent, for example, gadolinium-based contrast agent or iron-based nanoparticles. These agents are often administered for other purposes (perfusion or late enhancement) as part of routine clinical protocols, and 4D flow MR imaging is acquired afterward to benefit from improved image signal-to-noise ratio (SNR) and velocity-to-noise ratio (VNR) performance.[18,19] It should be noted, however, that all 4D flow MR imaging methods, such as 2D PC MR are inherently non–contrast-enhanced MR imaging methods and do not require the use of vascular contrast agents. When using such agents, the flip angle can be increased to capitalize on the increased SNR and VNR performance afforded by the T1-shortening effects.

## *Accelerated Imaging*

4D flow MR imaging was conceptualized in the early 1990s as "7D flow" by Firmin and colleagues.[20] However, fully sampled 4D flow MR imaging acquisitions were prohibitively lengthy for in vivo scanning because of the time penalties for 3D imaging, cardiac cine acquisitions, and reduced efficiency when gating to the respiratory

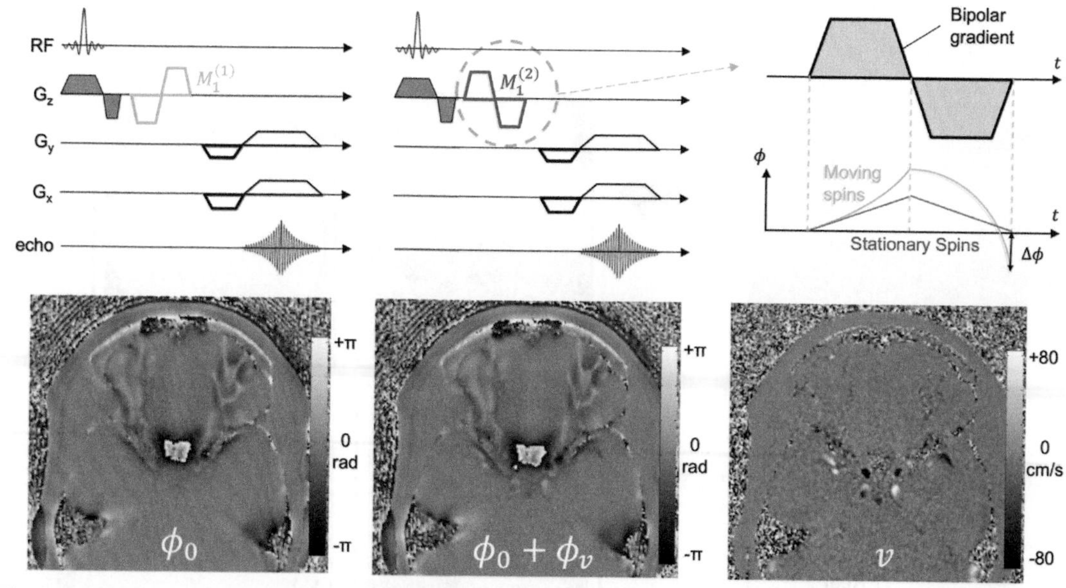


Fig. 2. PC-MR imaging principles. A 2D gradient echo sequence with velocity encoding in the through-plane direction (z). Motion can be encoded into the image phase by the addition of a bipolar gradient (*blue*). The phase of stationary spins does return to its original value after the bipolar gradient is played out (*yellow*). However, moving spins will experience different precession frequencies as they advance along the gradient and thus will gain a net phase that actually is proportional to their velocity. In order to account for background phase variations, 2 separate acquisitions are acquired in which the bipolar gradients are inverted (*red*). Subtracting the 2 images leads to an image that is directly proportional to velocity. Note that the velocity map differentiates between blood into and out of the imaging plane indicated by positive (*white*) and negative (*black*) greyscale.

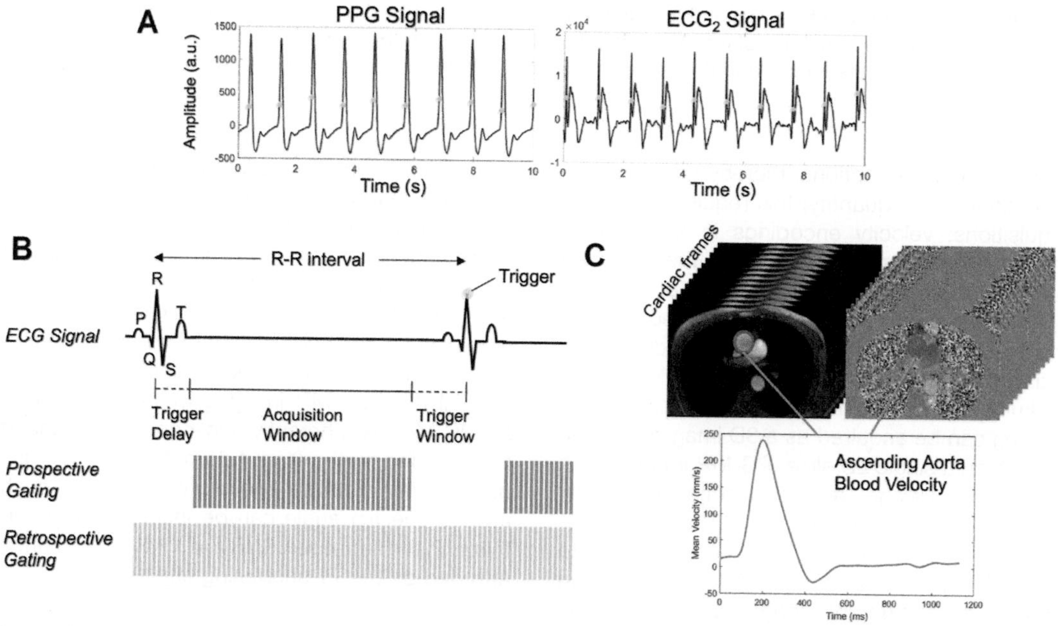


Fig. 3. Physiological gating and cine reconstruction: (*A*) pulse oximeter (PPG), and electrocardiogram (ECG) in a 65-year-old, healthy female subject. The trigger data (*green dots*) are detected by the scanner system and are used either during data acquisition for r prospective gating or after scan completion with retrospective gating. (*B*) Prospective cardiac gating (or triggering) acquires data within a predefined window of the cardiac cycle. Time delays are introduced for imaging specific parts of the cardiac cycle and to allow for slight variations in heart rate during the scan. Retrospective cardiac gating, on the other hand, continuously acquires data and retrospectively synchronizes acquired data to the cardiac cycle. (*C*) Cardiac gating allows for "cine" reconstructions, which create a series of time-resolved images, with each image representing data from a different part of the cardiac cycle. By drawing regions of interest around vessels, velocity or flow curves can be obtained from the time-resolved velocity images.

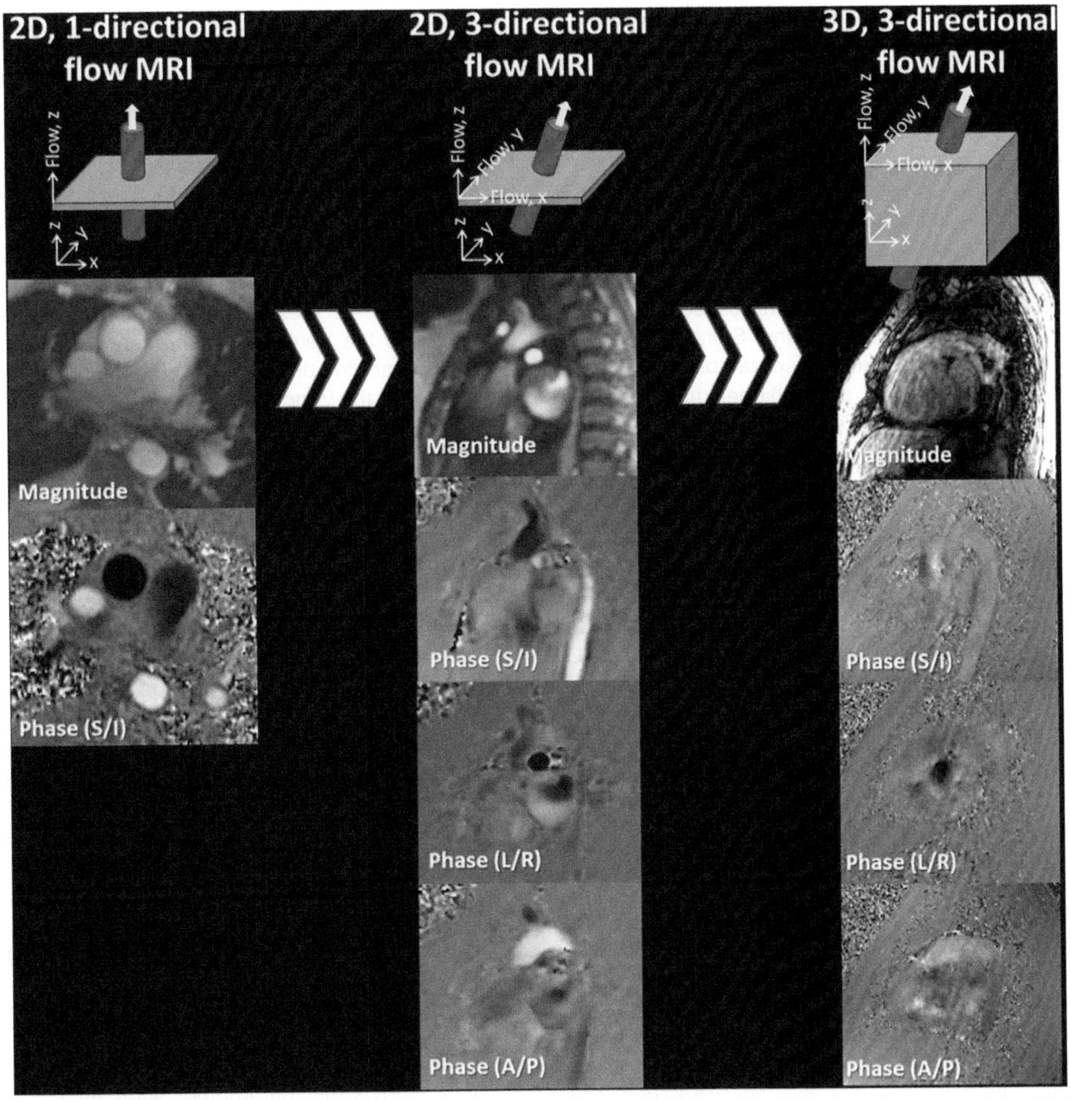


Fig. 4. Sample images showing the evolution from 2D PC-MR imaging with 1-directional velocity encoding (*left*) to 2D PC-MR imaging with 3-directional velocity encoding (*center*) and to a volumetric acquisition with 3-directional velocity encoding, aka 4D flow MR imaging. Note that each image shows a single time frame of a CINE series for simplicity.

cycle is required, the need for 4 acquisitions to resolve 3 velocity measures, and the addition of bipolar gradients. Initial feasibility studies required 30 minutes of scan time for compromised voxel sizes.[21] Advances in hardware design, especially higher performance gradients and multichannel receiver coils as well as methodology advances in accelerated cardiovascular MR imaging have been rapidly adopted to 4D flow MR imaging for reduced scan times acceptable in clinical settings. Initial approaches used methods such as view sharing[22] and improved respiratory gating efficiency.[23,24] The use of parallel imaging with multichannel receiver coils,[25] advanced reconstruction approaches that exploit redundancies in the acquired data such as k-t BLAST,[26] k-t SENSE,[27] and k-t GRAPPA[28]; and sparse sampling theory with compressed sensing[29] and local low rank[30] have been successfully exploited to further reduce scan times. Several of these approaches or combination thereof are used in practice today to routinely decrease scan times to 10 minutes or less in vascular territories that require respiratory gating, typically achieved with navigators or respiratory bellows, which is further reduced in regions that do not loose efficiency due to such gating.

Meanwhile, radial undersampling was introduced early as an effective method for accelerated

2D[31] and 4D flow acquisitions with stack of stars[31] and true 3D radial sampling trajectories[32,33] as illustrated in **Fig. 5**. The latter was introduced as PC vastly undersampled isotropic projection reconstruction and can be particularly in combination with temporal view sharing.[34] 3D radial acquisitions also have superior motion robustness, enable self-gating, and are better suited than traditional Cartesian sampling when used with state-of-the-art reconstruction algorithms that rely on sparse sampling such as compressed sensing or local low-rank reconstructions. Spiral trajectories were introduced for improved sampling efficiency with longer readouts and a higher duty cycle for sampling within each repetition time.[35]

## PREPROCESSING

4D flow cardiovascular magnetic resonance (CMR) data processing usually involves the use of automated or semiautomated corrections of known artifacts and often requires calculation of a geometric representation of the underlying 3D cardiac or vascular geometry through segmentation. Several sources of error can compromise 4D flow CMR analysis and need to be recognized and corrected. Several data corrections are necessary to prepare PC-MR imaging data for quantitative analysis, and their rationale and common approaches are well described in a consensus statement on cardiovascular 4D flow MR imaging.[36] The bipolar gradients cause concomitant gradient cross-terms, leading to phase sensitivity along the non–flow-encoded directions as well. These phase contributions can be predicted by Maxwell equations and are automatically corrected for during image reconstruction.[37] In practice, magnetic field gradients are nonlinear and fall off toward the edge of view. These nonlinearities do cause not only geometric distortions but also phase errors, which are automatically corrected during reconstruction.[38,39] Eddy currents unintentionally alter the gradient waveforms in any MR acquisitions. MR systems use preemphasis systems that seek to predict and counteract the eddy currents. However, this compensation is not perfect and can lead to significant velocity errors if unaccounted for.[40,41] Common remedies include manual or semiautomatic approaches that aim to fit background phase to tissues identified as stationary[42] and subsequently subtract that background phase. Velocity aliasing occurs when velocities in the acquired image volume exceed the Venc.[5] The correction is simple by properly adding or subtracting the offset velocity defined by the Venc. The challenging task is the identification of affected voxels, which can be done by user inspection while automated algorithms[43,44] have also been proposed.

## POSTPROCESSING

4D flow MR imaging provides datasets with comprehensive information on the vascular anatomy and function by means of angiograms and dynamic velocity vectors. As shown in **Fig. 6**, these data can be used for several purposes, including the generation of non–contrast-enhanced MR angiography (MRA) by generating velocity-weighted angiograms, commonly referred to as 3D PC-MRAs, from the final velocity and magnitude data[33] to display the vascular lumens. Advanced interactive velocity and flow analysis can be conducted in vessels across the imaging volume after the scan is completed. Complex flow patterns can be visualized in animations, for example, through dynamic velocity vector plots, streamlines, pathlines, and particles traces. Additional hemodynamic parameters such as PWV, wall shear stress, pressure gradients, KE, vorticity, ventricular flow compartments, and others can be derived from the dynamic velocity vector field. These rich data sets can also be used as patient-

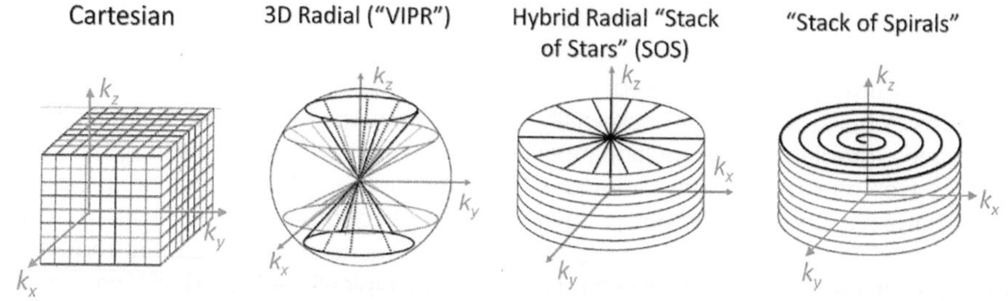


**Fig. 5.** Examples of k-space sampling trajectories for 3D acquisitions: traditional Cartesian sampling on a rectilinear grid, "true 3D" sampling where each echo traverses the center of k-space, a hybrid scheme called "stack of stars" with radial in-plane encoding and traditional Fourier encoding in the through-plane direction, and the "stack of spirals" trajectory with prolonged readouts.

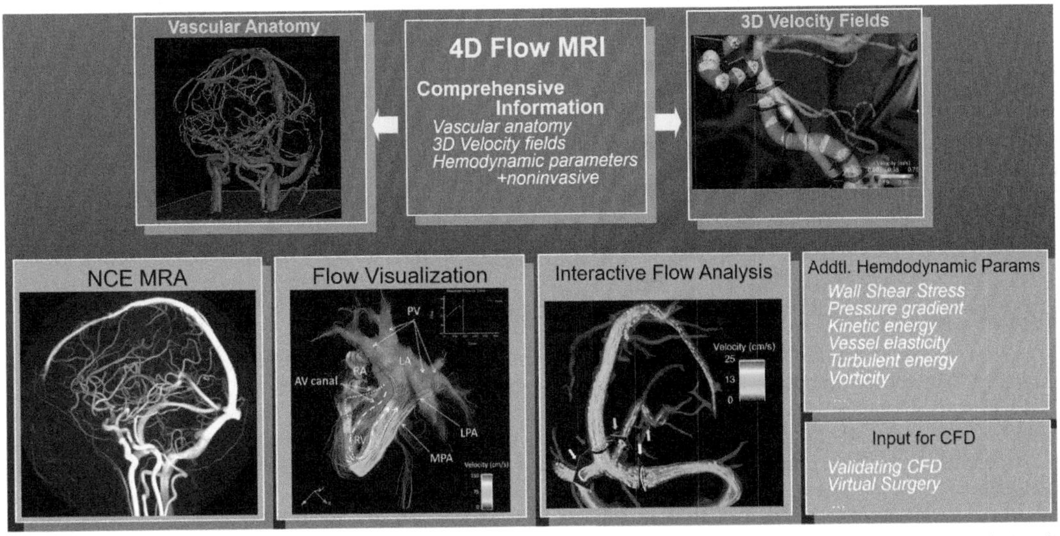


**Fig. 6.** 4D flow MR imaging provides a platform for comprehensive, patient-specific hemodynamic analysis. The availability of inherently coregistered vascular anatomy and 3D velocity fields throughout the cardiac cycle allow for the generation of PC-MRA (phase-contrast MR angiograms), static or dynamic flow visualizations such as particle traces, interactive flow analysis visualization and analysis, and the derivation of additional hemodynamic parameters such as wall shear stress, kinetic energy, pulse wave velocity, flow compartments, and more.

specific inputs for computational fluid dynamic modeling.

A representative workflow for 4D flow MR imaging processing using a freely available cerebrovascular analysis software package[45] is illustrated in **Fig. 7**. In the first step, velocity-weighted angiograms (also known as PC-MRA) are calculated from the final velocity and magnitude data for all time frames.[33] The velocity field within the vascular structures is displayed, for example, through velocity vectors, streamlines, pathlines, particle traces, or similar displays in an interactive 3D viewer that allows for rotations and zooming and manual placement of cut-planes perpendicular to the vessels of interest. Velocity and flow analysis is then performed for each cut-plane in a fashion similar to traditional 2D PC-MR imaging processing, including segmentation of the vessel lumen for all cardiac phases.

This workflow is particularly advantageous in cases where multiple vessels or vessel segments are of interest or the vascular anatomy is complex or unusual. In traditional 2D PC-MR imaging, such examinations would require the acquisition of a good-quality MRA to subsequently prescribe multiple 2D slices, all of which need to be determined at the time of data acquisition; this might require the presence of a highly skilled expert at the time of image acquisition. In comparison, 4D flow MR imagings are acquired over a large imaging volume, and analysis planes are selected after scan completion, thereby enabling a free choice of vessels or vessel segments to be analyzed that might become of interest during the patient specific analysis. **Fig. 8** shows an example of a multivessel analysis in the chest. Multiple dedicated 4D flow visualization and analysis packages are available for clinical and research purposes. A recent study compared quantitative results from a cross-over comparison in individuals examined on 2 scanners of different vendors analyzed with 4 such postprocessing software packages.[46]

## Second-Order Hemodynamic Parameters

In order to maximize and enhance the quantitative outcomes of 4D flow MR imaging, other more complex fluid dynamics (second-order hemodynamic) parameters can be derived from the acquired anatomical and flow velocity data. To illustrate one connected set of such parameters the authors present the analysis of the ventricular–vascular interaction in the systemic circulation, the left ventricle and aorta, in **Fig. 9**, reconstructed into 20 cardiac phases. First, the left ventricle and aorta are segmented from time-averaged 4D flow MR imaging magnitude and PC-MRA images, respectively. Subsequently, PWV, wall shear stress, and KE are derived.

### Pulse wave velocity

PWV is a biomarker directly related to vessel stiffness that has the potential to provide information on early atherosclerotic disease burden.[47] MR imaging can provide both measures needed for PWV assessment: the distance Dx between 2 analysis planes and the transit time Dt between the flow

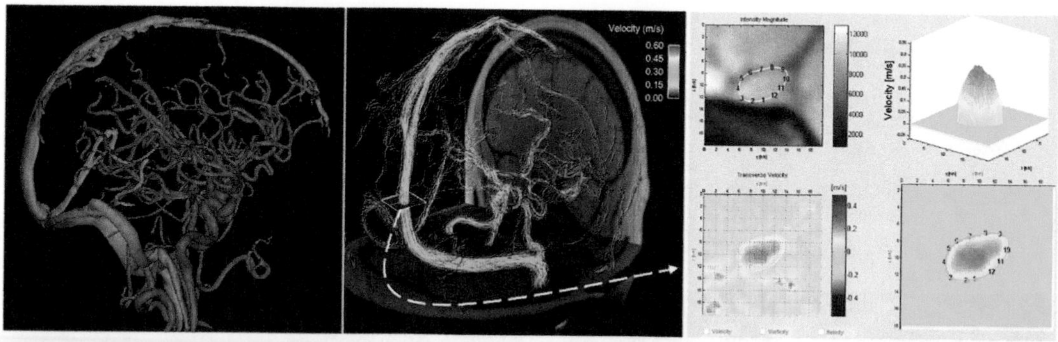


**Fig. 7.** Representative 4D flow MR imaging Postprocessing. A cranial 4D flow MR imaging was segmented based on the 3D PC angiogram, displayed here as a surface-shaded display for a cranial 4D flow MR imaging as an isosurface of veins (*blue*) and arteries (*red*). Using the segmented vessels, streamlines can be generated within vessels and can be color-coded by velocity. The middle image shows streamlines generated in a healthy, 54-year-old female subject. Cut-planes can be interactively placed in vessels of interest (eg, superior sagittal sinus), and region-specific vessel segmentation can be performed within the cut-plane, as shown on the right. This yields hemodynamic parameters of interest, such as vessel diameter mean velocity, peak velocity, velocity distribution, blood flow as the integral of the velocity x voxel area over the vessel cross-section, and others.

waveforms. 4D flow MR imaging can even provide local PWV, for example, along the aorta, but the temporal resolution is inferior to 2D PC-MR imaging. An example workflow is demonstrated in **Fig. 9**. A spline is placed as a centerline along the longitudinal axis of the aortic volume. 2D planes are automatically placed at equal distances from each other, normal to the created spline (see **Fig. 9**). Flow waveforms are obtained for the entire cardiac cycle in each 2D plane and the transit time Dt between flow at the first 2D cut plane and flow at each subsequent cut plane. The flow waveform changes with distance from the heart, and the systolic peak lowers and widens. Several algorithms have been proposed for the calculation of Dt,[48] including (1) cross-correlation (XCOR[49]), (2) point to point of 50% upstroke (TTM[49]), and (3) intersecting tangent (TTF[50]) algorithms. Here, transit

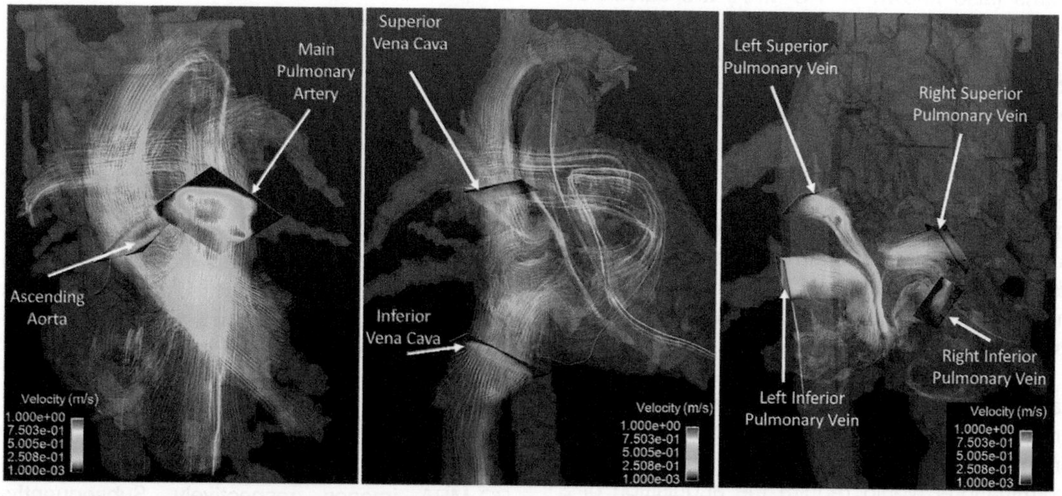


**Fig. 8.** Example of 4D flow visualization and analysis in the chest. The left image shows color-coded flow streamlines for the ascending aorta (AAo) and main pulmonary artery (MPA) superimposed on semitransparent magnitude data from the identical dataset for improved orientation. Cut-planes can be interactively placed perpendicular to the vessel path and analyzed to yield hemodynamic parameters of interest, such as vessel diameter mean velocity, peak velocity, velocity distribution, blood flow as the integral of the velocity x voxel area over the vessel cross-section, and others. The center image shows flow streamlines in the superior and inferior vena cava (SVC and IVC), and the right image shows flow streamlines in the pulmonary veins (LSPV, LIPV, RSPV, RIPV). Streamlines were generated in a peak systolic phase using Ensight (v2020 R1, Ansys, Inc., Canonsburg, PA, USA). LIPV, left inferior pulmonary vein; LSPV, left superior pulmonary vein; RIPV, right inferior pulmonary vein; RSPV, right superior pulmonary vein.

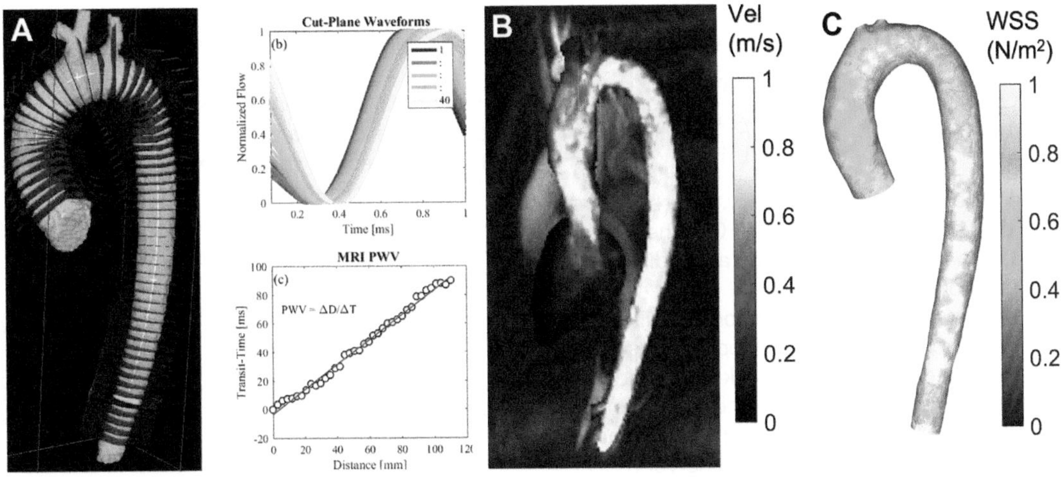


**Fig. 9.** Representative analysis of ventricular—vascular interaction in the left ventricle (LV) and aorta. (*A*) MR imaging PWV calculation: cut-planes placed along the aorta in EnSight; flow waveforms of each cut-plane; line fitted to transit-time versus distance data for PWV estimation. (*B*) Maximum intensity projection of LV and aorta velocity overlaid on the complex-difference angiogram, (*C*) contours of aorta wall shear stress.

time is plotted against the distance of each cut-plane to the first cut-plane, and PWV is expressed as the inverse slope of a line fitted to the transit time versus distance data (see **Fig. 9**A), as previously described by Markl and colleagues[51] A recent study has validated this PWV calculation using experimental fluid dynamics including invasive pressure measurements and optical imaging methods.[52]

### *Wall shear stress*

Wall shear stress (WSS) assesses the frictional force of the blood on the vessel wall,[53] and there is substantial evidence that WSS induced by the pulsatile blood flow plays a major role in endothelial function and structure and affects the atherogenic process.[54,55] 2D and 4D flow MR imaging enables the estimation of WSS from the measured arterial velocity field, and various approaches have been proposed for its implementation and use in vascular territories such as the aorta and intracranial aneurysms[56–60] and used to differentiate flow regimes characteristic of pathological conditions. For example, Stalder and colleagues[57] used a smooth spline fitting for improved robustness, whereas Bieging and colleagues used an approach where aortic WSS was calculated from triangulated surface meshes by taking the cross-product of the velocity vector and the surface normal vector and then averaged over the aorta surface,

$$\tau_w = \frac{1}{A}\int_A \mu \frac{\partial u_i}{\partial n_i} dA\# \qquad \textbf{(5)}$$

where $\mu$ is the viscosity of blood (4 cP) and $n_i$ is the surface normal vector. WSS was calculated both as a time-averaged value and as the peak systolic value (see **Fig. 9**C) and reported as a raw measurement and in dimensionless form:

$$\tau_w^* = \frac{\tau_w}{\mu Q A^{-\frac{3}{2}}}\# \qquad \textbf{(6)}$$

It has been well documented that accurate measurement of WSS is challenging with MR imaging because of some inherent limitations: the spatial and temporal resolution are limited, the VNR is low in the area of interest (low velocity at vessel wall region), and the vessel walls move throughput the cardiac cycle,[61,62] leading to a systematic underestimation of WSS.

### *Kinetic energy*

4D flow patterns are rich in information but it can be challenging to quantify them into metrics that can be easily reported and charted. KE has been proposed as a simple measure, represented as a scalar throughout the cardiac cycle, for example, to investigate ventricular efficiency as well as ventricular vascular coupling.[63–67]

Left ventricle (LV) and aortic KE is calculated as an integral over the analyzed volume:

$$KE(t) = \int_V \frac{\rho}{2} u_i(t)^2 dV \#(7)$$

where ρ is density (1060 kg/m3), ui is the velocity vector, and V is the segmented LV or aortic volume. LV KE is calculated at peak systole, and peak diastole and aorta KE is reported at peak systole. KE is normally reported as a raw value, normalized by stroke volume and in dimensionless form

$$KE^* = \frac{KE}{\rho Q^2 V^{-\frac{1}{3}}} \text{ or } KE^* = \frac{KE}{\rho\left(\frac{Q}{A}\right)^2 V} \# \quad (8)$$

for the LV and aorta, respectively, where * represents the dimensionless variable. Q is the cardiac output, V is volume, and A is the ascending aorta cross-sectional area (**Fig. 9**B).[64]

KE analysis has also been performed within the ventricle, where the KE of the blood represents a fundamental component of work performed by the heart, which results in the movement of the blood (**Fig. 10**). A key strength of this technique is its excellent intraobserver/interobserver repeatability.[68] Also, as it factors in the complete intracavity flow (x-, y-, and z-components throughout the entire ventricle), LV blood flow KE is a finer marker of diastolic function than standard diastolic parameters.[69] Several studies have since shown measures of KE to be altered in forms of congenital heart disease,[63,70] and KE normalized by end diastolic volume has been shown to decrease in patients with heart failure [71] and myocardial infarction.[72] Therefore, this emerging tool holds promise for phenotyping cardiac hemodynamics and potentially predicting disease course as evidenced in a systematic review.[73]

## *Vorticity*

4D flow MR imaging has be used to demonstrate the existence of rotational patterns that establish as vortex formations, for example, in the thoracic aorta[74,75] or as a vortex ring in the LV during diastole.[76] Vortices can usually be identified by a human observer but can be challenging to properly quantify in the presence of measurements that contain noise, such as PC-MR imaging. Vorticity is known as the local spinning motion of an element of fluid and represents a parallel quantitative measure of flow and its spatial distribution. Vorticity has recently been used to study ventricular hemodynamic efficiency.[63,77]

LV and aorta average vorticity (ωavg) were calculated as

$$\omega_{avg} = \frac{1}{V\,T_{HB}} \int_{T_{HB}} \int_{V} \nabla \times u_i dV dt \# \quad (9)$$

where $\nabla\times$ is the curl operator and THB is the heart beat duration. Vorticity is normally reported as a raw value and in dimensionless form

$$\omega^* = \frac{\omega}{QV^{-1}} \text{ or } \omega^* = \frac{\omega}{QA^{-\frac{3}{2}}} \# \quad (10)$$

for the LV and aorta, respectively. Ventricular-vascular coupling for both KE and vorticity were calculated by taking the ratio of the LV-to-aorta value.

## *Additional Hemodynamic Measures*

Several more advanced measures of hemodynamic function have shown promise in the research world but have not yet demonstrated utility in the clinical management of patients. For example, Bolger and colleagues used 4D flow MR imaging data to separate ventricular flow into 4 components based on the starting and ending position of flow pathlines (computed by integrating the velocity field with respect to time) over the cardiac cycle (**Fig. 11**): direct flow (DF; blood that enters the ventricle during diastole and leaves the ventricle during systole in the analyzed heartbeat), retained inflow (blood that enters the ventricle

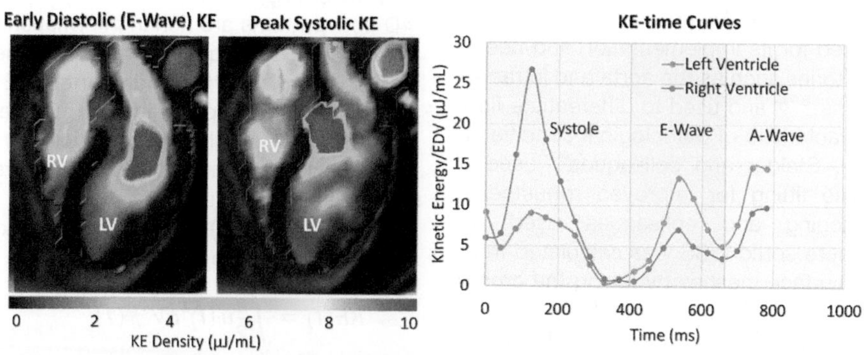


**Fig. 10.** Example case of KE measurement in the left and right ventricle. KE density (*left*) is computed based on the velocity of blood in each voxel and the density of blood (1060 kg/m$^3$) at each cardiac frame and time point within the ventricle. By integrating KE density over each ventricle, ventricular KE-time curves can be computed, yielding 3 characteristic peaks: systole, early diastole (E-wave), and late diastole (A-wave, also known as atrial contraction). LV, left ventricle; RV, right ventricle.

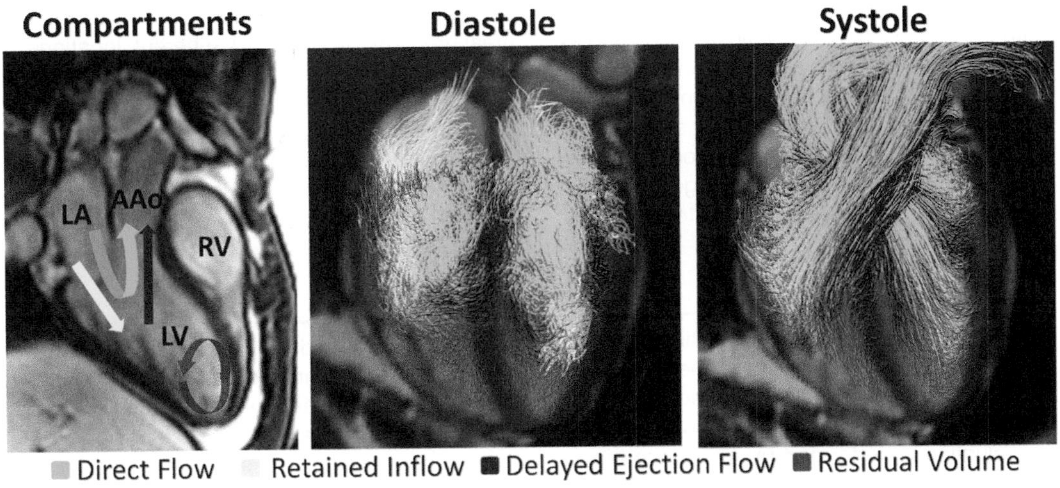


Fig. 11. Left ventricular flow compartment analysis showing direct flow (*green*), retained inflow (*yellow*), delayed ejection flow (*blue*) and residual volumes (*red*) in a concept visualization (*left*), and as color-coded streamlines in diastole (*center*) and systole (*right*).

during diastole but does not leave during systole in the analyzed heartbeat), delayed ejection flow (blood that starts and resides inside the ventricle during diastole and leaves during systole), and residual volume (blood that resides within the ventricle for at least 2 cardiac cycles).[78–81] The DF fraction, or the ratio of blood volume in the DF compartment to the ventricle's end diastolic volume, is reduced in patients with heart disease: LV DF fraction is lower in patients with dilated cardiomyopathy than in controls,[82] and patients with primary LV mild ischemic heart disease have reduced DF fraction even in the right ventricle.[83]

## VALIDATION

Th establishment of quantitative imaging markers requires validations. However, in vivo measurements of velocities, flow, and advanced hemodynamic parameters are difficult to validate because of the lack of a reliable gold standard. Instead, validation work can be performed in phantoms, in preclinical models that allow comparisons with invasive measures, and through consistency measures in vivo.

### *Flow Pumps, Three-Dimensional Printing, and Particle Image Velocimetry*

The rapid advances in 3D printing have enabled the onsite fabrication of anatomically realistic vascular models[84] with quick turnaround times. These models can be used for in vitro experiments for the validation of quantitative fluid dynamics markers using different 3D printing technologies including materials with elastic properties.[85] In addition, particle image velocimetry (PIV), a reference fluid dynamics method widely used in engineering applications, can be used as an external validation for quantitative MR imaging markers derived from 4D flow MR imaging data.[86–88]

**Fig. 12** shows an example of a patient-specific, anatomically realistic 3D printed model obtained from MRA images of a single ventricle patient with total cavopulmonary connection and the PIV results obtained for validation of 4D flow MR imaging.[86] In a more recent study, velocity measurements from 4D flow MR imaging were qualitatively and quantitatively compared with those from tomographic PIV using a patient-specific intracranial aneurysm model.[89] Velocity fluctuations were investigated by acquiring multiple cardiac cycles using tomographic PIV at a high image rate under pulsatile flow conditions. These cycles were later averaged to compare velocities and estimations of WSS with 4D flow MR imaging measurements. The purpose of this study

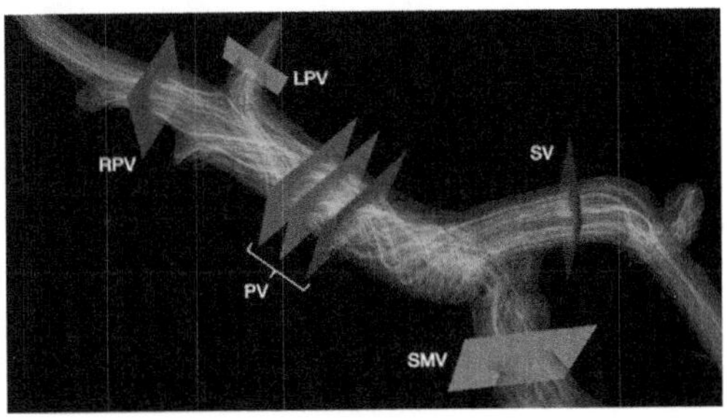


Fig. 12. PIV on an anatomically realistic model fabricated using 3D printing from an MRA on a total cavopulmonary (TCPC) connection single ventricle patient.

was to better understand aneurysm flow while taking into account cycle-to-cycle fluctuations and to analyze the ability of 4D flow MR imaging to assess complex flows in anatomical geometries. The quantitative results obtained in this study show good agreement between the velocity values measured with 4D flow MR imaging and those from the averaged data set from tomographic PIV.[89]

### Internal Consistency

In some 4D flow MR imaging examinations, the accuracy and internal consistency of the flow measurements can be indirectly validated based on the concept of continuity (conservation of mass). This evaluation is performed by measuring blood flow through 2 confluent vessels and the resulting daughter vessel, a parent vessel, and its branches or at 3 adjacent locations spaced at least 1 cm apart within the same vessel. For example, in a recent study, conservation of mass was tested at the portal vein by placing 3 consecutive planes (**Fig. 13**). In addition, consistency was also tested at the confluence and bifurcation by measuring blood flow in the splenic vein (QSV), superior mesenteric vein (QSMV), and right and left portal veins (QRPV) and (QLPV) respectively, such that

$$Q_{SV}+Q_{SMV} = Q_{PV} = Q_{RPV}+Q_{LPV} \quad \textbf{(11)}$$

as shown schematically in **Fig. 12**. In this study, measurement of $Q_{PV}$ at 3 different locations in the portal vein revealed an average absolute error of $4.2 \pm 3.9\%$. Second, comparison of flow into the portal confluence ($Q_{SV}$ + $Q_{SMV}$) with the flow in the portal vein ($Q_{PV}$) demonstrated an error of $5.9 \pm 2.5\%$ and the comparison of flow in the portal bifurcation ($Q_{RPV}$ + $Q_{LPV}$) showed an error of $5.8 \pm 3.1$.[90]

### Recent Advances

Over the last decade, 4D flow MR imaging has evolved from a research tool into a widely available approach with readily available acquisition and processing packages. It has also spurred additional research activities, some of which will likely find their way into clinical use. Machine learning (ML) has made great inroads into medical imaging and holds promise for 4D flow MR imaging as well.[91] ML can automate processes that are otherwise user intense and dependent, such as the segmentation of vessels and automated placement of analysis planes. ML has also been proposed to denoise velocity fields, for example, with the fusion of information from 4D flow MR imaging and computational fluid dynamics (CFD) using supervised learning, to provide high-resolution, physics-based, patient-specific flow fields in cerebrovascular anatomy.[92]

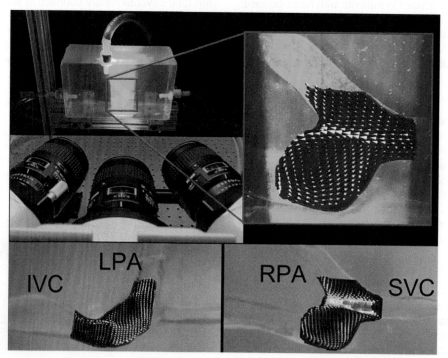


Fig. 13. Conservation of mass at the portal confluence, portal bifurcation, and within the main portal vein will provide indirect validation of flow measurement accuracy. Analysis planes were placed at the superior mesenteric vein (SMV), splenic vein (SV), portal vein (PV), right portal vein (RPV), and left portal vein (LPV).

The more widespread availability of 4D flow acquisition and analysis packages has enabled larger studies to establish normative data across genders and age, for example, for aortic pulse wave velocity[93] and cerebrovascular flow and pulsatility.[94] Atlas-based approaches have been implemented that allow for more consistent analysis across large cohorts, for example, for aortic wall shear stress.[95] Such normative datasets and atlas-based comparisons will be extraordinarily helpful in studying various pathologies, even in smaller cohorts.

Another exciting development is the added capability to resolve 4D flow data not only to the cardiac cycle but also to the respiratory cycle to investigate flow changes due to pressure changes in the chest, predominantly in the venous return.[96] This double-gating approach, also referred to as "5D flow MR imaging"[97] is typically implemented as a radially undersampled acquisition trajectory due to the flexibility offered for retrospective sorting of the data based on physiological gating information.

The pairing of 4D flow MR imaging and CFD also holds promise in complementing each other's strengths. For example, patient-specific models have been recently created to better understand the blood flow dynamics of cardiovascular conditions and more importantly predict the outcomes of therapeutical interventions. Briefly, patient-specific, anatomically realistic virtual geometries are generated from the PC-MRAs. In addition to the anatomical information, the velocity data are used to determine the boundary conditions and define the simulations parameters. Successful correlation of in vivo 4D flow MR imaging and validated CFD has the potential to provide a powerful noninvasive surveillance tool that will allow clinicians to follow-up patients with different cardiovascular conditions and evaluate their treatment outcomes over time, to identify potential hemodynamic deterioration and intervene in asymptomatic phases to improve their quality of life and increase their life span.[98–100]

## SUMMARY

4D flow MR imaging is an advanced phase contrast MR imaging technique that is now available on most MR systems. Methodology advances in data acquisition, image reconstruction, and postprocessing enable its use for clinical and research applications. This approach provides unique and otherwise unattainable noninvasive in vivo data with inherently coregistered anatomical and quantitative hemodynamic information in form of dynamic velocity vector field over a large imaging volume. The acquired data provide the basis for comprehensive hemodynamic analysis and non–contrast-enhanced MR angiography. The recent advances in scan time reductions and availability of postprocessing packages have established 4D flow MR imaging as a clinically available option and facilitates much needed multicenter, multivendor studies to demonstrate the maturity of this novel technique and ultimately, if successful, demonstrate clinical value.

## CLINICS CARE POINTS

- 4D Flow MR imaging is a lengthy scan, but enables velocity and flow measurements in multiple vessels as well as advanced hemodynamic analysis.
- 4D Flow MR acquisitions are performed during free breathing and as such do not require breathholds.
- 4D Flow MRI requires a careful selection of the velocity sensitivity encoding (Venc).

## DISCLOSURE

O. Wieben: GE Healthcare, United States: Grant Funding, NIH, United States: Grant Funding. G.S. Roberts: NIH: Grant Funding. P.A. Corrado: NIH: Grant Funding. Kevin M. Johnson, GE Healthcare: Grant Funding, NIH: Grant Funding. A. Roldán-Alzate: GE Healthcare: Grant Funding, NIH: Grant Funding.

## REFERENCES

1. Moran PR. A flow velocity zeugmatographic interlace for NMR imaging in humans. Magn Reson Imag 1982;1(4):197–203.
2. Bryant DJ, Payne JA, Firmin DN, et al. Measurement of flow with NMR imaging using a gradient pulse and phase difference technique. J Comput Assist Tomogr 1984;8(4):588–93.
3. van Dijk P. Direct cardiac NMR imaging of heart wall and blood flow velocity. J Comput Assist Tomogr 1984;8(3):429–36.
4. Firmin DN, Nayler GL, Klipstein RH, et al. In vivo validation of MR velocity imaging. J Comput Assist Tomogr 1987;11(5):751–6.
5. Lotz J, Meier C, Leppert A, et al. Cardiovascular flow measurement with phase-contrast MR imaging: basic facts and implementation. Radiographics 2002;22(3):651–71.
6. Markl M, Frydrychowicz A, Kozerke S, et al. 4D flow MRI. J Magn Reson Imaging 2012;36(5):1015–36.

7. Gorecka M, Bissell MM, Higgins DM, et al. Rationale and clinical applications of 4D flow cardiovascular magnetic resonance in assessment of valvular heart disease: a comprehensive review. J Cardiovasc Magn Reson 2022;24(1):49.
8. Ota H, Kamada H, Higuchi S, et al. Clinical Application of 4D Flow MR Imaging to Pulmonary Hypertension. Magn Reson Med Sci 2022;21(2):309–18.
9. Doyle CM, Orr J, Greenwood JP, et al. Four-Dimensional Flow Magnetic Resonance Imaging in the Assessment of Blood Flow in the Heart and Great Vessels: A Systematic Review. J Magn Reson Imaging 2022;55(5):1301–21.
10. Oechtering TH, Roberts GS, Panagiotopoulos N, et al. Clinical Applications of 4D Flow MRI in the Portal Venous System. Magn Reson Med Sci 2022;21(2):340–53.
11. Takahashi K, Sekine T, Ando T, et al. Utility of 4D Flow MRI in Thoracic Aortic Diseases: A Literature Review of Clinical Applications and Current Evidence. Magn Reson Med Sci 2022;21(2):327–39.
12. Oyama-Manabe N, Aikawa T, Tsuneta S, et al. Clinical Applications of 4D Flow MR Imaging in Aortic Valvular and Congenital Heart Disease. Magn Reson Med Sci 2022;21(2):319–26.
13. Wahlin A, Eklund A, Malm J. 4D flow MRI hemodynamic biomarkers for cerebrovascular diseases. J Intern Med 2022;291(2):115–27.
14. Kilner PJ, Gatehouse PD, Firmin DN. Flow measurement by magnetic resonance: a unique asset worth optimising. J Cardiovasc Magn Reson 2007;9(4):723–8.
15. Nayak KS, Nielsen JF, Bernstein MA, et al. Cardiovascular magnetic resonance phase contrast imaging. J Cardiovasc Magn Reson 2015;17(1):71.
16. Pelc NJ, Bernstein MA, Shimakawa A, et al. Encoding strategies for three-direction phase-contrast MR imaging of flow. J Magn Reson Imaging 1991;1(4):405–13.
17. Dumoulin CL, Souza SP, Darrow RD, et al. Simultaneous acquisition of phase-contrast angiograms and stationary-tissue images with Hadamard encoding of flow-induced phase shifts. J Magn Reson Imaging 1991;1(4):399–404.
18. Bock J, Frydrychowicz A, Stalder AF, et al. 4D phase contrast MRI at 3 T: effect of standard and blood-pool contrast agents on SNR, PC-MRA, and blood flow visualization. Magn Reson Med 2010;63(2):330–8.
19. Annual Meeting of the International Society for Magnetic Resonance in Medicine (ISMRM), 2011, Montreal, Quebec, Canada, 86.
20. Firmin DN, Gatehouse PD, Konrad JP, et al. Rapid 7-dimensional imaging of pulsatile flow. Computers in Cardiology IEEE Computer Society, London; 1993;14(2):353–6.
21. Wigstrom L, Sjoqvist L, Wranne B. Temporally resolved 3D phase-contrast imaging. Magn Reson Med 1996;36(5):800–3.
22. Markl M, Chan FP, Alley MT, et al. Time-resolved three-dimensional phase-contrast MRI. J Magn Reson Imaging 2003;17(4):499–506.
23. Markl M, Harloff A, Bley TA, et al. Time-resolved 3D MR velocity mapping at 3T: improved navigator-gated assessment of vascular anatomy and blood flow. J Magn Reson Imaging 2007;25(4):824–31.
24. Uribe S, Beerbaum P, Sorensen TS, et al. Four-dimensional (4D) flow of the whole heart and great vessels using real-time respiratory self-gating. Magn Reson Med 2009;62(4):984–92.
25. Bammer R, Hope TA, Aksoy M, et al. Time-resolved 3D quantitative flow MRI of the major intracranial vessels: initial experience and comparative evaluation at 1.5T and 3.0T in combination with parallel imaging. Magn Reson Med 2007;57(1):127–40.
26. Marshall I. Feasibility of k-t BLAST technique for measuring "seven-dimensional" fluid flow. J Magn Reson Imaging 2006;23(2):189–96.
27. Stadlbauer A, van der Riet W, Crelier G, et al. Accelerated time-resolved three-dimensional MR velocity mapping of blood flow patterns in the aorta using SENSE and k-t BLAST. Eur J Radiol 2010;75(1):e15–21.
28. Giese D, Schaeffter T, Kozerke S. Highly undersampled phase-contrast flow measurements using compartment-based k-t principal component analysis. Magn Reson Med 2013;69(2):434–43.
29. Hsiao A, Lustig M, Alley MT, et al. Evaluation of valvular insufficiency and shunts with parallel-imaging compressed-sensing 4D phase-contrast MR imaging with stereoscopic 3D velocity-fusion volume-rendered visualization. Radiology 2012;265(1):87–95.
30. Hutter J, Schmitt P, Aandal G, et al. Low-rank and sparse matrix decomposition for compressed sensing reconstruction of magnetic resonance 4D phase contrast blood flow imaging (loSDeCoS 4D-PCI). Med Image Comput Comput Assist Interv 2013;16(Pt 1):558–65.
31. Barger AV, Peters DC, Block WF, et al. Phase-contrast with interleaved undersampled projections. Magn Reson Med 2000;43(4):503–9.
32. Gu T, Korosec FR, Block WF, et al. PC VIPR: a high-speed 3D phase-contrast method for flow quantification and high-resolution angiography. AJNR Am J Neuroradiol 2005;26(4):743–9.
33. Johnson KM, Lum DP, Turski PA, et al. Improved 3D phase contrast MRI with off-resonance corrected dual echo VIPR. Magn Reson Med 2008;60(6):1329–36.
34. Liu J, Redmond MJ, Brodsky EK, et al. Generation and visualization of four-dimensional MR angiography data using an undersampled 3-D projection

trajectory. IEEE Trans Med Imaging 2006;25(2): 148–57.
35. Sigfridsson A, Petersson S, Carlhall CJ, et al. Four-dimensional flow MRI using spiral acquisition. Magn Reson Med 2012;68(4):1065–73.
36. Dyverfeldt P, Bissell M, Barker AJ, et al. 4D flow cardiovascular magnetic resonance consensus statement. J Cardiovasc Magn Reson 2015;17(1): 72.
37. Bernstein MA, Zhou XJ, Polzin JA, et al. Concomitant gradient terms in phase contrast MR: analysis and correction. Magn Reson Med 1998;39(2): 300–8.
38. Markl M, Bammer R, Alley MT, et al. Generalized reconstruction of phase contrast MRI: analysis and correction of the effect of gradient field distortions. Magn Reson Med 2003;50(4):791–801.
39. Peeters JM, Bos C, Bakker CJ. Analysis and correction of gradient nonlinearity and B0 inhomogeneity related scaling errors in two-dimensional phase contrast flow measurements. Magn Reson Med 2005;53(1):126–33.
40. Gatehouse PD, Rolf MP, Graves MJ, et al. Flow measurement by cardiovascular magnetic resonance: a multi-centre multi-vendor study of background phase offset errors that can compromise the accuracy of derived regurgitant or shunt flow measurements. J Cardiovasc Magn Reson 2010;12(1):5.
41. Minderhoud SCS, van der Velde N, Wentzel JJ, et al. The clinical impact of phase offset errors and different correction methods in cardiovascular magnetic resonance phase contrast imaging: a multi-scanner study. J Cardiovasc Magn Reson 2020;22(1):68.
42. Walker PG, Cranney GB, Scheidegger MB, et al. Semiautomated method for noise reduction and background phase error correction in MR phase velocity data. J Magn Reson Imaging 1993;3(3): 521–30.
43. Xiang QS. Temporal phase unwrapping for CINE velocity imaging. J Magn Reson Imaging 1995; 5(5):529–34.
44. Loecher M, Schrauben E, Johnson KM, et al. Phase unwrapping in 4D MR flow with a 4D single-step laplacian algorithm. J Magn Reson Imaging 2016; 43(4):833–42.
45. Roberts GS, Hoffman CA, Rivera-Rivera LA, et al. Automated hemodynamic assessment for cranial 4D flow MRI. Magn Reson Imaging 2023;97:46–55.
46. Oechtering TH, Nowak A, Sieren MM, et al. Repeatability and reproducibility of various 4D Flow MRI postprocessing software programs in a multi-software and multi-vendor cross-over comparison study. J Cardiovasc Magn Reson 2023;25(1):22.
47. Wentland AL, Wieben O, Francois CJ, et al. Aortic pulse wave velocity measurements with under-sampled 4D flow-sensitive MRI: comparison with 2D and algorithm determination. J Magn Reson Imaging 2013;37(4):853–9.
48. Ibrahim el SH, Johnson KR, Miller AB, et al. Measuring aortic pulse wave velocity using high-field cardiovascular magnetic resonance: comparison of techniques. J Cardiovasc Magn Reson 2010;12(1):26.
49. Dogui A, Redheuil A, Lefort M, et al. Measurement of aortic arch pulse wave velocity in cardiovascular MR: comparison of transit time estimators and description of a new approach. J Magn Reson Imaging 2011;33(6):1321–9.
50. Chiu YC, Arand PW, Shroff SG, et al. Determination of pulse wave velocities with computerized algorithms. Am Heart J 1991;121(5):1460–70.
51. Markl M, Wallis W, Brendecke S, et al. Estimation of global aortic pulse wave velocity by flow-sensitive 4D MRI. Magn Reson Med 2010;63(6):1575–82.
52. Ruesink T, Medero R, Rutkowski D, et al. In Vitro Validation of 4D Flow MRI for Local Pulse Wave Velocity Estimation. Cardiovasc Eng Technol 2018; 9(4):674–87.
53. Katritsis D, Kaiktsis L, Chaniotis A, et al. Wall shear stress: theoretical considerations and methods of measurement. Prog Cardiovasc Dis 2007;49(5): 307–29.
54. Reneman RS, Arts T, Hoeks AP. Wall shear stress–an important determinant of endothelial cell function and structure–in the arterial system in vivo. Discrepancies with theory. J Vasc Res 2006;43(3): 251–69.
55. Gijsen F, Katagiri Y, Barlis P, et al. Expert recommendations on the assessment of wall shear stress in human coronary arteries: existing methodologies, technical considerations, and clinical applications. Eur Heart J 2019;40(41):3421–33.
56. Bieging ET, Frydrychowicz A, Wentland A, et al. In vivo three-dimensional MR wall shear stress estimation in ascending aortic dilatation. J Magn Reson Imaging 2011;33(3):589–97.
57. Stalder AF, Russe MF, Frydrychowicz A, et al. Quantitative 2D and 3D phase contrast MRI: optimized analysis of blood flow and vessel wall parameters. Magn Reson Med 2008;60(5):1218–31.
58. Szajer J, Ho-Shon K. A comparison of 4D flow MRI-derived wall shear stress with computational fluid dynamics methods for intracranial aneurysms and carotid bifurcations - A review. Magn Reson Imaging 2018;48:62–9.
59. Iffrig E, Timmins LH, El Sayed R, et al. A New Method for Quantifying Abdominal Aortic Wall Shear Stress Using Phase Contrast Magnetic Resonance Imaging and the Womersley Solution. J Biomech Eng 2022;144(9):091011.
60. Kolipaka A, Illapani VS, Kalra P, et al. Quantification and comparison of 4D-flow MRI-derived wall shear stress and MRE-derived wall stiffness of the

abdominal aorta. J Magn Reson Imaging 2017; 45(3):771–8.
61. Cibis M, Potters WV, Gijsen FJ, et al. The Effect of Spatial and Temporal Resolution of Cine Phase Contrast MRI on Wall Shear Stress and Oscillatory Shear Index Assessment. PLoS One 2016;11(9): e0163316.
62. Petersson S, Dyverfeldt P, Ebbers T. Assessment of the accuracy of MRI wall shear stress estimation using numerical simulations. J Magn Reson Imaging 2012;36(1):128–38.
63. Rutkowski DR, Barton G, Francois CJ, et al. Analysis of cavopulmonary and cardiac flow characteristics in fontan Patients: Comparison with healthy volunteers. J Magn Reson Imaging 2019;49(6): 1786–99.
64. Pewowaruk R, Rutkowski D, Johnson C, et al. Assessment of sex differences in ventricular-vascular coupling of left ventricular and aortic flow derived from 4D flow MRI in healthy, young adults. J Biomech 2021;117:110276.
65. Hussaini SF, Rutkowski DR, Roldan-Alzate A, et al. Left and right ventricular kinetic energy using time-resolved versus time-average ventricular volumes. J Magn Reson Imaging 2017;45(3):821–8.
66. Cibis M, Bustamante M, Eriksson J, et al. Creating hemodynamic atlases of cardiac 4D flow MRI. J Magn Reson Imaging 2017;46(5):1389–99.
67. Bock J, Toger J, Bidhult S, et al. Validation and reproducibility of cardiovascular 4D-flow MRI from two vendors using 2 x 2 parallel imaging acceleration in pulsatile flow phantom and in vivo with and without respiratory gating. Acta Radiol 2019; 60(3):327–37.
68. Kamphuis VP, Westenberg JJM, van der Palen RLF, et al. Scan-rescan reproducibility of diastolic left ventricular kinetic energy, viscous energy loss and vorticity assessment using 4D flow MRI: analysis in healthy subjects. Int J Cardiovasc Imaging 2018;34(6):905–20.
69. Crandon S, Westenberg JJM, Swoboda PP, et al. Impact of Age and Diastolic Function on Novel, 4D flow CMR Biomarkers of Left Ventricular Blood Flow Kinetic Energy. Sci Rep 2018;8(1):14436.
70. Jeong D, Anagnostopoulos PV, Roldan-Alzate A, et al. Ventricular kinetic energy may provide a novel noninvasive way to assess ventricular performance in patients with repaired tetralogy of Fallot. J Thorac Cardiovasc Surg 2015;149(5):1339–47.
71. Kanski M, Arvidsson PM, Toger J, et al. Left ventricular fluid kinetic energy time curves in heart failure from cardiovascular magnetic resonance 4D flow data. J Cardiovasc Magn Reson 2015; 17:111.
72. Garg P, Crandon S, Swoboda PP, et al. Left ventricular blood flow kinetic energy after myocardial infarction - insights from 4D flow cardiovascular magnetic resonance. J Cardiovasc Magn Reson 2018;20(1):61.
73. Kaur H, Assadi H, Alabed S, et al. Left Ventricular Blood Flow Kinetic Energy Assessment by 4D Flow Cardiovascular Magnetic Resonance: A Systematic Review of the Clinical Relevance. J Cardiovasc Dev Dis 2020;7(3):37.
74. Bissell MM, Dall'Armellina E, Choudhury RP. Flow vortices in the aortic root: in vivo 4D-MRI confirms predictions of Leonardo da Vinci. Eur Heart J 2014;35(20):1344.
75. Catapano F, Pambianchi G, Cundari G, et al. 4D flow imaging of the thoracic aorta: is there an added clinical value? Cardiovasc Diagn Ther 2020;10(4):1068–89.
76. Arvidsson PM, Kovacs SJ, Toger J, et al. Vortex ring behavior provides the epigenetic blueprint for the human heart. Sci Rep 2016;6:22021.
77. Schafer M, Browning J, Schroeder JD, et al. Vorticity is a marker of diastolic ventricular interdependency in pulmonary hypertension. Pulm Circ 2016;6(1):46–54.
78. Bolger AF, Heiberg E, Karlsson M, et al. Transit of blood flow through the human left ventricle mapped by cardiovascular magnetic resonance. J Cardiovasc Magn Reson 2007;9(5):741–7.
79. Eriksson J, Carlhall CJ, Dyverfeldt P, et al. Semi-automatic quantification of 4D left ventricular blood flow. J Cardiovasc Magn Reson 2010;12(1):9.
80. Eriksson J, Dyverfeldt P, Engvall J, et al. Quantification of presystolic blood flow organization and energetics in the human left ventricle. Am J Physiol Heart Circ Physiol 2011;300(6):H2135–41.
81. Fredriksson AG, Zajac J, Eriksson J, et al. 4-D blood flow in the human right ventricle. Am J Physiol Heart Circ Physiol 2011;301(6):H2344–50.
82. Eriksson J, Bolger AF, Ebbers T, et al. Four-dimensional blood flow-specific markers of LV dysfunction in dilated cardiomyopathy. Eur Heart J Cardiovasc Imaging 2013;14(5):417–24.
83. Fredriksson AG, Svalbring E, Eriksson J, et al. 4D flow MRI can detect subtle right ventricular dysfunction in primary left ventricular disease. J Magn Reson Imaging 2016;43(3):558–65.
84. Falk KL, Medero R, Roldan-Alzate A. Fabrication of Low-Cost Patient-Specific Vascular Models for Particle Image Velocimetry. Cardiovasc Eng Technol 2019;10(3):500–7.
85. Medero R, Garcia-Rodriguez S, Francois CJ, et al. Patient-specific in vitro models for hemodynamic analysis of congenital heart disease - Additive manufacturing approach. J Biomech 2017;54: 111–6.
86. Rutkowski DR, Medero R, Ruesink TA, et al. Modeling Physiological Flow in Fontan Models With Four-Dimensional Flow Magnetic Resonance Imaging, Particle Image Velocimetry, and Arterial

Spin Labeling. J Biomech Eng 2019;141(12): 1210041–9.
87. Medero R, Hoffman C, Roldan-Alzate A. Comparison of 4D Flow MRI and Particle Image Velocimetry Using an In Vitro Carotid Bifurcation Model. Ann Biomed Eng 2018;46(12):2112–22.
88. Medero R, Falk K, Rutkowski D, et al. Correction: In Vitro Assessment of Flow Variability in an Intracranial Aneurysm Model Using 4D Flow MRI and Tomographic PIV. Ann Biomed Eng 2023;51(2):457.
89. Medero R, Falk K, Rutkowski D, et al. In Vitro Assessment of Flow Variability in an Intracranial Aneurysm Model Using 4D Flow MRI and Tomographic PIV. Ann Biomed Eng 2020;48(10): 2484–93.
90. Roldan-Alzate A, Frydrychowicz A, Niespodzany E, et al. In vivo validation of 4D flow MRI for assessing the hemodynamics of portal hypertension. J Magn Reson Imaging 2013;37(5):1100–8.
91. Peper ES, van Ooij P, Jung B, et al. Advances in machine learning applications for cardiovascular 4D flow MRI. Front Cardiovasc Med 2022;9:1052068.
92. Rutkowski DR, Roldan-Alzate A, Johnson KM. Enhancement of cerebrovascular 4D flow MRI velocity fields using machine learning and computational fluid dynamics simulation data. Sci Rep 2021;11(1):10240.
93. Jarvis K, Scott MB, Soulat G, et al. Aortic Pulse Wave Velocity Evaluated by 4D Flow MRI Across the Adult Lifespan. J Magn Reson Imaging 2022; 56(2):464–73.
94. Roberts GS, Peret A, Jonaitis EM, et al. Normative Cerebral Hemodynamics in Middle-aged and Older Adults Using 4D Flow MRI: Initial Analysis of Vascular Aging. Radiology 2023;307(3): e222685.
95. Ferdian E, Dubowitz DJ, Mauger CA, et al. WSSNet: Aortic Wall Shear Stress Estimation Using Deep Learning on 4D Flow MRI. Front Cardiovasc Med 2021;8:769927.
96. Schrauben EM, Anderson AG, Johnson KM, et al. Respiratory-induced venous blood flow effects using flexible retrospective double-gating. J Magn Reson Imaging 2015;42(1):211–6.
97. Ma LE, Yerly J, Piccini D, et al. 5D Flow MRI: A Fully Self-gated, Free-running Framework for Cardiac and Respiratory Motion-resolved 3D Hemodynamics. Radiol Cardiothorac Imaging 2020;2(6): e200219.
98. Fernandes JF, Gill H, Nio A, et al. Non-invasive cardiovascular magnetic resonance assessment of pressure recovery distance after aortic valve stenosis. J Cardiovasc Magn Reson 2023;25(1):5.
99. Ha H, Kvitting JP, Dyverfeldt P, et al. Validation of pressure drop assessment using 4D flow MRI-based turbulence production in various shapes of aortic stenoses. Magn Reson Med 2019;81(2): 893–906.
100. Shahid L, Rice J, Berhane H, et al. Enhanced 4D Flow MRI-Based CFD with Adaptive Mesh Refinement for Flow Dynamics Assessment in Coarctation of the Aorta. Ann Biomed Eng 2022;50(8):1001–16.

# Clinical Applications of Four-Dimensional Flow MRI

Anthony Maroun, MD*, Sandra Quinn, MD, PhD, David Dushfunian, MD, Elizabeth K. Weiss, BS, Bradley D. Allen, MD, MS, James C. Carr, MD[1], Michael Markl, PhD

**KEYWORDS**

• Phase contrast MR imaging • Flow imaging • 4D flow • Hemodynamics • Cardiovascular • Neurovascular • Abdominal

**KEY POINTS**

- Four-dimensional (4D) flow MRI can be advantageous in the evaluation of heart valve disease because it allows the identification of valve-mediated flow patterns and optimal corresponding placement of analysis planes for flow quantification, and can be combined with retrospective valve tracking to account for valve motion.
- By acquiring a time-resolved velocity field, numerous advanced hemodynamic parameters can be quantified (eg, wall shear stress, kinetic energy, pulse wave velocity, and so forth) that have the potential to improve disease monitoring and outcome prediction, particularly in aortic disease.
- In congenital heart disease, 4D flow MRI improves hemodynamic understanding through three-dimensional (3D) visualization of complex 3D blood flow dynamics and comprehensive retrospective flow assessment in multiple vessels.
- Applications of 4D flow MRI may also extend to the neurovascular and abdominal systems, for which studies have shown promise as a diagnostic and prognostic tool in conditions such as intracranial aneurysms, arteriovenous malformations, Alzheimer disease, and cirrhosis.

**Video content accompanies this article at http://www.mri.theclinics.com**

## INTRODUCTION

Phase contrast (PC) MR imaging (MRI) is a technique used to visualize and quantify moving fluid.[1] Since its introduction in the late 1980s, it has received broad clinical acceptance for the visualization and quantitative assessment of blood flow in patients with cardiac and vascular diseases.[2] This technique measures the velocity of blood by calculating changes in the MRI signal phase of moving blood subjected to a pair of bipolar magnetic field gradients. It was initially designated two-dimensional (2D) PC-MRI because it measured unidirectional velocities in a 2D plane perpendicular to the long axis of the vessel of interest.

In recent decades, 2D PC-MRI has emerged as an important alternative diagnostic tool to echocardiography. In fact, 2D-PC-MRI is as reliable as echocardiography but has better access to deep segments of the aortic and pulmonary systems and is not limited by individual acoustic window.[3] However, 2D PC-MRI has several constraints. First, it is typically limited to

Department of Radiology, Northwestern University, Feinberg School of Medicine, 737 North Michigan Avenue Suite 1600, Chicago, IL 60611, USA
[1] Present address. 676 N. Street. Clair Street, Suite 800, Chicago, Illinois 60611, USA
* Corresponding author.
*E-mail address:* anthony.maroun@northwestern.edu

Magn Reson Imaging Clin N Am 31 (2023) 451–460
https://doi.org/10.1016/j.mric.2023.04.005
1064-9689/23/

measuring blood flow velocity along a single direction, which may be inadequate for characterizing three-dimensional (3D) flow dynamics inside the heart and vessels with complex geometry.[4] Second, if flow must be measured at multiple sites, the acquisition must be repeated at each site with careful positioning of the 2D plane and repeated breath holding for cardiothoracic applications. As a result, the method depends on the experience of a trained operator to make accurate measurements, which limits its reproducibility.[5]

In contrast to standard 2D PC-MRI, time-resolved 3D PC-MRI with 3-directional velocity encoding (4D flow MRI) allows the measurement of blood flow velocities in all 3 spatial dimensions along the cardiac cycle, providing a time-resolved 3D velocity field.[6] Acquisition of 4D information (4D = 3D + time over the cardiac cycle) enables the visualization of multidirectional flow patterns inside the vessels and eliminates the need for precise plane positioning at the time of acquisition. Furthermore, by capturing a full volumetric velocity data set in a single acquisition, areas at any location within the 3D data can be retrospectively analyzed.[7] However, due to the large amount of information that must be collected, efficient data acquisition is necessary to achieve clinically practical scan times. Several recent developments in image acquisition have been applied to 4D flow MRI , such as parallel imaging, and compressed sensing.[8–10] These methods have contributed significantly to its clinical feasibility by reducing scan times to 5 to 12 minutes.

During the past decade, there has been increasing interest in the use of 4D flow MRI in a wide range of cardiac and vascular diseases. Recently, several commercial analysis software packages have been introduced, which have facilitated clinical translation and standardized analysis workflows enabling 4D flow MRI to become part of clinical routine in large medical centers. The purpose of this article is to provide an overview of the clinical applications of 4D flow MRI in cardiovascular, neurovascular, and abdominal diseases. The authors would like to emphasize, however, that this review is by no means complete or exhaustive but is a summary of the important applications that have accumulated in the literature. For more extensive overviews and insights into future research directions, the reader is referred to several recently published 4D flow MRI review articles.[4,11–18]

## Cardiovascular Applications

Four-dimensional flow MRI can image the heart and main vessels within clinically acceptable scan times of 5 to 12 minutes. In the past decade, many studies have demonstrated its role in developing a better understanding of the association between altered hemodynamics and disease progression. In this section, we present the clinical applications of 4D flow MRI in the setting of valvular, aortic, and congenital heart diseases (CHDs).

### Valvular disease

Flow quantification is central for the assessment of valvular disease severity and critical for treatment planning. Doppler echocardiography is the most commonly used technique for assessing valvular flow. However, it has limited acoustic window, depends on operator expertise, and relies on assumptions regarding the underlying flow profile, which can render it inaccurate in the presence of eccentric jets.[17] Two-dimensional PC-MRI can also be used to assess valvular flow; however, similar to echocardiography, it requires careful positing of the 2D acquisition plane by an experienced operator to avoid flow underestimation. Four-dimensional flow MRI offers several advantages over 2D techniques. First, by measuring the full 3D velocity field, 4D flow MRI enables the visualization of 3D flow patterns across the valves and the major arteries by using time-resolved pathlines and streamlines, color-coded according to the velocity magnitude. Pathlines are traces of the time-varying blood flow over the cardiac cycle and are best displayed in a video mode to fully appreciate the dynamic information that 4D flow MRI provides.[12] However, streamlines represent instantaneous curved lines tangential to the velocity direction at a single time-point and are used to characterize blood flow profiles. Particularly, 3D streamlines facilitate the identification of 3 distinguished flow forms: laminar flow, helical flow (when blood rotates around an axis while moving forward), or vortical flow (when blood particles rotate and curl back on themselves).[4] This is relevant in valvular disease because vortical flow has been shown to cause discrepancy in flow measurements and should be avoided when selecting analysis planes.[19]

In aortic stenosis (AS), the reliable and accurate quantification of peak aortic velocity and mean transvalvular pressure gradient are important in the clinical workup because they are used to score AS severity and guide treatment planning.[20] Four-dimensional flow MRI has been shown to be superior in assessing valvular flow in AS, particularly in patients with eccentric or angulated jets.[17] Several studies have demonstrated that 2D PC-MRI and echocardiography suffer from flow underestimation because they are limited by single-directional velocity encoding and lack the ability to accurately identify flow direction.[12,21] Four-dimensional flow MRI offers 3-directional velocity encoding and can guide the appropriate placement of 2D analysis planes by providing 3D streamlines that allow an operator to retrospectively place planes orthogonal to the eccentric jet direction and in a plane that corresponds to the highest velocity. Furthermore, regions with complex and deranged flow can be identified and avoided to limit flow discrepancies. **Fig. 1** shows an example of peak systolic streamlines in a patient with severe AS, which were used to guide plane placement. The patient has an associated mild aortic regurgitation that can be appreciated on the corresponding time-resolved 3D pathlines (see Video 1). Once accurate transvalvular peak velocity measurements have been made, mean pressure gradient can be derived using the simplified Bernoulli equation ($\Delta P = 4V^2_{max}$). In a study by Archer and colleagues, peak pressure gradient by 4D flow MRI was comparable to the invasive pressure assessment but superior to transthoracic echocardiography, which was limited by overestimation.[22] Furthermore, after surgical repair, left ventricular mass regression was better associated with 4D flow MRI-derived pressure gradient change.

Aortic regurgitation (AR) and pulmonary regurgitation (PR) also require accurate and consistent quantification of valve flow. In patients with eccentric jets or aneurysmal aorta or aneurysmal pulmonary artery, vortical flow may be observed and can lead to inaccurate measurements. Four-dimensional flow MRI can help to identify regions of more laminar and less turbulent flow for quantification and is a reliable technique. In AR, strong correlation with 2D PC-MRI and transthoracic echocardiography was observed, and 4D flow MRI was able to detect more than mild aortic valve regurgitation with a sensitivity of 100% and a specificity of 98%.[23,24] For PR, a prospective study showed that pulmonary flow can also be accurately quantified although peak systolic velocity may be underestimated.[25] However, this underestimation can be minimized by placing the plane at the level corresponding to the highest velocity in the pulmonary artery.

Four-dimensional flow MRI may also improve quantification of mitral and tricuspid flow. Although echocardiography is the clinical standard, direct measurement of regurgitant flow in the mitral and tricuspid valves is particularly difficult due to complex valve anatomy, valve plane motion during systole, and the often-associated eccentric jets. Similarly, 2D PC-MRI is imprecise because of through-plane motion.[17] In contrast, 4D flow MRI has the advantage to be combined with retrospective valve tracking (RVT) obtained from CINE-MRI acquisitions of the valve to improve the valvular flow assessment. By tracking the position and angulation of the moving valves during all phases

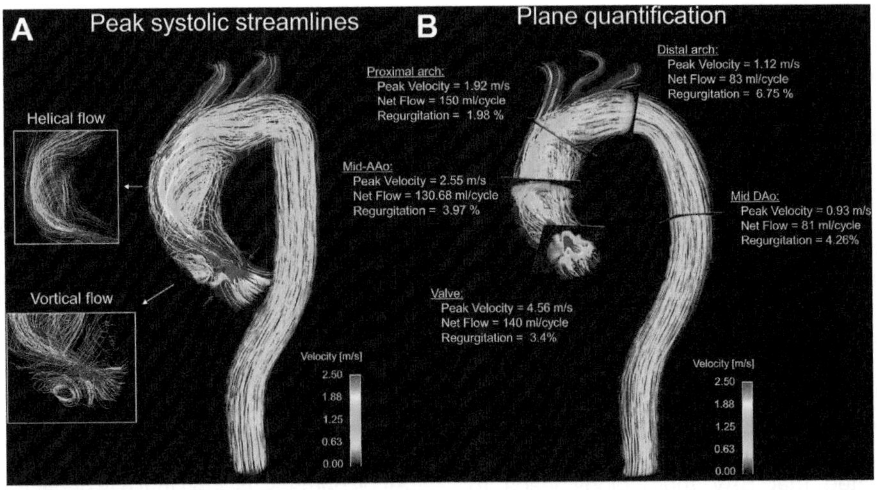


**Fig. 1.** Quantification of aortic flow in a 73-year-old patient with a severely calcified trileaflet aortic valve associated with severe aortic valve stenosis and mild regurgitation. Three-dimensional streamlines of peak systolic flow (*A*) showed the presence of a vortex and a helix formation in the ascending aorta (AAo). Streamlines were used to guide the placement of the valvular 2D analysis plane orthogonally to the outflow jet direction at the location corresponding to the highest velocity (*red arrows*) while avoiding vortex and helical flows. In addition to guiding plane placement, 4D flow MRI, through its full volumetric coverage, allows retrospective flow quantification at multiple locations (*B*). Notably, for this patient, the helical flow in the AAo caused discrepancy in net flow assessment at the mid-AAo and proximal arch levels. For reliable quantifications, such formations should be avoided when placing analysis planes.

of the cardiac cycle, 4D flow-MRI analysis planes can be retrospectively reformatted to follow the valve during systole and diastole. Planes can also be adjusted according to blood flow direction. This technique proved superior to 2D PC-MRI in mitral and tricuspid regurgitation quantification and had good intraobserver and interobserver agreement.[26,27] Interestingly, RVT can be applied to the 4 valves in a single scan and was shown to be reproducible and accurate for all valves, irrespective of scanner type and protocol.[28] To improve the utility of this technique, automated solutions have been developed and have reduced the time-consuming manual placement and tracking of multiplanar reformatting planes by half while improving reliability.[29] Four-dimensional flow MRI has not been extensively studied in mitral or tricuspid stenosis; however, in a recent case report, the pressure gradient derived from 4D flow MRI agreed with invasive assessment, whereas transthoracic echocardiography led to overestimation.[30]

### *Aortic disease*

Aortic coarctation is a congenital narrowing of the aorta that requires surgical repair when the systolic pressure gradient across the site of coarctation is greater than 20 mm Hg.[31] For accurate assessment of coarctation severity, 4D flow MRI provides streamlines visualization that can facilitate accurate positioning of the analysis plane at the location of the highest velocity inside the vessel narrowing. After peak velocity measurement, pressure can be calculated according to the Bernoulli equation. A study by Riesenkampff and colleagues compared 4D flow MRI against catheterization in a small group of patients and found that pressure fields can be accurately estimated using 4D flow MRI .[32] Furthermore, coarctation requires the quantification of collateral flow through intercostal vessels, which increases with coarctation severity. Four-dimensional flow MRI enables direct visualization and quantification of the collateral blood flow.

Bicuspid aortic valve (BAV) is the most common congenital cardiac malformation and is associated with an increased incidence of aortic aneurysms and dissections.[33] Four-dimensional flow studies have indicated that BAV morphology leads to abnormal transvalvular flow patterns, such as an eccentric outflow jets even in the absence of AS and aneurysmal degeneration.[34,35] Furthermore, 4D flow MRI studies have shown that different BAV leaflet fusion patterns are associated with distinct differences in ascending aortic flow ($Q_A$) jet directions.[36] These valve-mediated flow patterns have been shown to alter wall shear stress (WSS) in the ascending aorta, a known trigger of wall remodeling and aneurysmal formation (ie, aortic growth).[37] Further, Bollache and colleagues found that increased regional WSS is associated with decreased elastic fiber thickness, and Kiema and colleagues showed that WSS correlates with aortic media degeneration and aortic wall thickness.[38,39] These findings support the relationship between abnormal valve-mediated flow hemodynamics, as determined by 4D flow MRI , with biomechanical changes in the aortic wall and their implication in BAV aortopathy. Furthermore, they provided evidence that WSS is a key driver of aortic dilation and a promising risk measure. The potential of WSS from 4D MRI to serve as a baseline clinical measure was further validated in recent studies that demonstrated significant association between WSS and aortic growth, attesting that it could be used clinically to improve risk stratification.[40–42]

Aortic dissection is a life-threatening condition caused by a tear in the aortic intima leading to the formation of a true and false lumen. Four-dimensional flow MRI has the potential to become an integral part of dissection workup because it can improve the detection of hemodynamically active intimal fenestrations in chronic type B aortic dissection.[43] This is significant because dissection flow hemodynamics are thought to be a major driver of secondary complications such as rupture and progressive aortic dilatation (ie, aortic growth) which warrant immediate prophylactic thoracic endovascular aortic repair. In addition, there is evidence that 4D flow MRI-derived hemodynamic parameters in the true and false lumen can improve risk stratification (**Fig. 2**). For example, Marlevi and colleagues showed that pressure in the false lumen, estimated as retrograde flow and relative pressure, correlated independently with aortic growth, whereas Chu and colleagues found that the ratio between true and false lumen kinetic energy could be a potential predictor.[44,45] These results demonstrate that dissection hemodynamics may become an important determinant of adverse outcomes for improved risk stratification and thus treatment selection.

### *Congenital heart disease*

CHD is perhaps the area that has benefited the most from 4D MRI. Echocardiography and 2D PC-MRI are particularly challenging in the pediatric CHD population because of the often-complex anatomy and small vessel caliber.[15] CHD often requires quantification of flow at multiple sites to identify possible shunts or collaterals, which would require time-consuming plane positioning and acquisition with 2D techniques. Four-dimensional flow MRI

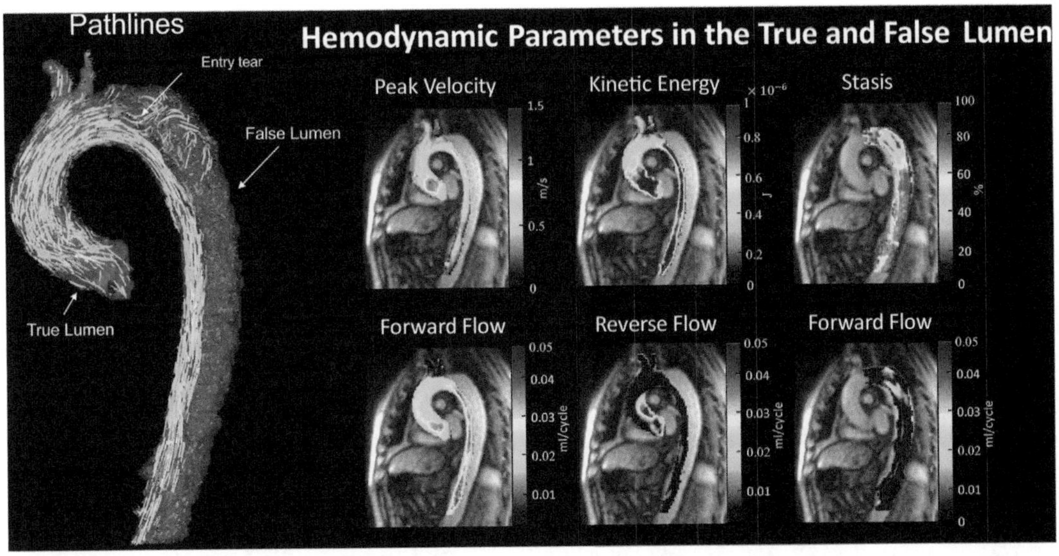


Fig. 2. Three-dimensional pathlines of a systolic time-point and voxelwise parametric flow maps in a chronic type B aortic dissection case. As shown by the pathlines, 4D flow MRI can be used for the visualization of 3D hemodynamics in dissected aortas. In this case, a small active entry tear in the proximal descending aorta was detected, with associated slow flow in the distal false lumen. Advanced 4D flow MRI-derived parameters can be also quantified and provide a better understanding of dissection hemodynamics. Although their use is currently limited to research, they have shown potential to predict outcomes and, hence, may see clinical acceptance in the future.

addresses all these limitations and allows the visualization of complex 3D blood flow patterns and pathways in complex CHD.

Four-dimensional flow MRI is used clinically to evaluate various conditions such as atrial septal defects, ventricular septal defects, patent ductus arteriosus, and anomalous pulmonary venous return. Three-dimensional pathlines allow intuitive identification of shunts and flow reversals in systole or diastole that are not always visible on echocardiography.[4] Permanent or transient shunt inversion is crucial to recognize because it may be a sign of secondary pulmonary hypertension. In addition, in this type of disease, it is important to quantify intracardiac left-to-right shunts because it may determine the choice of treatment. Four-dimensional flow MRI provides accurate shunt quantification by measuring the difference between the simultaneous pulmonic flow and $Q_A$ in the case of a single intracardiac shunt. However, in the presence of an extracardiac shunt (eg, patent ductus arteriosus), or to determine the contribution of each shunt in the case of multiple intracardiac shunts, flow is better assessed directly by placing a plane orthogonal to the shunt flow.[46] The comparability of 4D flow MRI with invasive cardiac catheterization, as well as the reproducibility and consistency between different readers for shunt assessment have been validated in several studies.[47,48] In Video 2, we provide an example of shunt quantification in a pediatric patient and illustrate the advantage of 3D visualization and quantification offered by 4D flow MRI.

Four-dimensional flow MRI is also an important postoperative tool. In patients with Fontan palliation, it can assess 3D blood flow dynamics in the cavopulmonary connections and detect uneven flow distribution from the caval veins to the right and left pulmonary arteries, which has been implicated as a driver of complications such as pulmonary arteriovenous malformations (AVMs).[49] **Fig. 3** illustrates an example of venous flow distribution assessment. Other uses of 4D flow MRI postoperatively include repaired teratology of Fallot. After surgical repair, the most important complications to evaluate are secondary PR or stenosis, which are very common and can be accurately assessed with 4D flow MRI.[50,51] As noted in several studies, repaired Fallot teratology is also associated with a higher incidence of vortical flow, which may affect the accuracy of flow measurements.[15,52] In such cases, 4D flow MRI can aid in plane selection and provide less erroneous measurements compared with 2D techniques.

A key feature of 4D flow MRI is the ability to select analysis planes and quantify flow in a post hoc fashion. This allows the selection of appropriate planes after determining the direction of flow and allows clinicians to quantify flow at locations that may not have been considered relevant before scan analysis. However, this feature can

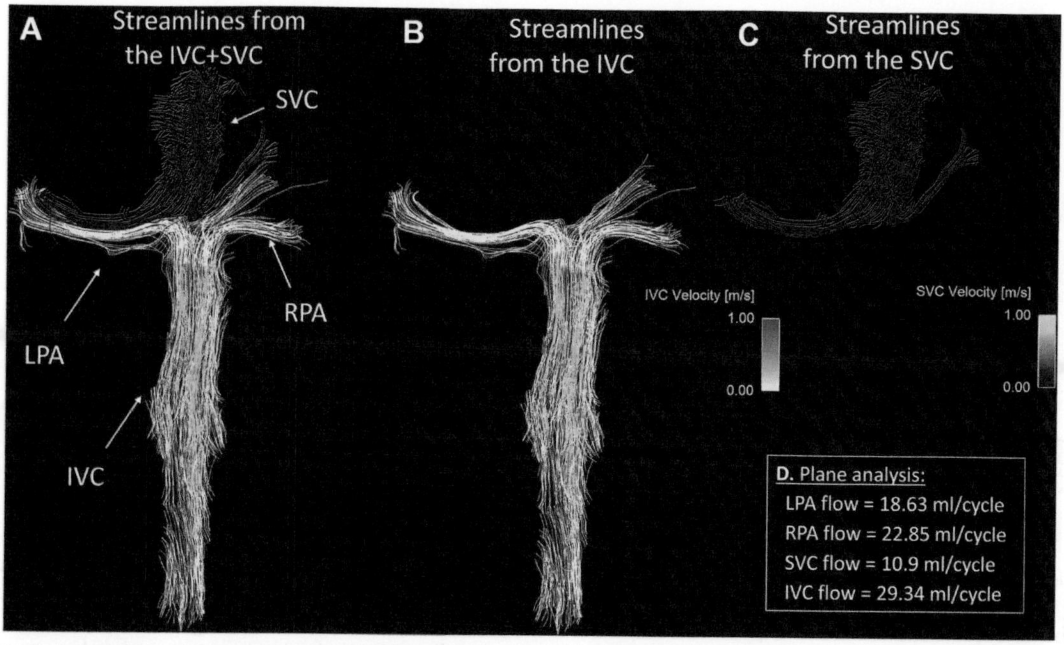


**Fig. 3.** Streamlines of a young male patient with hypoplastic left heart syndrome after Fontan operation. Streamlines originating from the inferior (IVC) and superior vena cava (SVC) show slow, evenly distributed flow into the right pulmonary artery (RPA) and left pulmonary artery (LPA) (*A*). Further flow partitioning indicated that IVC flow is evenly distributed to both sides, whereas SVC flow is predominantly directed toward the LPA (*B* and *C*). Quantification of flow confirmed the internal consistency of the data because caval and pulmonary flows were equal (*D*).

also be used for data quality control. In fact, by applying the principle of conservation of mass, pulmonary and aortic flows can be compared for equality. This is useful because it helps to identify erroneous data, but also, unnoticed shunts between circuits. Nonetheless, studies determined that 4D flow MRI provides excellent flow quantification results and is more consistent than 2D PC-MRI.[53,54]

## Neurovascular Applications

The first applications of 4D flow MRI focused on the large vessels, particularly the aorta. However, this technique has been extended to other vascular territories throughout the human circulatory system, such as the cerebral arteries and veins. Although these applications are currently limited to research, we briefly review some applications that have shown strong potential for use in clinical practice.

In patients with intracranial aneurysms, 4D flow MRI allows for the 3D visualization of complex intracranial flow patterns irrespective of aneurysm size or morphology and can identify distinct groups of hemodynamics that correlate with morphology subtypes.[55,56] Quantitative hemodynamics such as 3D velocity distribution and WSS can also be successfully acquired and were correlated with aneurysm size and morphology.[55] Furthermore, flow vortex cores can be identified and may help to stratify the risk of rupture.[57]

In AVMs, intricate and highly variable 4D flow MRI patterns have been identified.[58,59] Four-dimensional flow MRI may help in detecting AVMs at risk of rupture or assist in individualized planning of staged embolization treatment because it provides 3D visualization of complex AVM feeding and venous draining patterns (an example is shown in **Fig. 4**) and offers quantitative flow characterization of large intracranial AVM vessels.

In the context of intracranial or carotid stenosis, 4D flow MRI has the potential to identify patients at risk of cerebral hypoperfusion or stroke by providing in-depth understanding of complex intracranial hemodynamics. It can identify compromised hemodynamics in the region of intracranial artery stenosis and adjacent vascular territories due to redistribution of flow.[60,61] Pressure gradient estimation can also be performed using the modified Bernoulli equation.

Promising applications of 4D flow MRI also extend to Alzheimer disease (AD). In AD, there is a prevailing hypothesis that vascular dysfunction is an early feature in prodromal AD. Several recent

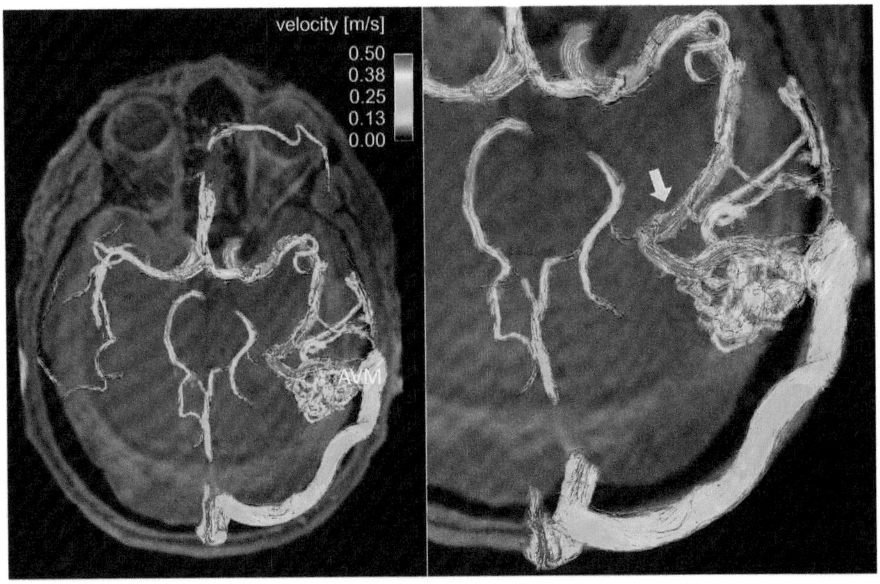


Fig. 4. Three-dimensional blood flow visualization in a patient with a large (Spetzler-Martin grade = 3) unruptured temporo-occipital AVM. Convoluted hemodynamics and high flow velocity in a main AVM feeding artery (*arrow*) are clearly visible using 4D flow MRI.

studies have demonstrated that AD is associated with altered venous blood flow and pulsatility, decreased spontaneous low-frequency oscillations in arterial blood flow, and higher transcranial pulse wave velocity, indicating that 4D flow parameters may serve as an early disease marker.[62–64]

### *Abdominal Applications*

Four-dimensional flow MRI is less commonly used in the abdomen compared with the heart, aorta, and brain. This is partly due to the complex abdominal anatomy and the small caliber of abdominal vessels. Nonetheless, abdominal 4D flow MRI has good scan rescan reproducibility and a low interobserver variability and could be used as a valuable assessment tool for certain abdominal pathologic conditions.[65]

Abdominal applications focus mostly on cirrhosis, where 4D flow MRI may be used to characterize portal blood flow after a meal challenge and predict hypersplenism in patients with portal hypertension.[66,67] Four-dimensional flow MRI can also offer volumetric and functional evaluation of transjugular intrahepatic portosystemic shunt with access to stent lumen and feasibility for long-term follow-up.[68,69] Additional applications include renal artery assessment for which 4D MRI allows quantification of blood flow before and after renal artery angioplasty, and assessment of intrarenal flow in kidney transplant patients during systole and diastole.[70,71]

## SUMMARY

Four-dimensional flow MRI is a relatively new technique that has not been widely used but has become part of clinical routine in large academic medical centers due to its superiority over echocardiography and 2D PC-MRI for assessing 3D blood flow dynamics. Studies during the past decade have demonstrated the usefulness of the technique to better diagnose and monitor various diseases spanning the cardiovascular, neurovascular, and abdominal systems. With faster acquisition techniques, more efficient postprocessing methods, and the introduction of commercial analysis solutions, 4D flow MRI can in the coming years see a broader clinical acceptance and expanded demand.

## CLINICS CARE POINTS

- 4D flow MRI enables precise placement of planes directed by streamlines, leading to superior assessment of valvular flow, especially for quantifying peak aortic velocity and mean transvalvular pressure gradient.
- Volumetric velocity data acquisition from 4D flow MRI allows compensation for valve motion through retrospective valve tracking, resulting in improved quantification of mitral and tricuspid flow.

- 4D flow MRI quantifies advanced hemodynamic parameters, such as wall shear stress, a key factor driving the progression of aortic dilation and aortopathy in patients with bicuspid aortic valve.
- In the pediatric population, 4D flow MRI provides the capability to visualize complex 3D blood flow patterns and conduct comprehensive evaluation of congenital heart diseases.
- The clinical utility of 4D flow extends to the neurological and abdominal vascular systems, demonstrating promising applications in the context of intracranial aneurysms, arteriovenous malformations, Alzheimer's disease, and cirrhosis.

## DISCLOSURE

B.D. Allen Circle Cardiovascular Imaging: Consultant. American Roentgen Ray Society: Grant Funding. American Heart Association: Grant Funding. J C. Carr: Siemens: Research Grant to Institution; Advisory Board. Bayer: Research Grant to Institution; Advisory Board; Speaker. Bracco: Advisory Board. Guerbet: Research Grant to Institution. M. Markl: Siemens: Grant Funding. Circle Cardiovascular Imaging: Consultant. A. Maroun, S. Quinn, D. Dushfunian, and E.K. Weiss: These Authors have nothing to disclose.

## SUPPLEMENTARY DATA

Supplementary data related to this article can be found online at https://doi.org/10.1016/j.mric.2023.04.005.

## REFERENCES

1. Pelc NJ, Herfkens RJ, Shimakawa A, et al. Phase contrast cine magnetic resonance imaging. Magn Reson Q 1991;7(4):229–54.
2. Stankovic Z, Allen BD, Garcia J, et al. 4D flow imaging with MRI. Cardiovasc Diagn Ther 2014;4(2):173–92.
3. Defrance C, Bollache E, Kachenoura N, et al. Evaluation of aortic valve stenosis using cardiovascular magnetic resonance: comparison of an original semiautomated analysis of phase-contrast cardiovascular magnetic resonance with Doppler echocardiography. Circ Cardiovasc Imaging 2012;5(5):604–12.
4. Azarine A, Garçon P, Stansal A, et al. Four-dimensional Flow MRI: Principles and Cardiovascular Applications. Radiographics 2019;39(3):632–48.
5. Lotz J, Meier C, Leppert A, et al. Cardiovascular flow measurement with phase-contrast MR imaging: basic facts and implementation. Radiographics 2002;22(3):651–71.
6. Markl M, Kilner PJ, Ebbers T. Comprehensive 4D velocity mapping of the heart and great vessels by cardiovascular magnetic resonance. J Cardiovasc Magn Reson 2011;13(1):7.
7. Dyverfeldt P, Bissell M, Barker AJ, et al. 4D flow cardiovascular magnetic resonance consensus statement. J Cardiovasc Magn Reson 2015;17(1):72.
8. Kilinc O, Baraboo J, Engel J, et al. Aortic Hemodynamics with Accelerated Dual-Venc 4D Flow MRI in Type B Aortic Dissection. Applied Sciences 2023;13:6202.
9. Stadlbauer A, van der Riet W, Crelier G, et al. Accelerated time-resolved three-dimensional MR velocity mapping of blood flow patterns in the aorta using SENSE and k-t BLAST. Eur J Radiol 2010;75(1):e15–21.
10. Kilinc O, Chu S, Baraboo J, et al. Hemodynamic Evaluation of Type B Aortic Dissection Using Compressed Sensing Accelerated 4D Flow MRI. J Magn Reson Imaging 2022. https://doi.org/10.1002/jmri.28432.
11. Vasanawala SS, Hanneman K, Alley MT, et al. Congenital heart disease assessment with 4D flow MRI. J Magn Reson Imaging 2015;42(4):870–86.
12. Garcia J, Barker AJ, Markl M. The Role of Imaging of Flow Patterns by 4D Flow MRI in Aortic Stenosis. JACC Cardiovasc Imaging 2019;12(2):252–66.
13. Catapano F, Pambianchi G, Cundari G, et al. 4D flow imaging of the thoracic aorta: is there an added clinical value? Cardiovasc Diagn Ther 2020;10(4):1068–89.
14. Zhuang B, Sirajuddin A, Zhao S, et al. The role of 4D flow MRI for clinical applications in cardiovascular disease: current status and future perspectives. Quant Imaging Med Surg 2021;11(9):4193–210.
15. Geiger J, Callaghan FM, Burkhardt BEU, et al. Additional value and new insights by four-dimensional flow magnetic resonance imaging in congenital heart disease: application in neonates and young children. Pediatr Radiol 2021;51(8):1503–17.
16. Takahashi K, Sekine T, Ando T, et al. Utility of 4D Flow MRI in Thoracic Aortic Diseases: A Literature Review of Clinical Applications and Current Evidence. Magn Reson Med Sci 2022;21(2):327–39.
17. Gorecka M, Bissell MM, Higgins DM, et al. Rationale and clinical applications of 4D flow cardiovascular magnetic resonance in assessment of valvular heart disease: a comprehensive review. J Cardiovasc Magn Reson 2022;24(1):49.
18. Soulat G, McCarthy P, Markl M. 4D Flow with MRI. Annu Rev Biomed Eng 2020;22:103–26.
19. Contijoch FJ, Horowitz M, Masutani E, et al. 4D Flow Vorticity Visualization Predicts Regions of Quantitative Flow Inconsistency for Optimal Blood Flow Measurement. Radiol Cardiothorac Imaging 2020;2(1):e190054.
20. Blanken CPS, Farag ES, Boekholdt SM, et al. Advanced cardiac MRI techniques for evaluation

of left-sided valvular heart disease. J Magn Reson Imaging 2018;48(2):318–29.
21. Rose MJ, Jarvis K, Chowdhary V, et al. Efficient method for volumetric assessment of peak blood flow velocity using 4D flow MRI. J Magn Reson Imaging 2016;44(6):1673–82.
22. Archer GT, Elhawaz A, Barker N, et al. Validation of four-dimensional flow cardiovascular magnetic resonance for aortic stenosis assessment. Sci Rep 2020; 10(1):10569.
23. Alvarez A, Martinez V, Pizarro G, et al. Clinical use of 4D flow MRI for quantification of aortic regurgitation. Open Heart 2020;7(1):e001158.
24. Chelu RG, van den Bosch AE, van Kranenburg M, et al. Qualitative grading of aortic regurgitation: a pilot study comparing CMR 4D flow and echocardiography. Int J Cardiovasc Imaging 2016;32(2):301–7.
25. Chelu RG, Wanambiro KW, Hsiao A, et al. Cloud-processed 4D CMR flow imaging for pulmonary flow quantification. Eur J Radiol 2016;85(10): 1849–56.
26. Westenberg JJ, Roes SD, Ajmone Marsan N, et al. Mitral valve and tricuspid valve blood flow: accurate quantification with 3D velocity-encoded MR imaging with retrospective valve tracking. Radiology 2008; 249(3):792–800.
27. Roes SD, Hammer S, van der Geest RJ, et al. Flow assessment through four heart valves simultaneously using 3-dimensional 3-directional velocity-encoded magnetic resonance imaging with retrospective valve tracking in healthy volunteers and patients with valvular regurgitation. Invest Radiol 2009;44(10):669–75.
28. Juffermans JF, Minderhoud SCS, Wittgren J, et al. Multicenter Consistency Assessment of Valvular Flow Quantification With Automated Valve Tracking in 4D Flow CMR. JACC Cardiovasc Imaging 2021; 14(7):1354–66.
29. Kamphuis VP, Roest AAW, Ajmone Marsan N, et al. Automated Cardiac Valve Tracking for Flow Quantification with Four-dimensional Flow MRI. Radiology 2019;290(1):70–8.
30. Wardley J, Swift A, Ryding A, et al. Four-dimensional flow cardiovascular magnetic resonance for the assessment of mitral stenosis. Eur Heart J Case Rep 2021;5(12):ytab465.
31. Baumgartner H, Bonhoeffer P, De Groot NM, et al. ESC Guidelines for the management of grown-up congenital heart disease (new version 2010). Eur Heart J 2010;31(23):2915–57.
32. Riesenkampff E, Fernandes JF, Meier S, et al. Pressure fields by flow-sensitive, 4D, velocity-encoded CMR in patients with aortic coarctation. JACC Cardiovasc Imaging 2014;7(9):920–6.
33. Verma S, Siu SC. Aortic dilatation in patients with bicuspid aortic valve. N Engl J Med 2014;370(20): 1920–9.
34. Rodríguez-Palomares JF, Dux-Santoy L, Guala A, et al. Aortic flow patterns and wall shear stress maps by 4D-flow cardiovascular magnetic resonance in the assessment of aortic dilatation in bicuspid aortic valve disease. J Cardiovasc Magn Reson 2018;20(1):28.
35. Hope MD, Meadows AK, Hope TA, et al. Images in cardiovascular medicine. Evaluation of bicuspid aortic valve and aortic coarctation with 4D flow magnetic resonance imaging. Circulation 2008;117(21): 2818–9.
36. Mahadevia R, Barker AJ, Schnell S, et al. Bicuspid aortic cusp fusion morphology alters aortic three-dimensional outflow patterns, wall shear stress, and expression of aortopathy. Circulation 2014; 129(6):673–82.
37. Hope MD, Hope TA, Crook SE, et al. 4D flow CMR in assessment of valve-related ascending aortic disease. JACC Cardiovasc Imaging 2011;4(7):781–7.
38. Bollache E, Guzzardi DG, Sattari S, et al. Aortic valve-mediated wall shear stress is heterogeneous and predicts regional aortic elastic fiber thinning in bicuspid aortic valve-associated aortopathy. J Thorac Cardiovasc Surg 2018;156(6):2112–20.e2.
39. Kiema M, Sarin JK, Kauhanen SP, et al. Wall Shear Stress Predicts Media Degeneration and Biomechanical Changes in Thoracic Aorta. Front Physiol 2022;13:934941.
40. Soulat G, Scott MB, Allen BD, et al. Association of Regional Wall Shear Stress and Progressive Ascending Aorta Dilation in Bicuspid Aortic Valve. JACC Cardiovasc Imaging 2022;15(1):33–42.
41. Guala A, Dux-Santoy L, Teixido-Tura G, et al. Wall Shear Stress Predicts Aortic Dilation in Patients With Bicuspid Aortic Valve. JACC Cardiovasc Imaging 2022;15(1):46–56.
42. Minderhoud SCS, Roos-Hesselink JW, Chelu RG, et al. Wall shear stress angle is associated with aortic growth in bicuspid aortic valve patients. Eur Heart J Cardiovasc Imaging 2022;23(12):1680–9.
43. Allen BD, Aouad PJ, Burris NS, et al. Detection and Hemodynamic Evaluation of Flap Fenestrations in Type B Aortic Dissection with 4D Flow MRI: Comparison with Conventional MRI and CTA. Radiol Cardiothorac Imaging 2019;1(1). https://doi.org/10.1148/ryct.2019180009.
44. Marlevi D, Sotelo JA, Grogan-Kaylor R, et al. False lumen pressure estimation in type B aortic dissection using 4D flow cardiovascular magnetic resonance: comparisons with aortic growth. J Cardiovasc Magn Reson 2021;23(1):51.
45. Chu S, Kilinc O, Pradella M, et al. Baseline 4D Flow-Derived in vivo Hemodynamic Parameters Stratify Descending Aortic Dissection Patients With Enlarging Aortas. Front Cardiovasc Med 2022;9:905718.
46. Jacobs K, Hahn L, Horowitz M, et al. Hemodynamic Assessment of Structural Heart Disease Using 4D

Flow MRI: How We Do It. AJR Am J Roentgenol 2021;217(6):1322–32.
47. Horowitz MJ, Kupsky DF, El-Said HG, et al. 4D Flow MRI Quantification of Congenital Shunts: Comparison to Invasive Catheterization. Radiol Cardiothorac Imaging 2021;3(2):e200446.
48. Chelu RG, Horowitz M, Sucha D, et al. Evaluation of atrial septal defects with 4D flow MRI-multilevel and inter-reader reproducibility for quantification of shunt severity. Magma 2019;32(2):269–79.
49. Imoto Y, Sese A, Joh K. Redirection of the hepatic venous flow for the treatment of pulmonary arteriovenous malformations after Fontan operation. Pediatr Cardiol 2006;27(4):490–2.
50. Oosterhof T, Vriend JW, Mulder BJ. Letter regarding article by Frigiola et al, "pulmonary regurgitation is an important determinant of right ventricular contractile dysfunction in patients with surgically repaired tetralogy of Fallot". Circulation 2005;111(8): e112. author reply e112.
51. Isorni MA, Martins D, Ben Moussa N, et al. 4D flow MRI versus conventional 2D for measuring pulmonary flow after Tetralogy of Fallot repair. Int J Cardiol 2020;300:132–6.
52. François CJ, Srinivasan S, Schiebler ML, et al. 4D cardiovascular magnetic resonance velocity mapping of alterations of right heart flow patterns and main pulmonary artery hemodynamics in tetralogy of Fallot. J Cardiovasc Magn Reson 2012;14(1):16.
53. Gabbour M, Schnell S, Jarvis K, et al. 4-D flow magnetic resonance imaging: blood flow quantification compared to 2-D phase-contrast magnetic resonance imaging and Doppler echocardiography. Pediatr Radiol 2015;45(6):804–13.
54. Hsiao A, Alley MT, Massaband P, et al. Improved cardiovascular flow quantification with time-resolved volumetric phase-contrast MRI. Pediatr Radiol 2011;41(6):711–20.
55. Schnell S, Ansari SA, Vakil P, et al. Three-dimensional hemodynamics in intracranial aneurysms: influence of size and morphology. J Magn Reson Imaging 2014;39(1):120–31.
56. Zhang M, Peng F, Li Y, et al. Associations between morphology and hemodynamics of intracranial aneurysms based on 4D flow and black-blood magnetic resonance imaging. Quant Imaging Med Surg 2021;11(2):597–607.
57. Futami K, Uno T, Misaki K, et al. Identification of Vortex Cores in Cerebral Aneurysms on 4D Flow MRI. AJNR Am J Neuroradiol 2019;40(12):2111–6.
58. Wu C, Ansari SA, Honarmand AR, et al. Evaluation of 4D vascular flow and tissue perfusion in cerebral arteriovenous malformations: influence of Spetzler-Martin grade, clinical presentation, and AVM risk factors. AJNR Am J Neuroradiol 2015;36(6):1142–9.
59. Hope MD, Purcell DD, Hope TA, et al. Complete intracranial arterial and venous blood flow evaluation with 4D flow MR imaging. AJNR Am J Neuroradiol 2009;30(2):362–6.
60. Wu C, Schnell S, Vakil P, et al. In Vivo Assessment of the Impact of Regional Intracranial Atherosclerotic Lesions on Brain Arterial 3D Hemodynamics. AJNR Am J Neuroradiol 2017;38(3):515–22.
61. Vali A, Aristova M, Vakil P, et al. Semi-automated analysis of 4D flow MRI to assess the hemodynamic impact of intracranial atherosclerotic disease. Magn Reson Med 2019;82(2):749–62.
62. Rivera-Rivera LA, Cody KA, Eisenmenger L, et al. Assessment of vascular stiffness in the internal carotid artery proximal to the carotid canal in Alzheimer's disease using pulse wave velocity from low rank reconstructed 4D flow MRI. J Cereb Blood Flow Metab 2021;41(2):298–311.
63. Rivera-Rivera LA, Cody KA, Rutkowski D, et al. Intracranial vascular flow oscillations in Alzheimer's disease from 4D flow MRI. Neuroimage Clin 2020;28: 102379.
64. Rivera-Rivera LA, Schubert T, Turski P, et al. Changes in intracranial venous blood flow and pulsatility in Alzheimer's disease: A 4D flow MRI study. J Cereb Blood Flow Metab 2017;37(6):2149–58.
65. Stankovic Z, Jung B, Collins J, et al. Reproducibility study of four-dimensional flow MRI of arterial and portal venous liver hemodynamics: influence of spatio-temporal resolution. Magn Reson Med 2014; 72(2):477–84.
66. Roldán-Alzate A, Frydrychowicz A, Said A, et al. Impaired regulation of portal venous flow in response to a meal challenge as quantified by 4D flow MRI. J Magn Reson Imaging 2015;42(4): 1009–17.
67. Keller EJ, Kulik L, Stankovic Z, et al. JOURNAL CLUB: Four-Dimensional Flow MRI-Based Splenic Flow Index for Predicting Cirrhosis-Associated Hypersplenism. AJR Am J Roentgenol 2017;209(1): 46–54.
68. Stankovic Z, Blanke P, Markl M. Usefulness of 4D MRI flow imaging to control TIPS function. Am J Gastroenterol 2012;107(2):327–8.
69. Bannas P, Roldán-Alzate A, Johnson KM, et al. Longitudinal Monitoring of Hepatic Blood Flow before and after TIPS by Using 4D-Flow MR Imaging. Radiology 2016;281(2):574–82.
70. Ishikawa T, Takehara Y, Yamashita S, et al. Hemodynamic assessment in a child with renovascular hypertension using time-resolved three-dimensional cine phase-contrast MRI. J Magn Reson Imaging 2015;41(1):165–8.
71. Motoyama D, Ishii Y, Takehara Y, et al. Four-dimensional phase-contrast vastly undersampled isotropic projection reconstruction (4D PC-VIPR) MR evaluation of the renal arteries in transplant recipients: Preliminary results. J Magn Reson Imaging 2017;46(2): 595–603.

# MR Imaging for Intracranial Vessel Wall Imaging: Pearls and Pitfalls

Laura B. Eisenmenger, MD[a,*], Alma Spahic, MS[a], Joseph Scott McNally, MD, PhD[b], Kevin M. Johnson, PhD[a], Jae W. Song, MD, MS[c], Jacqueline C. Junn, MD[d]

**KEYWORDS**

• Vessel wall imaging • Intracranial atherosclerotic disease • Vasculopathy • Vasculitis

**KEY POINTS**

- While conventional luminal imaging provides evaluation of the intracranial arterial lumen (computed tomography angiography, magnetic resonance angiography, digital subtraction angiography), vessel wall imaging provides noninvasive evaluation of the site where pathology occurs, the vessel wall.
- It can be used to differentiate among and monitor disease response in intracranial vasculopathies and potentially risk stratify patients with vascular pathology.
- Intracranial vessel wall imaging has technical requirements including high spatial resolution, multiplanar acquisitions, multiple tissue weighting, and suppression of intraluminal blood and cerebrospinal fluid flow.

## INTRODUCTION

Conventional vascular imaging methods, including computed tomography angiography, magnetic resonance angiography (MRA), and digital subtraction angiography, have primarily focused on evaluating the vascular lumen. However, these techniques are not intended to evaluate abnormalities within the vessel wall where many cerebrovascular pathologies reside. With increased interest for the visualization and study of the vessel wall, high-resolution vessel wall imaging (VWI) has gained traction.

Since intracranial VWI was first reported in 1994, there has been a progressive rise in its use. The first article that reported intracranial vessel wall characteristics was in intramural hematomas, which was followed by evaluation of cerebral atherosclerosis in 1995.[1,2] Over the past two decades, there has been a rapid increase in the number of vessel wall publications.[3] In 2018, Song and colleagues[3] performed a systematic review on intracranial vessel wall studies and found that many VWI studies focus on steno-occlusive disease including intracranial atherosclerosis followed by arterial dissection, vasculitis, Moyamoya disease (MMD), post-endovascular changes, and reversible cerebral vasoconstriction syndrome (RCVS). Other vascular pathologies investigated by VWI include vascular malformations with intracranial aneurysms as the most frequently investigated pathology.[4–11]

With increasing utility and interest in VWI, application of proper protocols and understanding imaging characteristics identified thus far are important for the interpreting radiologists. Although more work needs to be done in this area, this review will first discuss currently proposed technical aspects and considerations to optimize VWI studies then illustrate imaging

[a] University of Wisconsin – Madison, 1111 Highland Avenue, Madison, WI 53705, USA; [b] University of Utah, 50 N Medical Dr, Salt Lake City, UT 84132, USA; [c] University of Pennsylvania, 3400 Spruce Street, Philadelphia, PA 19104, USA; [d] Icahn School of Medicine at Mount Sinai, 1 Gustave Levy Place, Box 1234, New York City, NY 10029, USA
* Corresponding author.
*E-mail address:* LEisenmenger@uwhealth.org

Magn Reson Imaging Clin N Am 31 (2023) 461–474
https://doi.org/10.1016/j.mric.2023.04.006
1064-9689/23/

manifestations of vascular pathologies including atherosclerosis, vasculitis, aneurysm, and other vascular malformations.

### MR Imaging Technique

To accurately evaluate intracranial vessels, many technical factors need to be considered. A multidisciplinary study group was formed by the American Society of Neuroradiology in 2012 to assist in the development and implementation of VWI in clinical setting.[12] First, both high spatial resolution and contrast-to-noise ratio (CNR) are needed to visualize the vessel wall and to evaluate wall pathology in detail.[13] Both signal-to-noise ratio (SNR) and CNR are affected by the magnetic field strength, with 3T preferred over 1.5 T and even some studies investigating the use of 7T.[14] Second, different tissue weighted sequences (T1 precontrast, T1 postcontrast, and T2-weighted, and proton density) can be obtained. Additionally, luminal-based imaging, such as time-of-flight or contrast-enhanced MRA, is also often included. Third, both multiplanar 2D or 3D acquisitions can be used, each of which has their own advantages and disadvantages.

### Spatial Resolution

Histopathologic vessel wall thickness varies from 0.2 to 0.3 mm for middle cerebral arteries (MCAs) and 0.2 to 0.4 mm for distal internal carotid arteries[15] whereas radiologic evaluations have shown thicker vessel walls for MCAs and internal carotid arteries, measuring approximately 1 mm.[16] Differences in the measurements can be due to histopathologic preparation technique that results in cell shrinkage, overestimation on imaging from partial volume averaging effect due to large voxels, or a combination of both.[17,18] Although vessel wall thickness is smaller than reasonably achievable VWI voxel dimensions, VWI can still be acquired as one can suppress intraluminal blood and surrounding cerebrospinal fluid (CSF) signal within the voxel.

Higher field strength provides better SNR. According to the Study Group of the American Society of Neuroradiology on VWI, a 2D sequence with $2.0 \times 0.4 \times 0.4$ mm is sufficient for adequate balance between spatial resolution and SNR at 3T and 0.5 mm for 3D sequence.[12]

### Contrast-to-Noise Ratio/Blood and Cerebrospinal Fluid Suppression Techniques

High CNR is needed to visualize and characterize the vessel walls. CNR is dependent on sequence parameters and magnetic field strength. In general, it increases with increased field strength. For VWI, CNR consists of signal contrast of the vessel wall compared with its surroundings, particularly blood and CSF. Therefore, achieving high CNR requires suppressing luminal blood and surrounding CSF signal.

Black–blood sequences are used to suppress the incoming blood signal. These techniques take advantage of the different properties of flowing blood and the stationary vessel wall, utilizing 3D turbo spin echo (TSE) with variable flip-angle refocusing pulses.[13,19] Other techniques take advantage of pre-pulses to suppress the blood, such as double inversion recovery sequence by suppressing both the flow and the longitudinal relaxation time (T1) properties of blood.[20] Both CSF and blood can be suppressed with double inversion recovery technique. Delay alternating with nutation for tailored excitation (DANTE) is used to null the CSF signal.[21] Postreadout anti-driven equilibrium modules are also used to suppress CSF signal.[22–24]

### Multiple Tissue Weightings

Assessment of the intracranial vessel walls also includes obtaining different pulse sequences with varying tissue contrast weighting (T1 precontrast, T1 postcontrast, and T2-weighted, and proton density) as well as luminal images (time-of-flight or contrast-enhanced MRA). For intracranial VWI, T1 precontrast and T1 postcontrast are the most commonly used across different pathologies intracranially, T2-weighted images can be particularly useful for atherosclerotic disease and proton density-weighted images for evaluating arterial dissections.

### Multiplanar 2D or 3D Acquisitions

Both 2D and 3D acquisitions have been used in VWI protocols although 3D is increasingly being adopted for intracranial artery assessment. 2D sequences may require multiple acquisitions in the desired orthogonal planes. It is best suited for a known area of abnormality (ie, stenosis) with adequate field-of-view over the specific area. The 2D acquisitions can result in partial volume averaging as vessels are tortuous[25] whereas 3D images can generate reformatted images from isotropic data. Variable flip angle refocusing pulse with fast spin echo is commonly used 3D sequences.[26] These include volume isotropic TSE acquisition (Philips Healthcare, Best, the Netherlands), volumetric isotropically reconstructed turbo spin-echo acquisition (Philips Healthcare, Best, the Netherlands), sampling perfection with application-optimized contrast by using different flip angle evolutions (Siemens,

Erlangen, German), and CUBE (GE Healthcare, Milwaukee, Wisconsin).

### Peripheral Pulse Gating

Peripheral pulse gating is not routinely used in intracranial VWI. However, it has potential benefit when evaluating dilated intracranial arteries or large aneurysms.[12]

### Clinical Use

#### Intracranial Atherosclerosis

Previously, atherosclerotic plaque characterization was mainly examining the degree of stenosis; however, lipids, thrombotic substances (platelets and fibrin), and connective tissue matrix comprise atherosclerotic plaques. Plaque core volume increase, fibrous cap rupture, and intraplaque hemorrhage are associated with plaque progression.[27] Because of this, there is increasing interest in evaluating plaque composition and inflammation to identify vulnerable plaques,[28] and VWI is a noninvasive imaging modality for studying intracranial plaque composition.[29]

Imaging features of high-risk plaque include plaque enhancement, vessel wall remodeling (positive remodeling), intraplaque hemorrhage (T1 hyperintensity), and surface irregularity/thickness; T2 hyperintensity was not associated with downstream ischemic events in a meta-analysis pooling six studies, recognizing a T2w signal intensity threshold may be more specific.[30] Atherosclerotic plaques typically show eccentric, nonuniform arterial wall thickening and enhancement, which is thought to be secondary to neovascularization, inflammation, and endothelial dysfunction resulting in gadolinium leakage (**Fig. 1**).[12,31] The plaque adjacent to the lumen often shows T2 hyperintensity and may enhance; however, the component adjacent to the enhancement shows T2 hypointensity without enhancement. There may also be a third thinner peripheral enhancing layer. This imaging appearance corresponds to carotid endarterectomy specimens that showed fibrous cap that corresponds to the enhancing layer adjacent to the lumen, then the lipid core that does not enhance, and the third thinner peripheral layer that is due to increased vasa vasorum in the adventitia.[12,32] However, not all intracranial plaques show all three components, possibly due to technical limitations of spatial resolution. Furthermore, variability in the VWI appearance of plaques, regardless of stroke acuity, suggests further studies are warranted. Nevertheless, presence of contrast enhancement of a presumed intracranial plaque on VWI has been showing to be strongly associated with downstream acute ischemia accounting for sources of bias and variability in study design and instrumentation[30] (**Fig. 2**) and studies suggest lack of enhancement or decreasing enhancement on follow-up imaging after an ischemic event suggests the plaque is not culprit.[33] Taken together, contrast enhancement may be a valuable imaging biomarker for culprit plaques.

Vessel walls can undergo positive, negative, or no remodeling (**Fig. 3**). Positive remodeling is when atherosclerotic plaque results in outward bulging of the outer surface of the artery, often secondary to hemorrhage or inflammation.[34] In coronary arteries, positive remodeling is more common in plaques with hemorrhage and inflammation which indicate higher-risk vessel wall pathology.[35] In addition, identifying positive remodeling is important as positive remodeling has been shown to be a specific vulnerability marker in intracranial plaques.[36,37] Negative remodeling is when plaques show reduction in outer diameter, which is thought to be due to a fibrotic healing response.[38] Although MCA remodeling studies, on average, have shown positive remodeling for symptomatic plaques and negative remodeling for asymptomatic plaques, no definite consensus has been made as some studies showed no significant difference.[12,39] More studies are needed to evaluate the relationship between the location of plaques and the ones at a higher risk for downstream ischemic events.

T1 hyperintensity, reflecting intraplaque hemorrhage, and surface irregularity were more commonly seen in symptomatic plaque than the asymptomatic ones, which was also verified by carotid endarterectomy specimen.[40,41] Most VWI studies have shown that symptomatic plaques are thicker than asymptomatic plaques.[42,43] In addition, symptomatic plaques showed surface irregularity more frequently than the asymptomatic ones.[44]

Assessing the location of the atherosclerotic plaques and determining plaque inflammation are important for risk assessment. Similar to the coronary circulations, MCA plaques are more commonly seen opposite of branch artery ostium at the ventral or inferior aspects (45% and 32%, respectively) as opposed to the superior or dorsal aspects where penetrating arterial branches arise from (14% and 9%, respectively).[45] However, superior wall involvement was more commonly associated with infarctions in MCA plaques than those plaques without infarction.[45]

#### Vasculitis

Vessel wall inflammation leading to a beaded appearance of the arteries with varying degrees

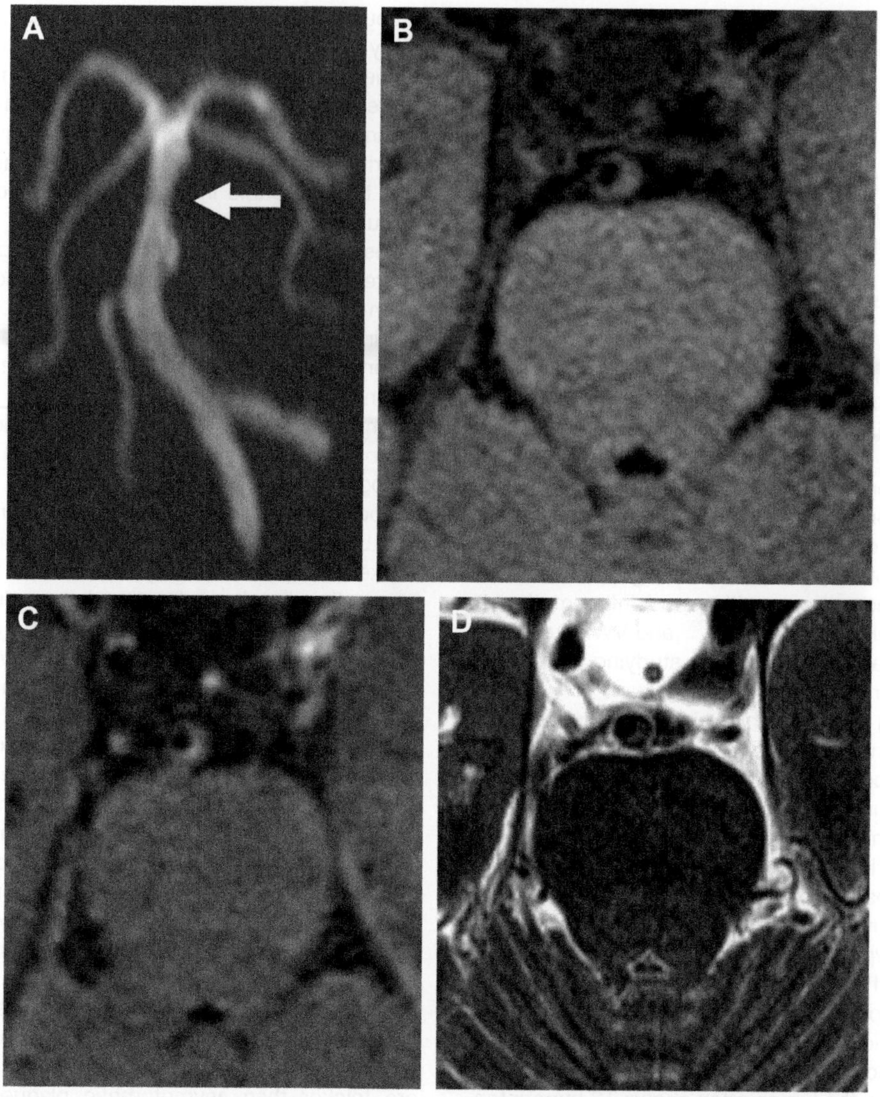


**Fig. 1.** Atherosclerotic plaque: (*A*) 60 year old woman with mild narrowing of the mid-basilar artery on TOF MRA (*arrow*). (*B*) Precontrast T1 vessel wall imaging shows eccentric wall thickening and enhancement on the postcontrast T1 image (*C*). (*D*) There is also juxtaluminal T2 signal intensity at the site of eccentricity. The findings favored an atherosclerotic plaque.

of stenosis and ectasia are often seen in vasculitis with luminal imaging. Central nervous system (CNS) vasculitis is challenging to diagnose both clinically and radiologically. It can be divided into the idiopathic primary form or be secondary to systemic vasculitis. VWI has been used to facilitate a diagnose CNS vasculitis, which often shows smooth concentric wall thickening and enhancement, whereas atheromatous plaque typically shows eccentric enhancement (**Figs. 4** and **5**).[46] However, eccentric wall enhancement has also been shown in vasculitis.[47] Vasa vasorum can be a route of delivery for inflammatory cytokines and lead to vasculitis, which can contribute to enhancement beyond the vessel wall extending into the perivascular tissue, especially for extracranial vessels.[48,49] In addition to perivascular enhancement, additional features that may help characterize vasculitis include concentric vessel wall thickening and edema.[49]

### *Aneurysms*

Unruptured intracranial aneurysms are found in 3% to 5% of the adult population worldwide, and while the majority will never rupture, 27% of patients who develop aneurysmal subarachnoid hemorrhage may die within 12 months.[50,51] Early recognition of aneurysms with high rupture risk is crucial in

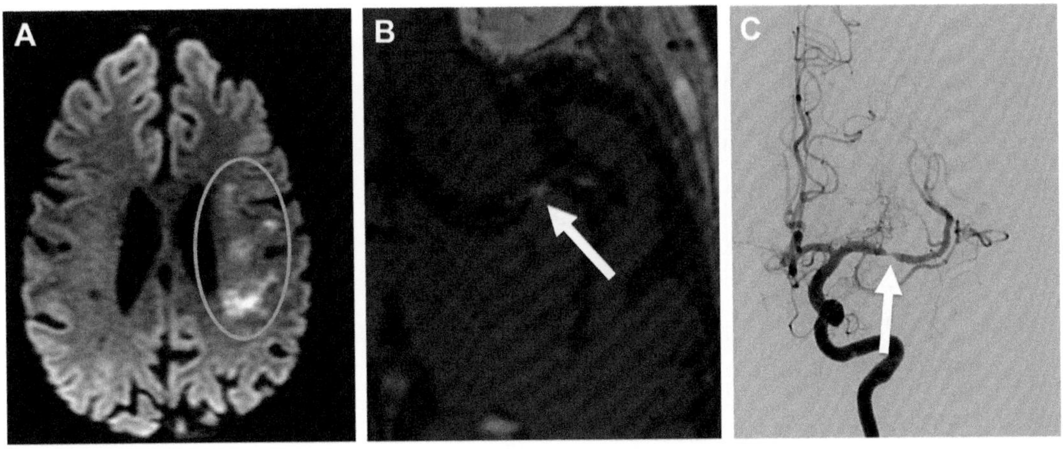


Fig. 2. VWI of culprit plaque. (*A*) Diffusion-weighted imaging shows restricted diffusion within the white matter of the left corona radiata (*pink oval*), consistent with acute ischemia (*B*). Contrast-enhanced T1 vessel wall imaging shows enhancement of the wall of the left middle cerebral artery (*white arrow*) (*C*), corresponding to the most likely culprit atherosclerotic plaque and vascular narrowing (*white arrow*).

stratification, and VWI may be a tool that could assist in this process. VWI has been used to evaluate ruptured and unruptured aneurysms to identify imaging biomarkers for unstable aneurysms.

Currently, the risk of rupture of intracranial aneurysms is evaluated based on size, location, shape, patient's ethnicity, age, hypertension, and history of previous aneurysmal rupture, which has its

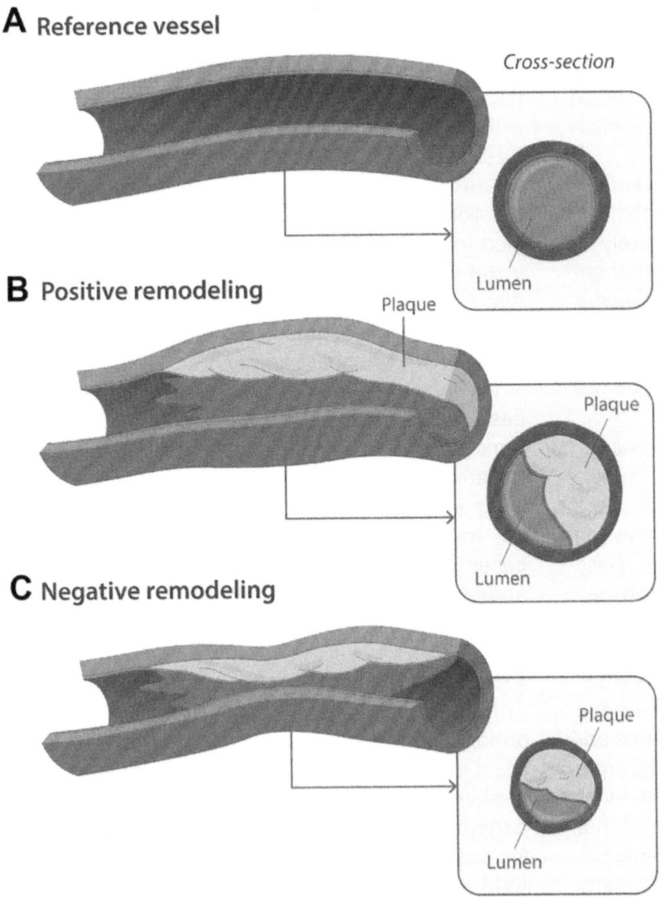


Fig. 3. Vascular remodeling: (*A*) In normal vessels, the vessel wall is smooth and covered by endothelium. But in atherosclerotid disease, vessels can undergo positive or negative remodeling, depending on atherosclerotic plaque growth pattern. (*B*) Positive remodeling results when atherosclerotic plaque leads to outward bulging of the outer surface of the artery. (*C*) Negative remodeling results when there is a decrease in outer diameter thought to be due to fibrotic healing response from the atheromatous plaque.

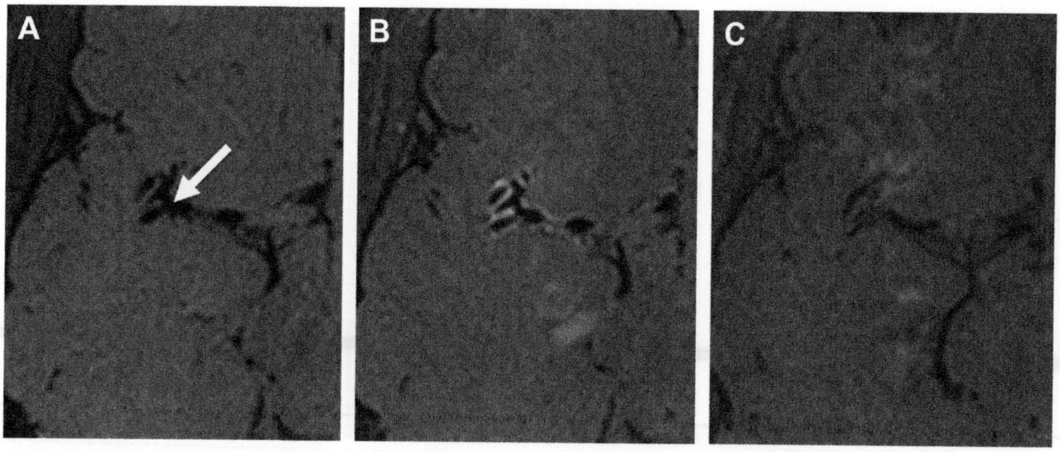


**Fig. 4.** Vasculitis: T1 SPACE black blood MR imaging precontrast (*A*) and postcontrast (*B*) in a patient with right MCA (*arrow*) vasculitis and stroke. Vessel wall enhancement (middle) indicates endothelial contrast leakage. Repeat postcontrast imaging (*C*) at 1 month after steroid treatment demonstrates resolution of the right MCA wall enhancement.

limitations. Therefore, it is important to identify imaging features of high-risk aneurysms for risk-stratification. Based on histopathology, vessel wall structure and inflammatory changes are important in the aneurysm's life cycle.[52] Histologic studies have shown an association between aneurysm enhancement and vessel wall inflammation.[6,53] However, other studies have shown that aneurysm wall enhancement is a nonspecific finding, which can be due to other factors such as neovascularization and presence of vasa vasorum.[54]

Most studies have been done on ruptured aneurysms which have thick peripheral enhancement, whereas unruptured aneurysms are less likely to enhance.[4,6,7] Additionally, vessel wall enhancement was more frequently seen in unstable aneurysms (ruptured, symptomatic, or morphologically changing), and this principle has been applied to evaluate unruptured intracranial aneurysms for risk stratification (**Fig. 6**).[4,6,7,54]

Evaluating aneurysm stability is very helpful, especially for unruptured aneurysms. Meta-analyses of unruptured aneurysm studies were performed to evaluate the association between aneurysm wall enhancement and rupture risk. These studies showed a significant association between aneurysm wall enhancement and aneurysm rupture.[55,56] When looking at circumferential wall enhancement, circumferential wall enhancement in small aneurysms was associated with aneurysm rupture, whereas this finding was limited in large aneurysms.[55] An important finding from Molenberg's meta-analysis was that aneurysm wall enhancement had a high negative predictive value in that most nonenhancing aneurysms were stable,[56] which can then be used to identify stable aneurysms that do not need close follow-up or intervention.

Assessment of aneurysm wall enhancement needs further prospective and longitudinal studies as studies have shown both unstable and stable aneurysms can enhance; therefore, resulting in low positive predictive value.[56] An important imaging aspect to be cognizant of aneurysmal flow artifact can mimic enhancement. Utilizing techniques such as motion-sensitized driven-equilibrium (MSDE) and DANTE can be used to address this artifact to evaluate for true enhancement. Voxel sizes are also important when selecting appropriate imaging parameters of aneurysms as smaller voxel sizes result in better signal suppression for higher flowing aneurysms whereas larger voxel sizes are better for aneurysms with slower flow.[57] Additionally, quantification of enhancement should be investigated rather than qualitative assessment of enhancement.[58]

VWI has also been used to identify culprit sources of hemorrhage in patients with computed tomography or catheter cerebral angiogram-negative subarachnoid hemorrhage.[59] Study by Jung and colleagues showed VWI was able to identify the source of subarachnoid hemorrhage in cases without a culprit on conventional cerebral angiogram, which included dissection, blister aneurysm, and fusiform aneurysms.[60]

## *Arteriovenous Malformations*

Arteriovenous malformations (AVMs) are due to abnormal connections between arteries and veins (via a nidus formed of pathological, immature vessels) without intervening capillaries within the brain parenchyma. VWI is useful to evaluate thrombus formation in a nidus and potentially in assessing AVM rupture risk. A case series with 13 patients by Matouk and colleagues[5] showed that VWI

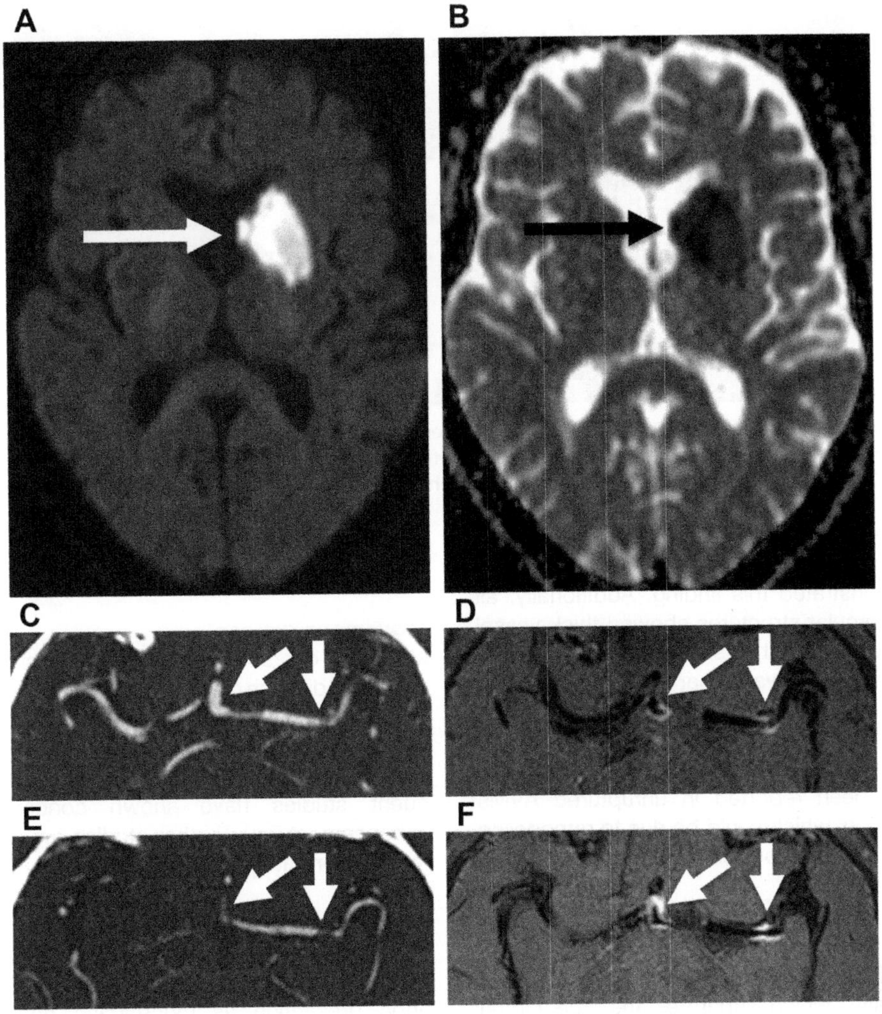


Fig. 5. Varicella Zoster Virus (VZV) vasculitis: 71 year old woman underwent imaging workup for a recent stroke shown on diffusion-weighted imaging (DWI) (*A*) and apparent diffusion coefficient (ADC) map (*B*) in the left lenticulostriate distribution (*arrows*). Initial computed tomography angiography (CTA) showed subtle lumen irregularity in the A1 segment of the left anterior cerebral artery (ACA) and in the M1 segment of the left middle cerebral artery (MCA) (*C, arrows*). Initial vessel wall MR imaging showed avid enhancement on T1 SPACE in the ACA and MCA vessel walls (*D, arrows*). Initial cerebrospinal fluid (CSF) was positive for VZV on polymerase chain reaction (PCR) analysis. Despite treatment, 1-month follow-up imaging showed progressive ACA and MCA lumen narrowing on CTA (*E, arrows*) and worsened vessel wall enhancement on vessel wall MR imaging (*F, arrows*). VZV PCR also remained positive on follow-up CSF sampling.

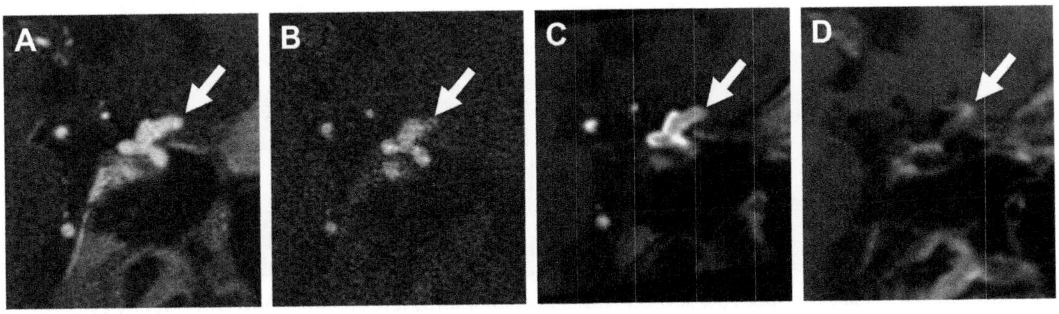


Fig. 6. Aneurysm: Contrast enhanced MRA (*A*), 4D-Flow MRA (*B*), and 3D-TOF MRA (*C*) show an internal carotid artery aneurysm with secondary outpouching (*white arrow*). Postcontrast T1-weighted "black blood" VWI (*D*) depicts arterial wall enhancement at the tip of the secondary pouch (*white arrow*).

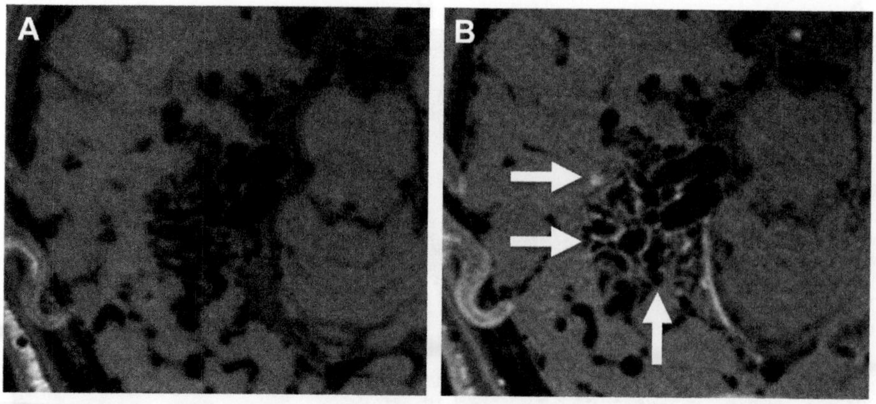


Fig. 7. Arteriovenous malformation: (*A*) T1 precontrast vessel wall imaging shows a large right temporoparietal AVM without any evidence of old hemorrhage on susceptibility-weighted imaging (not shown). (*B*) On postcontrast T1 VWI, there were multiple areas of vessel wall enhancement within the nidus (*white arrows*).

was helpful in identifying the rupture site in ruptured intracranial AVMs, although not all patients demonstrated this finding. Additionally, all ruptured vascular structures showed thick vessel wall enhancement in their study. Other case series also showed vessel wall enhancement in ruptured AVMs involving intranidal aneurysms.[61–63] Furthermore, vessel wall enhancement within the nidus and adjacent to the nidus (perivascular enhancement) has been reported in unruptured AVMs (**Figs. 7** and **8**), which could be due to remodeling or complex blood flow patterns as opposed to active inflammation.[64]

### Dissection

Intracranial dissection appears as a curvilinear T2 hyperintensity, which separates the true lumen from the false lumen with eccentric wall thickening.[65] VWI has also been shown to depict the intimal flap better than luminal imaging with hematoma visible on both T1 and T2-weighted images and wall enhancement.[66,67] When evaluating intramural hematoma, the signal characteristics can change with time as with other intracranial hemorrhage.[1]

### Moyamoya disease

MMD is characterized by progressive steno-occlusive disease classically involving the distal internal carotid arteries or proximal MCAs. Initial studies on MMD showed a lack of arterial wall thickening and enhancement.[68] However, subsequent studies have shown concentric wall enhancement.[69,70] Further studies are needed to resolve contradicting findings (see **Fig. 8**).

### Reversible cerebral vasoconstriction syndrome

RCVS is characterized by diffuse, multifocal arterial constriction that resolves in about 3 months, often presenting as thunderclap headaches.[71] VWI has been useful in differentiating it from other arteriopathies.[72,73] While both RCVS and vasculitis show vessel wall thickening, RCVS has typically no or little enhancement (**Fig. 9**), as the cause is result of a sudden constriction or tightening of the vessels that supply blood to the brain, not

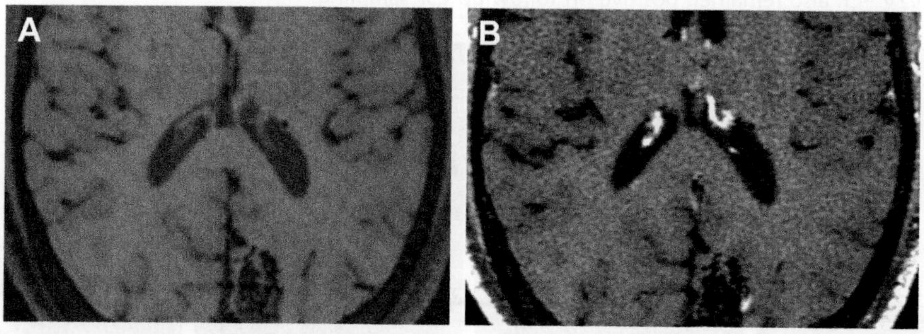


Fig. 8. Arteriovenous malformation: (*A*) Subject with a predominantly left occipital AVM without any evidence of old hemorrhage on susceptibility-weighted imaging (not shown). (*B*) On postcontrast VWI, there was only one area of vessel wall enhancement (*white arrow*), possibly related to complex or slow flow. No perivascular enhancement was present.

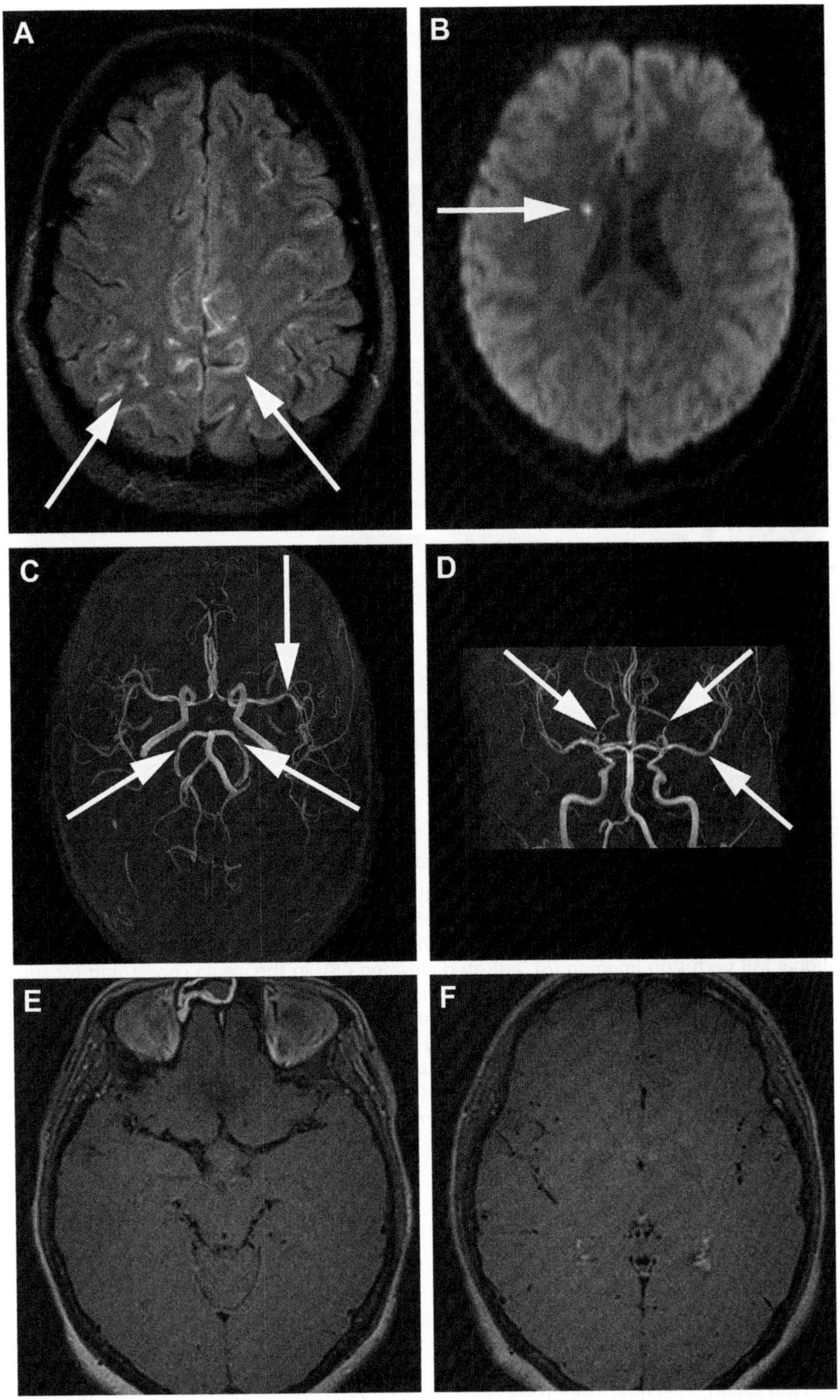


**Fig. 9.** Postpartum RCVS. A teenage postpartum woman with history of eclampsia and hemolysis, elevated liver enzymes, and low platelet count syndrome underwent stroke workup. MR imaging of the brain demonstrated posterior predominant blood–brain barrier breakdown and sulcal hyperintensity on T2 fluid attenuated inversion recovery (FLAIR) sequence (*A*, *arrows*) coupled with an acute punctate right corona radiata infarct on diffusion-weighted imaging (DWI) (B, *arrow*). TOF MRA MIP axial (*C*) and coronal (*D*) showed diffuse arterial narrowing (*arrows*). Postcontrast vwMR imaging T1 SPACE showed no vessel wall enhancement (*E* and *F*).

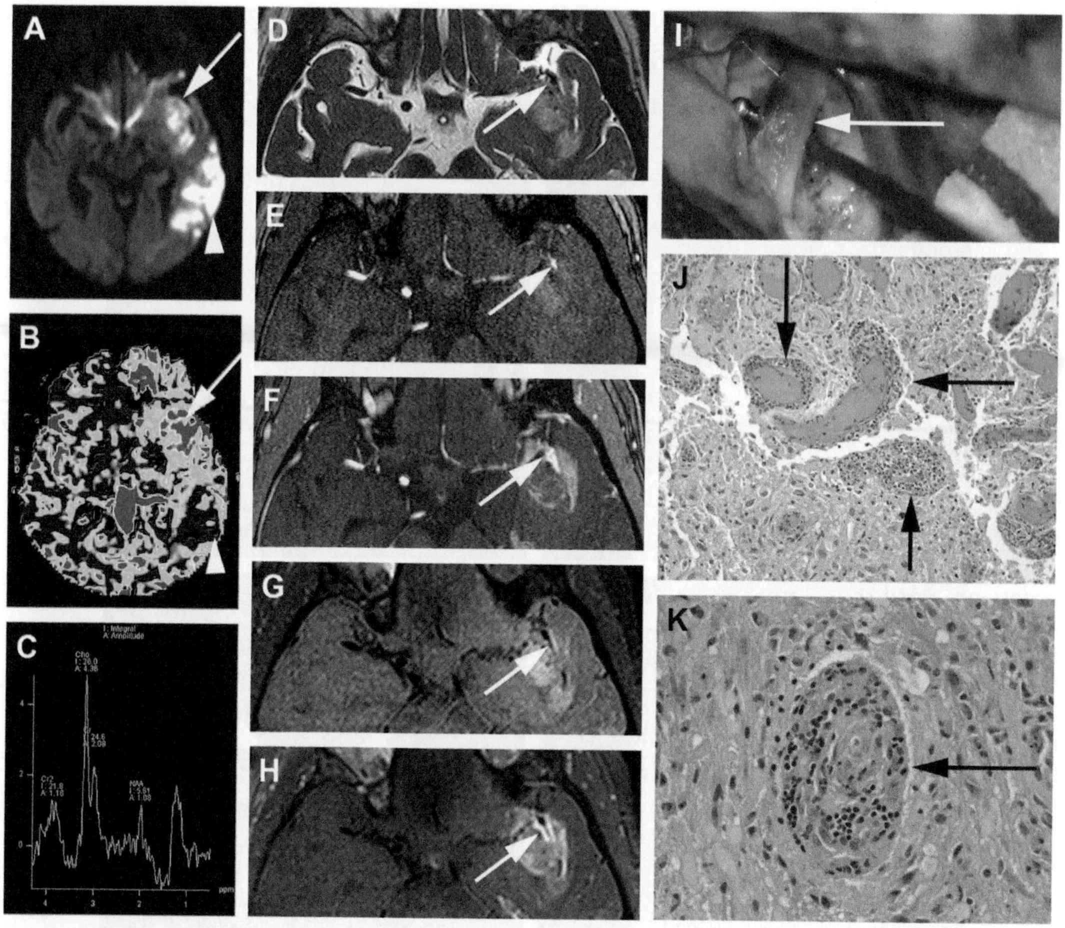


**Fig. 10.** Intravascular tumor invasion in patient with glioblastoma. A 59 year old woman undergoing stroke workup for slurred speech and an expressive aphasia. DTI trace imaging (*A*) revealed two areas of diffusion restriction, one appeared tumefactive in the insula (*arrow*) whereas the other appeared more infarct-like (*arrowhead*). Additional MR perfusion imaging (*B*) indicated elevated CBV in the insula concerning for tumor (*arrow*) but decreased CBV in the posterior temporal lobe which fit with infarct (*arrowhead*). MR spectroscopy (*C*) confirmed elevated choline and reversal of Hunter's angle in the insula, compatible with high grade tumor. Vessel wall MR imaging (*D–H*) showed tumor in close proximity to the left MCA flow void on T2 SPACE (*D, arrow*), narrowing of the MCA on TOF precontrast and postcontrast MRA (*E* and *F, arrow*), and thick vessel wall enhancement based on precontrast and postcontrast T1 SPACE (*G* and *H, arrow*). Intraoperative inspection confirmed tumor along the surface of the MCA at the Sylvian fissure (*I, arrow*). Pathology confirmed grade IV GBM with pseudopalisades of cellular tumor and whorled pattern on H&E staining at 200X and 400X (*J* and *K, arrows*).

inflammation; however, isolated cases with enhancement have been reported.[12]

### *Tumor invasion*

Some tumors have been associated with aneurysm development, possibly due to an increase in the directional blood flow due to a higher blood supply toward the lesion. This may induce secondary changes in the arterial wall and thus facilitate the formation of aneurysms.[74] Direct vessel wall invasion by tumor cells may also occur in glial tumors, lymphomas, and pituitary tumors, altering and potentially weakening the vessel wall.[75] Even if a rapid growth of the tumor does not give enough time to produce mechanisms for the formation of an aneurysm,[74,76] other consequences from treatment complications, such as radiation sequela, can lead to vasculopathies and stroke (**Fig. 10**).

## ARTIFACTS/LIMITATIONS

VWI relies on blood flow to suppress signal. However, blood flow is often laminar with slower flow near the vessel wall as opposed to center of the lumen. Utilizing inflow and outflow suppression of the lumen can result in incomplete suppression at the periphery of the vessel, which can mimic vessel wall thickening or hyperintensity and may be misinterpreted as "enhancement."[12] These artifacts are often more obvious in slow flow within an aneurysm, dilated arteries, or retrograde filling from collateral vessels.[77] Different techniques have been developed to decrease artifactual "enhancement" associated with slow flow and turbulent flow including DANTE and MSDE.[78]

Free-induction decay artifact can also hinder imaging interpretation, which results from repeated refocusing radiofrequency pulses with short echo times.[79] This artifact results in a linear dashed, "zigzag" pattern that may mimic pathology. Being aware of these limitations is essential to preventing misinterpretation.

## SUMMARY

VWI is noninvasive means to evaluate to the location of intracranial vascular pathology, the vessel wall. VWI can provide a useful adjunct to conventional luminal imaging. This includes differentiating among causes of intracranial arterial narrowing such as intracranial atherosclerotic plaque, vasculitis, RCVS, and arterial dissection as well as identifying symptomatic, nonstenotic disease of the intracranial arteries. More prospective studies are needed to further evaluate VWI imaging techniques, determine the sensitivity and specificity of VWI for different vascular pathologies, and the clinical implications to further refine the best clinical applications for these techniques.

## CLINICS CARE POINTS

- High spatial resolution and contrast-to-noise ratio (CNR) are needed to evaluate and visualized vessel wall and its pathology.
- Achieving high CNR requires suppresing luminal blood and surrounding CSF signal.
- High-risk plaque imaging features include plaque enhancement, vessel wall remodeling, intraplaque hemorrhage, and surface irregularity/thickness.
- Atherosclerotic plaques are typically eccentric, nonuniform arterial wall thickening and enhancement.
- Vasculitis often shows smooth, concentric wall thickening and enhancement although eccentric enhancement has also been shown in vasculitis.
- Aneurysm wall assessment needs further investigataion as both unstable and stable aneurysm can enhance.

## DISCLOSURE

L.B. Eisenmenger: This work is supported by the Clinical and Translational Science Award program, United States/NIH, United States, National Center for Advancing Translational Sciences, United States UL1TR002373 and KL2TR002374 (LE), and Wisconsin Alzheimer's Disease Research Center grant P30-AG062715 (LE). A. Spahic: Nothing to disclose. J. Scott McNally: Nothing to disclose. K.M. Johnson: Nothing to disclose. J. Song: Dr Song is supported by the American Heart Association Career Development Award (938082) and NINDS, United States, NIH (L30 NS118632). J.C. Junn: Nothing to disclose.

## REFERENCES

1. Kitanaka C, Tanaka J, Kuwahara M, et al. Magnetic resonance imaging study of intracranial vertebrobasilar artery dissections. Stroke 1994;25:571–5.
2. Aoki S, Shirouzu I, Sasaki Y, et al. Enhancement of the intracranial arterial wall at MR imaging: relationship to cerebral atherosclerosis. Radiology 1995; 194:477–81.
3. Song JW, Guiry SC, Shou H, et al. Qualitative assessment and reporting quality of intracranial vessel wall MR imaging studies: a systematic review. Am J Neuroradiol 2019;40:2025–32.
4. Matouk CC, Mandell DM, Gunel M, et al. Vessel wall magnetic resonance imaging identifies the site of rupture in patients with multiple intracranial aneurysms: proof of principle. Neurosurgery 2013;72: 492–6 [discussion:6].
5. Matouk CC, Cord B, Yeung J, et al. High-resolution vessel wall magnetic resonance imaging in intracranial aneurysms and brain arteriovenous malformations. Top Magn Reson Imaging 2016;25:49–55.
6. Edjlali M, Gentric JC, Regent-Rodriguez C, et al. Does aneurysmal wall enhancement on vessel wall MRI help to distinguish stable from unstable intracranial aneurysms? Stroke 2014;45:3704–6.
7. Nagahata S, Nagahata M, Obara M, et al. Wall enhancement of the intracranial aneurysms revealed by magnetic resonance vessel wall imaging using three-dimensional turbo spin-echo sequence with motion-sensitized driven-equilibrium: a sign of ruptured aneurysm? Clin Neuroradiol 2016;26: 277–83.
8. Tian B, Toossi S, Eisenmenger L, et al. Visualizing wall enhancement over time in unruptured intracranial aneurysms using 3D vessel wall imaging. J Magn Reson Imaging 2019;50:193–200.
9. Wang X, Zhu C, Leng Y, et al. Intracranial aneurysm wall enhancement associated with aneurysm rupture: a systematic review and meta-analysis. Acad Radiol 2019;26:664–73.

10. Liu X, Zhang Z, Zhu C, et al. Wall enhancement of intracranial saccular and fusiform aneurysms may differ in intensity and extension: a pilot study using 7-T high-resolution black-blood MRI. Eur Radiol 2020;30:301–7.
11. Zhu C, Wang X, Eisenmenger L, et al. Wall enhancement on black-blood MRI is independently associated with symptomatic status of unruptured intracranial saccular aneurysm. Eur Radiol 2020; 30:6413–20.
12. Mandell DM, Mossa-Basha M, Qiao Y, et al. Intracranial vessel wall MRI: principles and expert consensus recommendations of the American Society of Neuroradiology. AJNR Am J Neuroradiol 2017;38:218–29.
13. Qiao Y, Steinman DA, Qin Q, et al. Intracranial arterial wall imaging using three-dimensional high isotropic resolution black blood MRI at 3.0 Tesla. J Magn Reson Imaging 2011;34(1):22–30.
14. De Cocker LJ, Lindenholz A, Zwanenburg JJ, et al. Clinical vascular imaging in the brain at 7T. Neuroimage 2018;168:452–8.
15. Gutierrez J, Elkind MS, Petito C, et al. The contribution of HIV infection to intracranial arterial remodeling: a pilot study. Neuropathology 2013;33(3): 256–63.
16. Qiao Y, Guallar E, Suri FK, et al. MR Imaging Measures of Intracranial Atherosclerosis in a Population-based Study. Radiology 2016;280(3): 860–8.
17. Dobrin PB. Effect of histologic preparation on the cross-sectional area of arterial rings. J Surg Res 1996;61(2):413–5.
18. Xie Y, Yang Q, Xie G, et al. Improved black-blood imaging using DANTE-SPACE for simultaneous carotid and intracranial vessel wall evaluation. Magn Reson Med 2016;75(6):2286–94.
19. Weigel M, Henning J. Diffusion sensitivity of turbo spin echo sequences. Mag Reson Med 2012; 67(6):1528–37.
20. Edelman RR, Chien D, Kim D. Fast selective black blood MR imaging. Radiology 1991;181:655–60.
21. Wang J, Helle M, Zhou Z, et al. Joint blood and cerebrospinal fluid suppression for intracranial vessel wall MRI. Magn Reson Med 2016;75:831–8.
22. Dieleman N, Yang W, Abrigo JM, et al. Magnetic resonance imaging of plaque morphology, burden, and distribution in patients with symptomatic middle cerebral artery stenosis. Stroke 2016;47:1797–802.
23. Yang H, Zhang X, Qin Q, et al. Improved cerebrospinal fluid suppression for intracranial vessel wall MRI. J Mag Reson Imaging 2016;44:665–72.
24. Fan Z, Yang Q, Deng Z, et al. Whole-brain intracranial vessel wall imaging at 3 Tesla using cerebrospinal fluid-attenuated T1 weighted 3D turbo spin echo. Magn Reson Med 2017;77(3):1142–50.
25. Antiga L, Wasserman BA, Steinman DA. On the overestimation of early wall thickening at the carotid bulb by black blood MRI, with implications for coronary and vulnerable plaque imaging. Magn Reson Med 2008;60(5):1020–8.
26. Busse RF, Hariharan H, Vu A, et al. Fast spin echo sequences with very long echo trains: design of variable refocusing flip angle schedules and generation of clinical T2 contrast. Magn Reson Med 2006;55(5): 1030–7.
27. Fuster V, Moreno PR, Fayad ZA, et al. Atherothrombosis and high-risk plaque: part I: evolving concepts. J Am Coll Cardiol 2005;46(6):937–54.
28. Qureshi AI, Feldmann E, Gomez CR, et al. Consensus conference on intracranial atherosclerotic disease: rationale, methodology, and results. J Neuroimaging 2009;19:1S–10S.
29. Bodle JD, Feldmann E, Swartz RH, et al. High-resolution magnetic resonance imaging: an emerging tool for evaluating intracranial arterial disease. Stroke 2013;44(1):287–92.
30. Song JW, Pavlou A, Xiao J, et al. Vessel Wall Magnetic Resonance Imaging Biomarkers of Symptomatic Intracranial Atherosclerosis: A Meta-Analysis. Stroke 2021;52(1):193–202.
31. Millon A, Boussel L, Brevet M, et al. Clinical and histological significance of gadolinium enhancement in carotid atherosclerotic plaque. Stroke 2012;43(11): 3023–8.
32. Toussaint JF, LaMuraglia GM, Southern JF, et al. Magnetic resonance images lipid, fibrous, calcified, hemorrhagic, and thrombotic components of human atherosclerosis in vivo. Circulation 1996;94(5): 932–8.
33. Kwee RM, Qiao Y, Liu L, et al. Temporal course and implications of intracranial atherosclerotic plaque enhancement on high-resolution vessel wall MRI. Neuroradiology 2019;61(6):651–7.
34. Glagov S, Weisenberg E, Zarins CK, et al. Compensatory enlargement of human atherosclerotic coronary arteries. N Engl J Med 1987;316(22):1371–5.
35. Burke AP, Kolodgie FD, Farb A, et al. Morphological predictors of arterial remodeling in coronary atherosclerosis. Circulation 2002;105(3):297–303.
36. Zhang DF, Wu XY, Zhang WD, et al. The Relationship between Patterns of Remodeling and Degree of Enhancement in Patients with Atherosclerotic Middle Cerebral Artery Stenosis: A High-Resolution MRI Study. Neurol India 2021;69(6):1663–9.
37. Won SY, Cha J, Choi HS, et al. High-Resolution Intracranial Vessel Wall MRI Findings Among Different Middle Cerebral Artery Territory Infarction Types. Korean J Radiol 2022;23(3):333–42.
38. Pasterkamp G, Wensing PJ, Post MJ, et al. Paradoxical arterial wall shrinkage may contribute to luminal narrowing of human atherosclerotic femoral arteries. Circulation 1995;91(5):1444–9.
39. Lam WW, Wong KS, So NM, et al. Plaque volume measurement by magnetic resonance imaging as

an index of remodeling of middle cerebral artery: correlation with transcranial color Doppler and magnetic resonance angiography. Cerebrovasc Dis 2004;17(2–3):166–9.
40. Xu WH, Li ML, Gao S, et al. Middle cerebral artery intraplaque hemorrhage: prevalence and clinical relevance. Ann Neurol 2012;71(2):195–8.
41. Derksen WJ, Peeters W, van Lammeren GW, et al. Different stages of intraplaque hemorrhage are associated with different plaque phenotypes: a large histopathological study in 794 carotid and 276 femoral endarterectomy specimens. Atherosclerosis 2011;218(2):369–77.
42. Xu WH, Li ML, Gao S, et al. In vivo high-resolution MR imaging of symptomatic and asymptomatic middle cerebral artery atherosclerotic stenosis. Atherosclerosis 2010;212(2):507–11.
43. Ryu CW, Jahng GH, Kim EJ, et al. High resolution wall and lumen MRI of the middle cerebral arteries at 3 tesla. Cerebrovasc Dis 2009;27(5):433–42.
44. Chung GH, Kwak HS, Hwang SB, et al. High resolution MR imaging in patients with symptomatic middle cerebral artery stenosis. Eur J Radiol 2012; 81(12):4069–74.
45. Xu WH, Li ML, Gao S, et al. Plaque distribution of stenotic middle cerebral artery and its clinical relevance. Stroke 2011;42(10):2957–9.
46. Mossa-Basha M, Shibata DK, Hallam DK, et al. Added Value of Vessel Wall Magnetic Resonance Imaging for Differentiation of Nonocclusive Intracranial Vasculopathies. Stroke 2017;48(11):3026–33.
47. Obusez EC, Hui F, Hajj-Ali RA, et al. High-resolution MRI vessel wall imaging: spatial and temporal patterns of reversible cerebral vasoconstriction syndrome and central nervous system vasculitis. AJNR Am J Neuroradiol 2014;35(8):1527–32.
48. Hamaoka-Okamoto A, Suzuki C, Yahata T, et al. The involvement of the vasa vasorum in the development of vasculitis in animal model of Kawasaki disease. Pediatr Rheumatol Online J 2014;12:12.
49. Arnett N, Pavlou A, Burke MP, et al. Vessel wall MR imaging of central nervous system vasculitis: a systematic review. Neuroradiology 2022;64(1):43–58.
50. Vlak MH, Algra A, Brandenburg R, et al. Prevalence of unruptured intracranial aneurysms, with emphasis on sex, age, comorbidity, country, and time period: a systematic review and meta-analysis. Lancet Neurol 2011;10:626–36.
51. Karamanakos PN, von Und Zu Fraunberg M, Bendel S, et al. Risk factors for three phases of 12-month mortality in 1657 patients from a defined population after acute aneurysmal subarachnoid hemorrhage. World Neurosurg 2012;78:631–9.
52. Chalouhi N, Hoh BL, Hasan D. Review of cerebral aneurysm formation, growth, and rupture. Stroke 2013;44:3613–22.
53. Hu P, Yang Q, Wang DD, et al. Wall enhancement on high-resolution magnetic resonance imaging may predict an unsteady state of an intracranial saccular aneurysm. Neuroradiology 2016;58:979–85.
54. Larsen N, von der Brelie C, Trick D, et al. Vessel Wall Enhancement in Unruptured Intracranial Aneurysms: An Indicator for Higher Risk of Rupture? High-Resolution MR Imaging and Correlated Histologic Findings. AJNR Am J Neuroradiol 2018;39(9): 1617–21.
55. Wang X, Zhu C, Leng Y, et al. Intracranial Aneurysm wall enhancement associated with aneurysm rupture: a systematic review and meta-analysis. Acad Radiol 2019;26(5):664–73.
56. Molenberg R, Aalbers MW, Appelman APA, et al. Intracranial aneurysm wall enhancement as an indicator of instability: a systematic review and meta-analysis. Eur J Neurol 2021;28(11):3837–48.
57. Pravdivtseva MS, Gaidzik F, Berg P, et al. Pseudo-enhancement in intracranial aneurysms on black-blood mri: effects of flow rate, spatial resolution, and additional flow suppression. J Magn Reson Imaging 2021;54(3):888–901.
58. Zhu C, Mossa-Basha M. Wall enhancement as an emerging marker of intracranial aneurysm stability: Roadmap toward a potential target for clinical trials. Eur J Neurol 2021;28(11):3550–1.
59. Coutinho JM, Sacho RH, Schaafsma JD, et al. High-Resolution Vessel Wall Magnetic Resonance Imaging in Angiogram-Negative Non-Perimesencephalic Subarachnoid Hemorrhage. Clin Neuroradiol 2017; 27(2):175–83.
60. Jung HN, Suh SI, Ryoo I, et al. Usefulness of 3D High-resolution Vessel Wall MRI in Diffuse Nonaneurysmal SAH Patients. Clin Neuroradiol 2021;31(4): 1071–81.
61. Omodaka S, Endo H, Fujimura M, et al. High-grade cerebral arteriovenous malformation treated with targeted embolization of a ruptured site: wall enhancement of an intranidal aneurysm as a sign of ruptured site. Neurol Med -Chir 2015;55:813–7.
62. Komatsu K, Takagi Y, Ishii A, et al. Ruptured intranidal aneurysm of an arteriovenous malformation diagnosed by delay alternating with nutation for tailored excitation (DANTE)-prepared contrast-enhanced magnetic resonance imaging. Acta Neurochir 2018;160:2435–8.
63. Bhogal P, Lansley J, Wong K, et al. Vessel wall enhancement of a ruptured intra-nidal aneurysm in a brain arteriovenous malformation. Int Neuroradiol 2019;25:310–4.
64. Eisenmenger LB, Junn JC, Cooke D, et al. Presence of vessel wall hyperintensity in unruptured arteriovenous malformations on vessel wall magnetic resonance imaging: pilot study of AVM vessel wall "Enhancement. Front Neurosci 2021;15:697432.

65. Iwama T, Andoh T, Sakai N, et al. Dissecting and fusiform aneurysms of vertebro-basilar systems. MR imaging Neuroradiology 1990;32(4):272–9.
66. Wang Y, Lou X, Li Y, et al. Imaging investigation of intracranial arterial dissecting aneurysms by using 3 T high-resolution MRI and DSA: from the interventional neuroradiologists' view. Acta Neurochir 2014; 156(3):515–25.
67. Arai D, Satow T, Komuro T, et al. Evaluation of the Arterial Wall in Vertebrobasilar Artery Dissection Using High-Resolution Magnetic Resonance Vessel Wall Imaging. J Stroke Cerebrovasc Dis 2016; 25(6):1444–50.
68. Aoki S, Hayashi N, Abe O, et al. Radiation-induced arteritis: thickened wall with prominent enhancement on cranial MR images report of five cases and comparison with 18 cases of Moyamoya disease. Radiology 2002;223(3):683–8.
69. Wang M, Yang Y, Zhou F, et al. The Contrast Enhancement of Intracranial Arterial Wall on High-resolution MRI and Its Clinical Relevance in Patients with Moyamoya Vasculopathy. Sci Rep 2017;7: 44264.
70. Ryoo S, Cha J, Kim SJ, et al. High-resolution magnetic resonance wall imaging findings of Moyamoya disease. Stroke 2014;45(8):2457–60.
71. Calabrese LH, Dodick DW, Schwedt TJ, et al. Narrative review: reversible cerebral vasoconstriction syndromes. Ann Intern Med 2007;146(1):34–44.
72. Edjlali M, Qiao Y, Boulouis G, et al. Vessel wall MR imaging for the detection of intracranial inflammatory vasculopathies. Cardiovasc Diagn Ther 2020;10(4):1108–19.
73. Mandell DM, Matouk CC, Farb RI, et al. Vessel wall MRI to differentiate between reversible cerebral vasoconstriction syndrome and central nervous system vasculitis: preliminary results. Stroke 2012; 43(3):860–2.
74. Pia HW, Obrador S, Martin JD. Association of brain tumors and arterial intracranial aneurysms. Acta Neurochir 1972;27:189–204.
75. De Paulis D, Nicosia G, Taddei G, et al. Intracranial aneurysms and optic glioma – an unusual combination: a case report. J Med Case Rep 2016;10:78.
76. Licata C, Pasqualin A, Freschini A, et al. Management of associated primary cerebral neoplasms and vascular malformations. Acta Neurochir 1986; 82:28–38.
77. Hui FK, Zhu X, Jones SE, et al. Early experience in high-resolution MRI for large vessel occlusions. J Neurointerv Surg 2015;7(7):509–16.
78. Cornelissen BMW, Leemans EL, Coolen BF, et al. Insufficient slow-flow suppression mimicking aneurysm wall enhancement in magnetic resonance vessel wall imaging: a phantom study. Neurosurg Focus 2019;47(1):E19.
79. Lindenholz A, van der Kolk AG, Zwanenburg JJM, et al. The Use and Pitfalls of Intracranial Vessel Wall Imaging: How We Do It. Radiology 2018; 286(1):12–28.

# MR Angiography of Pulmonary Vasculature

Liisa L. Bergmann, MD, MBA[a,b,*], Jeanne B. Ackman, MD[c], Jitka Starekova, MD[d], Alexander Moeller, MD[d], Scott Reeder, MD, PhD[d], Scott K. Nagle, MD, PhD[d], Mark L. Schiebler, MD[d,*]

**KEYWORDS**

• MR angiography (MRA) • Pulmonary arteries • Pulmonary embolism • Pulmonary hypertension • Gadolinium • Ferumoxytol

**KEY POINTS**

- Pulmonary MR angiography for pulmonary embolism (MRA-PE) has similar accuracy and outcomes to computed tomographic angiography for pulmonary embolism (CTA-PE) at 6 months.
- More ancillary findings are found in MRA-PE examinations than CTA-PE examinations, as the field of view is larger.
- The Gibb's ringing artifact is frequently seen as a confounder to PE on MRA-PE examinations.
- The anatomy and physiology of pulmonary hypertension and partial anomalous pulmonary venous return are well demonstrated by pulmonary MRA.

## INTRODUCTION

In this review, the authors discuss the methods of lung perfusion using magnetic resonance imaging (MRI) and magnetic resonance angiography (MRA) methodology, the various contrast agents that are used, and major pulmonary arterial disorders. The authors start with pulmonary embolism (PE) and then discuss pulmonary hypertension providing representative figures illustrating these entities. References will be provided, should the reader seek additional depth regarding each subject.

### *Lung Perfusion*

Contrast-enhanced computed tomography (CT) methods for the determination of lung perfusion are well characterized. This is because the slope of the Hounsfield unit attenuation values scales linearly with contrast concentration. Thus, a simple application of the arterial input function for the pulmonary artery can be used for the first component of the equation, and the time density curves for various lobes can be derived to show the contrast passage through the lung parenchyma from the pulmonary arteries. The lungs have a second source of perfusion: the bronchial arteries. To evaluate their contribution to lung perfusion, a second arterial input function needs to be applied to the time density curve for the aorta. Pulmonary parenchymal density less the bronchial artery contribution determines the attenuation that can be attributed to pulmonary arterial perfusion alone. As larger detector array CT hardware becomes readily available, these perfusion maps will become much easier to obtain, as the helical scanner can perform multiple acquisitions at the same location.

For contrast-enhanced MRA, the situation is not as simple. The signal intensity of the contrast agent

[a] Department of Radiology, University of Kentucky College of Medicine, 800 Rose Street, HX332E, Lexington, KY 40536-0293, USA; [b] Department of Medicine, University of Kentucky College of Medicine, 800 Rose Street, HX332E, Lexington, KY 40536-0293, USA; [c] Massachusetts General Hospital, Department of Radiology, Division of Thoracic Imaging and Intervention Austin Building 202, 55 Fruit Street, Boston, MA 02114, USA; [d] Department of Radiology, University of Wisconsin School of Medicine and Public Health, 600 Highland Avenue, Madison, WI 53705, USA
* Corresponding authors.
*E-mail addresses:* Liisa.B@uky.edu (L.L.B.); mschiebler@uwhealth.org (M.L.S.)

Magn Reson Imaging Clin N Am 31 (2023) 475–491
https://doi.org/10.1016/j.mric.2023.05.004
1064-9689/23/

does not scale linearly with concentration.[1] Thus, the signal obtained must be corrected for these changes in T1 known to occur with increasing concentrations. Bell and colleagues have shown that a 3D radial method for lung structure and perfusion is possible in a single breath-hold.[2]

Interestingly, non-contrast MR methods for pulmonary perfusion and ventilation have been developed. Perfusion and ventilation are now being investigated using Fourier decomposition of the vascular signal variation with each heartbeat and the respiratory variation from each breath, respectively.[3,4] A variant of this method (phase-resolved functional lung) has recently been described by Voskrebenzev and colleagues.[5,6] This method has been used clinically to show differences in lung perfusion in children after COVID-19 infection, without exposing them to gadolinium-based contrast agent (GBCA) or to ionizing radiation.[7]

## *Contrast Agents*

Gadolinium-based contrast agents (GBCAs) are commonly used for pulmonary MRA. They are safe,[8,9] have a very low incidence of allergic reaction,[10] and macrocyclic and ionic (group II gadolinium agents) have been sanctioned for use by the American College of Radiology in the setting of severe renal insufficiency, with infinitesimal-to-no risk of nephrogenic systemic fibrosis (NSF) if patients have only received group II gadolinium agents previously.[11] The incidence of nephrogenic systemic fibrosis has plummeted with knowledge of its causes.[12,13] There is some concern about gadolinium retention, though there has never been proof of harm to patients from gadolinium retention over the past 3 decades. Another advantage of the use of ionic macrocyclic GBCAs is the reduction of free gadolinium chelate and resultant decrease in gadolinium retention. The advantages of GBCAs for MRA include ease of use; lower occurrence of adverse and allergic reactions than iodinated contrast for CT; ready availability for bulk purchase by medical facilities for cost savings; well-known, agent-specific biodistribution and plasma $T_{1/2}$ clearance profiles; and well-understood artifacts associated with the bolus injection of these agents.[14]

Ferumoxytol is an intravenously administered iron agent used to supplement iron stores in patients with refractory anemia, including pregnant women. This agent also has a very high relaxivity and can be used as a long-acting intravenous contrast agent. Nguyen and colleagues have shown that the administration of this agent by slow infusion is safe in the MR suite and has important advantages over GBCAs.[15] Recently, Starekova and colleagues have shown that this agent had good image quality when used for the primary diagnosis of PE in the setting of pregnancy.[16] The advantages of this agent for MRA examinations over GBCAs are numerous: higher T1 relaxivity; rapid T2 shortening; prolonged intravascular retention with long plasma $T_{1/2}$; inability to cross the placenta; good source of iron; different allergy profile from GBCAs; no association with NSF; and no deposition in the brain. The disadvantages include the following: higher cost; not tolerated as a bolus infusion; may give rise to the transient Fishbane reaction in 1/200 patients, described in detail below; may be associated with a change in heart rate and blood pressure; and deposition in the reticuloendothelial system with repeated use. The Fishbane reaction is transient flushing, chest tightness, abdominal pain, and/or back pain with infusion, which typically resolves with a brief pause in infusion and does not recur when the infusion is restarted.

GBCAs are commonly used for pulmonary MRA.[17,18] American College of Radiology group II GBCAs[19] are safe[8] and have a very low incidence of allergic reaction (0.01%–0.22%; severe adverse events 0.008%). These are also rapidly excreted.[10] The only remaining group II agent, gadoxetic acid, a linear agent, has yet to demonstrate any cases of NSF.[20] The use of macrocyclic gadolinium-based contrast agents (GBCAs) reduces free serum gadolinium chelate with a resultant decrease in gadolinium retention.

The incidence of nephrogenic systemic fibrosis (NSF), a potentially fatal debilitating condition associated with GBCAs and advanced kidney disease or acute kidney injury, has plummeted with better understanding of its potential risk factors.[12,13]

There is some concern about gadolinium retention. Aside from the known issue of NSF, there has never been proof of harm to patients from gadolinium retention over the past 3 decades of use.[21] Another advantage of the use of ionic macrocyclic GBCAs is the reduction of free gadolinium chelate and resultant decrease in gadolinium retention.[22,23]

The main advantages of GBCAs for MRA include:

- Low occurrence of allergic reactions and adverse events
- Ease of use
- Relatively low cost
- Well-known, agent-specific biodistribution and plasma $T_{1/2}$ clearance profiles
- Well understood artifacts associated with the bolus injection of these agents[14]

***Additional recommendations regarding use of gadolinium-based contrast agents for some patients***

- GBCAs are relatively contraindicated in pregnancy.[19,24]
- Group 1 GBCAs are contraindicated in patients with advanced renal disease (chronic kidney disease (CKD) 4–5 or patients on dialysis) or acute kidney injury.[19]

Ferumoxytol (Feraheme, AMAG) is an FDA-approved intravenously administered iron agent used to supplement iron stores in patients with refractory anemia and is recommended for treatment of iron-deficiency in pregnant women by some of the obstetric medical societies.[25] Ferumoxytol contains supermagnetic iron oxide nanoparticles with favorable MR imaging properties such as high T1-relaxivity and prolonged intravascular half-life (about 15 hour) and can be used off-label as an intravenous contrast agent. These attributes allow for homogenous enhancement of pulmonary vasculature and repeat acquisitions if needed without additional contrast injections.

Ferumoxytol showed an excellent safety profile as an off-label contrast agent, if administered diluted, in the form of a slow parenteral infusion (1.8% mild, 0.2% moderate allergic reactions).[15] Ferumoxytol is a useful gadolinium-free contrast alternative for pulmonary MRA in pregnancy. In to date a largest case-series study in pregnant women, ferumoxytol-enhanced MRA performed for diagnosis of pulmonary embolism (PE) showed an excellent image quality with short examination times (median 8 minute).[16] According to the Food and Drug Administration (FDA), a US Federal Agency, there are insufficient human data to evaluate adverse outcomes of ferumoxytol in pregnancy[26]; however, its increasing therapeutic use during pregnancy[25] and inability to cross the placenta in primate studies[27] are reassuring regarding its safety.

The main advantages of off-label use of ferumoxytol for MRA include:

- Low occurrence of severe allergic reactions
- High T1-relaxivity and prolonged intravascular half-life
- Possible use in pregnancy, patients with hyperdynamic state or those allergic to GBCA
- No association with NSF

**Additional considerations regarding the off-label use of ferumoxytol for MR angiography include:**

- Bolus administration should be avoided to heed the FDA black box warning.[28]
- Contraindicated in patients with a history of allergic reaction to intravenous iron or Feraheme components and in those with iron overload.
- Transient alteration of following MR imaging studies that may persist up to 3 months with maximal alteration reported 1 to 2 days following ferumoxytol administration.[29]
- Higher cost in comparison to GBCAs
- Longer preparatory time with slow infusion and monitoring of at least 30 minute

Finally, the combination of GBCA injected into the lymphatics and intravascular ferumoxytol allows for improved delineation of the lymphatics from the veins via venous blood suppression.[30] MR lymphangiogram using only GBCA often demonstrates signal intensity higher in the veins than in the lymphatics due to extensive contamination. Dual-contrast agent MR lymphangiogram could be used in the chest for post-Fontan patients as they are prone to lymphatic dysfunction; however, most studies have just used T2W imaging for this disorder.[31]

## DISEASES OF PULMONARY VASCULATURE

### *Pulmonary Embolism*

The incidence of PE varies by age, sex, and comorbidities. It is important to understand that PE and deep venous thrombosis (DVT) together are lumped under the broader definition of venous thromboembolic disease (VTE). For the general public, the Worcester, MA, population study for VTE showed an overall annual incidence of 0.1% (104/100,000).[32] In a second population-based study in Olmstead County, MN, the annual incidence of VTE was 0.12% (117/100,000), with 0.048% PE (48/100,000) and .089% DVT.

In the acute setting, there are few clinical scenarios that generate more cross-sectional chest imaging studies than the emergency department's quest to identify pulmonary embolism (PE). This places a burden on most hospital centers, as few of these examinations are positive for PE. Over the years, the incidence of positive CT angiography examinations has dropped. In an older study, Prologo and colleagues showed that from 1998 to 2003, the number of examinations went up in the emergency department (81–349) and the positivity rate went down (27.1% to 5.7%).[33]

In the evaluation of clinical study performance, there are three major categories. The first one is the efficacy study. In this analysis, a new test is compared with a reference standard to determine its overall utility, which is expressed in several ways. These include area under the curve, sensitivity, specificity, positive predictive value, negative predictive value, true positives, true negatives, false positives, and false negatives. The second type of study is outcomes-driven and is called an effectiveness study (or trial, if prospective). The third is a cost–benefit analysis. For the determination of test accuracy, most centers rely on prospective randomized and controlled efficacy trials. However, such trials are expensive, and funding is difficult to secure for them. Of more importance for patient outcomes are the effectiveness studies and employing a cost–benefit analysis to determine the relative value of one test versus another.

In 2010, Stein and colleagues published their results of the multicenter PIOPED III study.[34] This efficacy study had a design that featured MRA in the trial arm with several reference standards. These included CT angiography, venography, ventilation / perfusion (V/Q) scan, deep venous ultrasound, d-dimer, and clinical assessment for the determination of PE. They found the following: (1) MRA was technically inadequate in 25% (92 of 371 patients), (2) the range of technically inadequate examinations was high (11% –52%), (3) for MRA examinations of acceptable image quality, only 57% (59 of 104 patients) with PE were identified, (4) in the technically adequate examinations, MRA had a high specificity (99%), but only an intermediate sensitivity of 78%.[34] This publication had a chilling effect on any further publications and clinical trials that sought to confirm these findings.

At our institution, we were performing MRA-PE before the PIOPED III results came out and have continued to use this examination as an alternative to CTA-PE when appropriate.[35–37]

We primarily started to use MRA-PE to limit radiation exposure to young women and girls[38] and in patients with iodinated contrast allergies. Repplinger and colleagues performed a retrospective case-controlled analysis of 1173 (MRA or CTA) patients.[36] The primary endpoint was major adverse PE-related event (MAPE) within 6 months of the index examination. The term MAPE was defined as major bleeding, VTE, or death following the index imaging test. The overall 6-month MAPE rate following MRA (5.4%) was lower than following CTA (13.6%, $P < .01$). In evaluating just outpatients, the MAPE rate was lower for MRA (3.7%) than for CTA (8.0%, $P = .01$). Accounting for age, sex, referral source, BMI, and Wells' score, the MRA patients were less likely to suffer MAPE than those who underwent CTA (odds ratio of 0.44 [99% CI, 0.24–0.80]). Technical success rate did not differ significantly between MRA (92.6%) and CTA (90.5%) groups. They concluded that the rate of MAPE was lower for patients following pulmonary MRA than following CTA in the primary examination for PE.[36] These two effectiveness studies stand in direct opposition to the results of the PIOPED III efficacy trial.

How can these two very different interpretations of the utility of MRA-PE examinations for the primary diagnosis of PE be reconciled? One way is to assume that both are correct. This can be done if we agree that MRA may not demonstrate the subsegmental vasculature in a certain percentage of patients and thus is less sensitive for demonstrating small pulmonary emboli. This was in effect the conclusion of the PIOPED III study. Then, making the second assumption that subsegmental pulmonary emboli do not matter for MAPE, as determined in a meta-analysis[39] and the two effectiveness studies,[35,36] it now becomes possible to understand these two very different results. Although MRA-PE is less sensitive for the diagnosis of small PE, this is a nonissue in terms of patient outcomes after 6 months of follow-up.[36]

In counter point to this thesis that subsegmental emboli may be safely ignored is the current idea about the pathogenesis of Chronic Thromboembolic Pulmonary Hypertension (CTEPH). The current thinking is that CTEPH begins with one embolus and therefore all emboli should be treated aggressively with anticoagulation to prevent further emboli. The problem with this approach is that serious bleeding complications and death can occur from anticoagulation treatment, particularly in an elderly patient population. As with all treatment decisions in medicine, there must be careful consideration of what choices are best for a given patient.

## *Pulmonary MR Angiography Methodology*

Most MR imaging scanner hardware is capable of 3D MRA techniques, as this is the mainstay of brain imaging. Adapting these techniques to the chest requires limiting the acquisition to a breath-hold or relying on free breathing acquisitions. With the patient's arms above the head, an initial scout image is performed followed by a bolus triggered examination to the pulmonary arteries, a delayed examination and then a low flip angle delayed examination in an equilibrium phase of contrast enhancement (**Tables 1** and **2**).

## *Direct and Indirect Findings for Pulmonary Embolism*

The direct findings of PE at MRA include the following observations: occlusion of a pulmonary artery, partial occlusion or filling defect, web in the pulmonary artery, pulmonary artery cutoff, high T1W signal in a pulmonary artery on pre-contrast scans, and the double bronchus sign (**Figs. 1–4**). The indirect findings of PE at MRA include the following: atelectasis, pleural effusion, decreased perfusion, pulmonary infarction, and the black-white-black sign.

**Table 1**
**Gadolinium-enhanced pulmonary MR angiography protocol**

| Parameter | T1W 3D MRA Pre-contrast | T1W 3D CE-MRA Pulmonary Arterial Phase | T1W 3D CE-MRA Early Delayed Phase | T1W 3D CE-MRA Intermediate FA Early Delayed Phase | FS T1W 2D SGRE | CINE SSFP |
|---|---|---|---|---|---|---|
| Field of view (cm) | 36 × 28 | 36 × 28 | 36 × 28 | 36 × 28 | 36 × 28 | 400 × 320 |
| TR (ms) | 3.0 | 3.3 | 2.9 | 3.2 | 110 | 3.2 |
| TE (ms) | 1.0 | 1.2 | 1.0 | 1.1 | 4.2 | 1.1 |
| Flip angle (degrees) | 28 | 28 | 28 | 15 | 90 | 45 |
| Slice thickness (mm) | 2.0 | 2.0 | 2.0 | 2.0 | 5.0 | 8.0 |
| Acquisition matrix | 256 × 192 | 256 × 192 | 256 × 192 | 256 × 192 | 320 × 192 | 224 × 160 |
| Scan plane | Coronal | Coronal | coronal | coronal | axial | axial |

Protocol for 1.5 T MR imaging system. Contrast: 0.1 mmol/kg of gadobenate dimeglumine (Multihance, bracco diagnostics, Princeton, NJ), diluted to a total volume of 30 mL with saline and injected at 1.5 mL/s. Total table time: approximately 13 minute.

*Abbreviations:* CE-MRA, contrast-enhanced MR angiography; FA, flip angle; FS, fat-sat; SGRE, spoiled gradient echo; SSFP, steady-state free precession MR imaging; T1W, T1-weighted; TE, time to echo; TR, repetition time.

Tsuchiya and colleagues evaluated eight direct and eight indirect findings of PE on 66 MRA-PE examinations that were all positive for PE (**Tables 3** and **4**).[40] Each examination was interpreted separately by two radiologists with different experience levels. The reference PE was determined in consensus with a third reader. There was a training session of 10 cases before the interpretation started. The prevalence and intra- and inter-reader agreement for the direct and indirect findings of PE were recorded. The largest PE for each of the remaining 56 cases was included. The highest interobserver agreement for the direct findings were vessel cutoff (kappa = 0.52, 95% CI 0.30–0.74, $P < .0001$) and T1-hyperintense clot (kappa = 0.51, 95% CI 0.26–0.78, $P = .0001$). The highest interobserver agreement for the indirect findings were for atelectasis (kappa = 0.67, 95% CI 0.49–0.87, $P < .0001$), pleural effusions (kappa = 0.56, 95% CI 0.32–0.79, $P = 001$), and blank slate sign (kappa = 0.56, 95% CI 0.18–0.94, $P < .0001$). The investigators concluded that the indirect findings of atelectasis and pleural effusion had better interobserver reproducibility

**Table 2**
**Ferumoxytol-enhanced pulmonary MR angiography protocol**

| Scan Parameters | T1W 3D CE-MRA | T1W 3D CE-MRA Intermediate FA | FS T1W 3D SGRE | FS T1W 2D SGRE |
|---|---|---|---|---|
| Field of view (cm) | 44 × 44 | 44 × 44 | 42 × 42 | 36 × 28 |
| TR (ms) | 3.3 | 3.6 | 6.2 | 34 |
| TE (ms) | 1.1 | 1.1 | 4.2 | 1.6 |
| Flip angle | 25 | 15 | 12 | 90 |
| Slice thickness (mm) | 2.0 | 2.0 | 4.0 | 5.0 |
| Acquisition matrix | 256 × 192 | 256 × 192 | 288 × 192 | 288 × 192 |
| Scan plane | Coronal | Coronal | Axial | axial |

Protocol for 1.5 T MR imaging system. Contrast: 3 mg/kg of ferumoxytol (Feraheme, AMAG), max 510 mg (one bottle); 5-fold dilution in saline, infused over 15 min; blood pressure monitoring before and 5 and 30 minute after infusion. Total table time: approximately 8 minute.

*Abbreviations:* CE-MRA, contrast-enhanced MR angiography; FA, flip angle; FS, fat-sat; SGRE, spoiled gradient echo; T1W, T1-weighted; TE, time to echo; TR, repetition time.

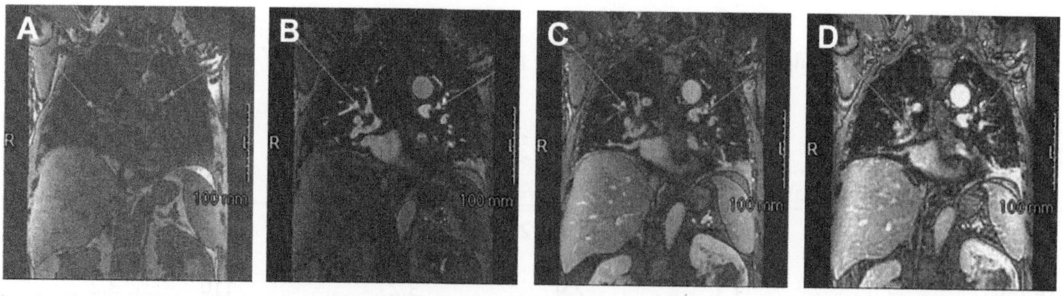


**Fig. 1.** Classic bilateral pulmonary emboli with high signal intensity thrombi on the non-contrast T1W image. From left to right: (*A*) arrows show high signal intensity thrombi in the right interlobar artery and left main pulmonary artery (*arrows*), (*B*) bolus phase of the pulmonary MRA shows the low signal intensity filling defects (*arrows*). Filling defects consistent with PE (*arrows*) persist in (*C*) equilibrium phase pulmonary MRA and (*D*) low flip angle delayed phase MRA.

than direct findings of vessel cutoff and T1-hyperintense clot on MRA-PE examinations.[40]

### *Actionable Findings*

Schiebler and colleagues performed a study of MRA-PE examinations that were negative for PE but had other findings that were actionable.[41] The findings, based on the final radiology report in the radiology information system (Powerscribe, Nuance), were divided into three types: those requiring further action (actionable-Type 1), those not requiring follow-up (non-actionable-Type 2) (**Figs. 5–7**), and normal examinations (normal-Type 3). There were 561/580 (97%) technically adequate examinations. Of these, 47/580 (8%) were positive for PE. In the PE negative group (514/580), Type 1 actionable findings were identified

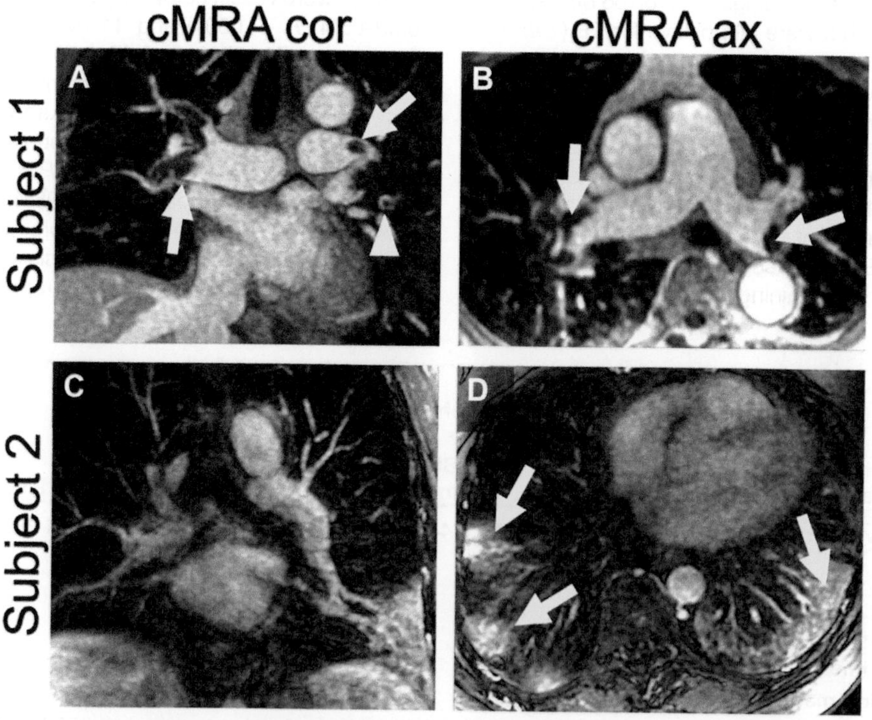


**Fig. 2.** Gadolinium-enhanced MR angiography (MRA) enables detection of pulmonary embolus and pulmonary findings. Shown are multiplanar reformatted 3D contrast-enhanced (cMRA) images in coronal (cor) and axial (ax) planes: Subject 1 (63-year-old man, A and B) with multifocal bilateral pulmonary emboli. The pulmonary emboli begin in both the left and right distal main pulmonary arteries (arrows) and extend into segmental branches (arrowhead). Subject 2 (70-year-old man, C and D) with bibasilar pneumonia (arrows). No pulmonary embolus was detected in this subject.

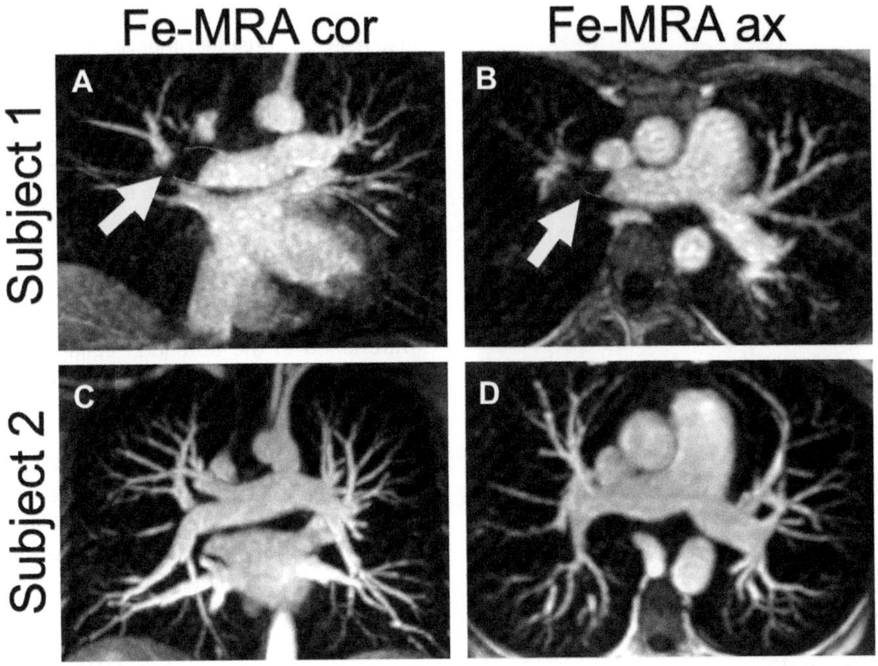


Fig. 3. Pulmonary ferumoxytol-enhanced MR angiography (Fe-MRA) is a feasible alternative to CT angiography and gadolinium-enhanced MRA for the diagnosis of pulmonary embolism. Shown are multiplanar reformatted 3D contrast-enhanced images in coronal (cor) and axial (ax) view: Subject 1 (22-year-old pregnant patient, 7 gestational weeks, A and B) with...Subject 2 (29-year-old pregnant patient, 35 gestational weeks, C and D) without pulmonary embolism.

85/514 (17%) of the examinations. There were 188/514 (36%) cases with Type 2 findings and 241/514 (47.0%) were Type 3-normal. There was no significant difference between the incidence of Type 1 and the combination of Type 2 and Type 3 findings on MRA and the published[42] incidence of actionable findings derived from negative CTA examinations for PE. We concluded that MRA as a first-line test for PE was able to identify actionable findings in those patients without PE, with an incidence similar to CTA.[41]

## *Artifacts*

There are several artifacts to consider when studying MRA-PE examinations.[43] The first to consider is the effect of intravascular contrast concentration on signal intensity and k-space acquisition order in 3D MRA examinations, also colloquially known as the "Maki" artifact.[14] When the signal intensity of the vessel is low during the acquisition of the center of k-space, there will be low signal intensity in the vessel as well. If the bolus finally catches up with the k-space acquisition, then there will be high signal for those portions of k-space that are being filled in. This artifact will look suspiciously like a large central defect and could simulate a PE on a single imaging pass. However, with multiple acquisitions this artifact is not an issue as the bolus finally arrives for the later acquisitions (delayed immediate post-bolus contrast administration and equilibrium contrast phases).

The second is Gibbs artifact or Gibbs-ringing (**Fig. 8**).[44] In general, approximately 50% of all MRA-PE examinations will have a Gibbs artifact on them. These artifacts are much more common than a PE. The Bannas' criteria based on quantitative signal drop can be used to objectively differentiate between Gibbs artifact and PE.[44]

The third artifact to discuss is phase wrap from selection of a field of view that is too small for patient size. This can be ameliorated by increasing the field of view. The downside of increasing the field of view is that the breath-hold is longer. If needed, the slice thickness can be increased to compensate for the larger field of view and to help keep the examination time within a reasonable breath-hold for the patient. Whenever possible, having the patient raise his/her arms above his/her head can reduce the likelihood of wrap.

## *Confounders for Pulmonary Embolism*

There are many possible confounders that can limit the accuracy of MRA-PE examinations. The major

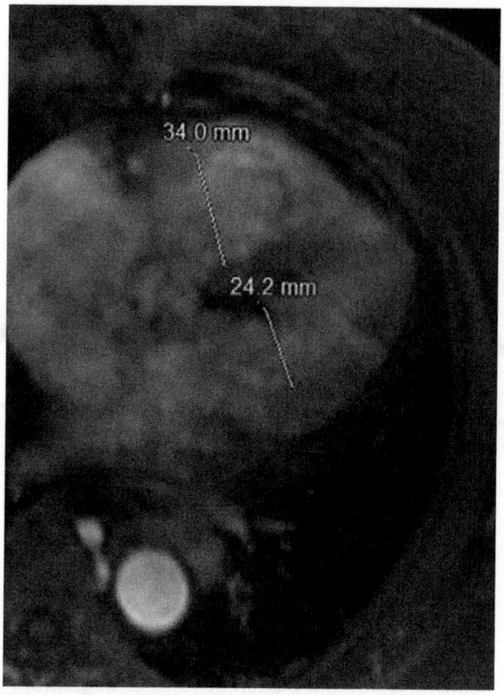


Fig. 4. Abnormal right ventricle to left ventricle ratio (RV:LV ratio) in a patient with submassive pulmonary emboli (not shown). Axial bSSFP electrocardiogram (ECG)-gated examination in a patient with bilateral obstructive pulmonary emboli shows an elevated right ventricle short axis (3.4 cm) to left ventricle short axis (2.4 cm) ratio of 1.42. A ratio greater than 1.0 is abnormal and is associated with right heart strain. A benefit of using the ECG-gated cine bSSFP images is the ability to identify the septal flattening or inversion that occurs with an increase in right heart pressures over the complete cardiac cycle.

one is a Gibbs artifact located centrally in vessels of a certain size and can be recognized by application of Bannas' criteria.[44] A true embolus should have a 50% or lower signal intensity than the surrounding contrast-filled lumen. These artifacts can be found centrally in pulmonary veins as well.[44] The second major confounder is an old PE that has totally occluded the pulmonary artery causing a cutoff sign (risks misinterpretation as a new PE). This is problematic for interpretation, but old examinations, history of prior PE that was treated, and a smaller lobe without perfusion can be helpful signs that can indicate the presence of old disease causing these findings. The third confounder is CTEPH. In these cases, webs in the pulmonary arteries and irregular pulmonary arterial walls may be identified. An enlarged main pulmonary artery and slow flow in the right and left pulmonary arteries can also be clues.[45] The fourth confounder is pulmonary arterial neoplasm, such as sarcoma or metastatic disease.[46–50] We also need to consider other diseases of the pulmonary vasculature that may mimic PE vasculitis and some syndromes, including granulomatosis with polyangiitis, Behcet's disease, Takayasu's arteritis, and Hughes-Stovin syndrome, which can also cause amputation of the pulmonary arterial vasculature.[51]

### *Programmatic Champions*

CT pulmonary angiography (CTPA) is firmly entrenched in the american college of radiology (ACR) clinical standards for the workup of PE, as it should be.[52] It is fast, reliable and has a long track record of high efficacy. In contrast, the ACR Appropriateness Criteria ratings for MRA-PE are low for the three clinical presentations evaluated: (1) intermediate probability with a negative D-dimer (rating 2/10), (2) intermediate probability with a positive D-dimer (rating 6/10), and (3) the pregnant patient (rating 3/10).

Why make the effort to build an MRA-PE program at your center, when CTPA is so easy to do? There are three major reasons: (1) the approach to "image wisely" (adults) and "image gently" (pediatric patients) by minimizing medical exposure to ionizing radiation are espoused by multiple entities, including the American College of Radiology and the Radiological Society of North America—less overall medical ionizing radiation is better than more; (2) for patients with iodinated contrast allergies, MRA-PE is a good alternative; and (3) the multiplicity of contrast phases on MRA provides multiple opportunities to achieve a high-quality examination without the need for further intravenous contrast administration.

Building a successful MRA for PE program is feasible when radiologists partner with clinical champions, from emergency medicine, internal medicine, obstetrics and gynecology (OB-Gyn), and/or pediatrics.[53] It is all is achievable with education and enthusiasm.

## PULMONARY HYPERTENSION

### *Background*

Pulmonary hypertension is a silent disease, frequently only discovered at a late stage.[54,55] The central problem with this disorder is that the right heart is not designed to generate high pressures. It is designed for accommodating the changes in volume associated with exercise (acute changes in volume) and pregnancy (slow changes in volume). When faced with the problem of acutely increased pressures in the pulmonary vasculature, the right ventricle fails. This situation occurs with massive pulmonary emboli, and sudden death

**Table 3**
**Observer agreement for direct findings of pulmonary embolism on 56 positive MR angiography for pulmonary embolism examinations**

| Finding | Interobserver Agreement Kappa Value (95% CI) [*P*-Value] | Intra-Reader Agreement Reader 1 (Novice) Kappa Value (95% CI) _[*P*-Value]_ | Intra-Reader Agreement Reader 2 (Experienced) Kappa Value (95% CI) _[*P*-Value] _ | N Findings at Consensus Read for 56 Positive MRA-PE Examinations |
|---|---|---|---|---|
| Nonocclusive filling defect | 0.36 (0.10–0.62) [.006] | 0.88 (0.75–1.00) [<.0001] | 0.46 (0.19–0.72) [.0006] | 12 |
| Occlusive filling defect | 0.44 (0.20–0.69) [.0009] | .88 (0.76–1.0) [<.0001] | 0.44 (0.20–0.69) [<.0001] | 43 |
| Vessel cutoff | 0.52 (0.30–74) [.0001] | 0.44 (.20–0.68) [.001] | 0.48 (0.25–0.70) [.0002] | 42 |
| Double bronchus sign | 0.45 (0.24–0.65) [.0001] | 0.53 (0.31–0.75) [<.0001] | 0.77 (0.51–0.95) [<.0001] | 26 |
| Bright T1W clot | 0.51 (0.26–78) [.0001] | 0.67 (0.45–0.89) [<.0001] | 0.64 (0.41–0.86) [<.0001] | 18 |
| Ghost vessel sign | 0.48 (0.27–0.69) [<.0001] | 0.54 (0.31–0.76) [<.0001] | 0.53 (0.39–0.83) [<.0001] | 31 |
| Central dot sign | 0.34 (0.12–0.57) [<.0001] | 0.32 (0.07–0.58) [.01] | 0.54 (0.33–0.75) [<.005] | 34 |
| Post-Gd fat-saturated images | 0.19 (−0.20–0.58) [NS] | 0.62 (0.24–1.00) [.0001] | 0.60 (0.24–0.95) [.0005] | 28 |

*Abbreviations:* NS, not significant; T1W, T1-weighted.
*Data adapted from* Tsuchiya and et al.[40]

**Table 4**
**Observer agreement for indirect findings of pulmonary embolism on 56 MR angiography for pulmonary embolism examinations**

| Finding | Interobserver Agreement Kappa Value (95% CI) [*P*-value] | Intra-Reader Agreement Reader 1 (Novice) Kappa Value (95% CI) [*P*-value] | Intra-Reader Agreement Reader 2 (Experienced) Kappa Value (95% CI) [*P*-value] | *N* Findings at Consensus Read for 56 Positive MRA-PE Examinations |
|---|---|---|---|---|
| Pulmonary venous stasis | 0.06 (−0.18–0.31) [NS] | 0.40 (0.11–0.69) [.003] | 0.37 (−0.18–0.93) [.004] | 10 |
| Atelectasis | 0.67 (0.49–0.87) [.0001] | 0.54 (0.32–0.76) [.0001] | 0.81 (0.66–0.97) [.0001] | 21 |
| Perfusion defect | 0.51 (0.27–0.75) [.0001] | 0.59 (0.37–0.82) [.0001] | 0.66 (0.45–0.87) [.0001] | 42 |
| Pleural effusion | 0.56 (0.32–0.79) [<.0001] | 0.79 (0.62–0.97) [<.0001] | 0.88 (0.75–1.0) [<.0001] | 21 |
| Visceral pleural enhancement | 0.31 (0.09–0.54) [.006] | 0.47 (0.20–0.75) [.0003] | 0.31 (0.009–0.54) [.006] | 22 |
| White-black-white sign | 0.47 (0.23–0.71) [.0005] | 0.60 (0.39–0.81) [<.0001] | 0.67 (0.4–0.86) [<.0001] | 34 |
| Pulmonary infarct | 0.52 (0.22–0.82) [<.0001] | 0.94 (0.84–1.0) [<.0001] | 0.74 (0.46–1.0) [<.0001] | 12 |
| Blank slate sign | 0.56 (0.18–0.94) [.0001] | 0.64 (0.26–1.0) [<.0001] | 1.0 (1.0–1.0) [<.0001] | 5 |

*Data adapted from* Tsuchiya et al.[40]

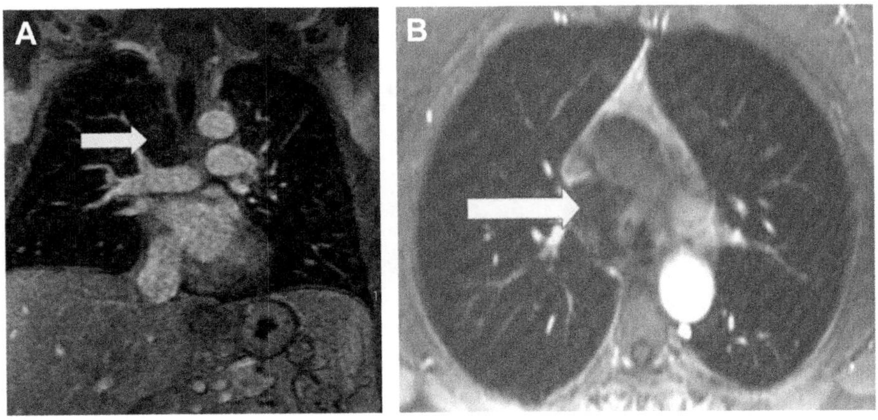


Fig. 5. Ancillary finding of mediastinal lymphadenopathy: From left to right, (*A*) coronal equilibrium phase MRA examination showing a low signal intensity right paratracheal mass (*arrow*) representing a calcified azygos lymph node and (*B*) axial post-gadolinium Lava Flex water-only image shows a low signal intensity mass representing a calcified azygous lymph node (*arrow*).

may result. Most of the time, it does not occur in patients with PE who make it to the hospital.

With the new definition of pulmonary hypertension of 20 mm Hg mean pulmonary artery pressure measured at right heart catheterization, more individuals will be diagnosed with this disorder.[56] Thus, the only direct finding of pulmonary hypertension are the pressure measurements of the main pulmonary artery at right heart catheterization. The new classification system for pulmonary hypertension is no longer based on the physiology of precapillary and postcapillary locations of the physiological underpinnings of this disease. In the previous iterations, one could categorize pulmonary hypertension based on causes and where in the cardiopulmonary system the disease etiology occurred. Now the classification system is based first on treatment options and secondarily on the anatomic/pathologic causes, if known. The role of imaging is to help stage the degree of cardiopulmonary impairment, determine a possible cause that can be corrected, and exclude some of the well-defined anatomic disorders associated with pulmonary hypertension, such as partial anomalous pulmonary venous return.

The following discussion will highlight some of the findings that can be seen with pulmonary hypertension involving the pulmonary arterial vasculature. This discussion will be an overview and will allow the reader to access other publications that deal with this subject in greater detail.[54]

## Pathophysiology

Pulmonary hypertension is directly related to dysfunction of the heart-lung axis (blood flow

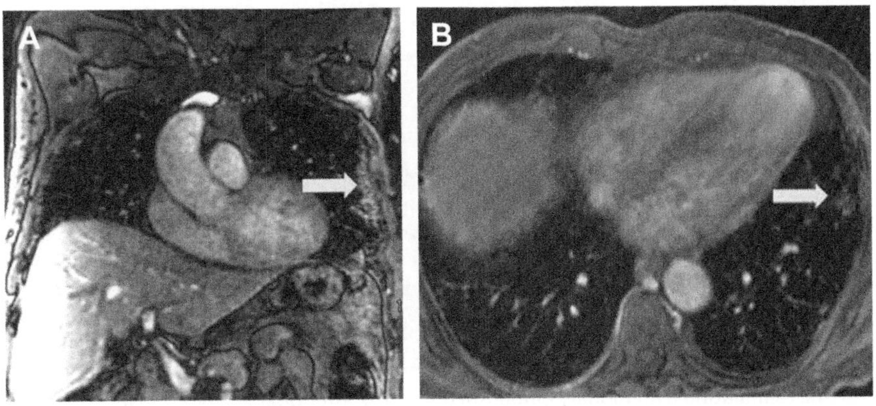


Fig. 6. Ancillary findings in the lungs of a patient with known COVID-19 pneumonia: From left to right (*A*) coronal equilibrium phase pulmonary MRA shows peripheral enhancing left lung opacities from an organizing pneumonia in a patient with active COVID-19 infection (*arrow*), (*B*) axial Lava Flex post-contrast MR imaging of the chest shows peripheral opacities in the lingula (*arrow*) consistent with the patient's known COVID-19 infection.

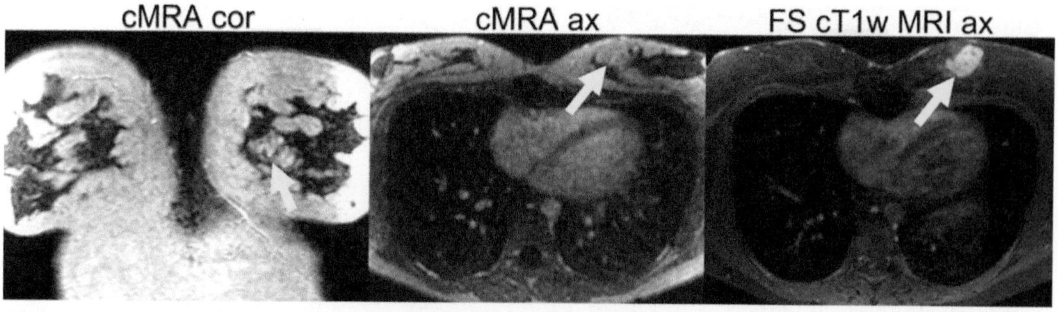


**Fig. 7.** Although most findings can be easily detected by MRA, some are better visible on fat suppressed T1W images. A left breast fibroadenoma (*arrows*) is seen best on the fat-suppressed contrast-enhanced T1-weighted (FS cT1W) images.

and oxygenation). A common cause of pulmonary hypertension is lung disease. Examples include chronic obstructive pulmonary disease/emphysema, idiopathic pulmonary fibrosis, and adult respiratory distress syndrome. With the increased obesity rate, the role of obstructive sleep apnea as a cause should be kept in mind while interpreting cross-sectional imaging of the chest.

In addition, the role of the kidneys and liver should not be discounted. Chronic volume overload from renal failure leads to pulmonary hypertension. Liver dysfunction is also associated with pulmonary vascular diseases. First is the issue of portopulmonary hypertension that occurs in cirrhotic patients, an entity which is problematic if not recognized before liver transplantation. Second is hepatopulmonary syndrome. Although the latter is not a cause of pulmonary hypertension, this disorder can be identified with CT or MRA because of dilation the peripheral pulmonary arteries and veins. Third, in classic (atrial pulmonary) Fontan patients, the liver is not able to metabolize vasoactive substances in the plasma and intrapulmonary arteriovenous malformations occur.

## Compliance

Kinetic energy is stored in the pulmonary arteries by vessel wall compliance. As vessel wall compliance is lost, there is a more direct relationship between the pressure in the pulmonary arteries and

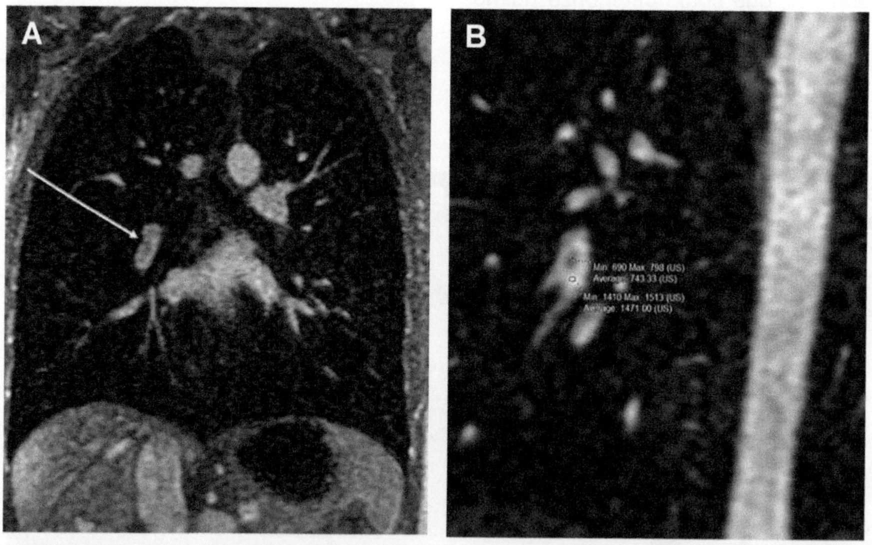


**Fig. 8.** Gibbs artifact simulating a pulmonary embolism (PE) in the interlobar artery. From left to right, (*A*) coronal equilibrium phase MRA showing a central linear area of low signal intensity simulating a filling defect (*arrow*), (*B*) Bannas' method for distinguishing Gibbs artifact from PE. The signal intensity (SI) of the "filling defect" is measured and becomes the numerator and the surrounding enhanced vessel lumen signal intensity is the denominator (SI of filling defect/SI of lumen, Bannas' ratio). Gibb's artifact will have a ratio of greater than 50%, whereas PE will have a ratio of less than 50%.

**Table 5**
**Pulmonary artery measurements suspicious for pulmonary hypertension based on the clinical suspicion for pulmonary hypertension**

| CT Measures | Low Clinical Suspicion for Pulmonary Hypertension | Medium Clinical Suspicion for Pulmonary Hypertension | High Clinical Suspicion for Pulmonary Hypertension |
|---|---|---|---|
| Pulmonary artery Diameter | > 3.4 cm | > 3.2 cm | > 3.0 cm |
| Pulmonary artery diameter/Aortic Diameter | > 1.1 | > 1.0 | > 0.9 |

*Adapted from* Remy-Jardin et al.[55]

in the right ventricle. As the pressure increases over time, the right ventricle hypertrophies and ultimately fails, leading to cor pulmonale.

Measurement of pulmonary arterial compliance is possible with standard electrocardiogram (ECG)-gated two-dimensional balanced steady-state free precession (bSSFP) MR methodology that is angled orthogonal to the pulmonary trunk.[57,58]

### *Chronic Thromboembolic Pulmonary Hypertension*

CTEPH is an insidious and slowly progressive disease.[55] One hypothesis regarding the etiology of CTEPH is that this requires years of subclinical thromboembolic disease during which multiple small emboli obstruct the peripheral pulmonary capillary bed. This raises the mean pulmonary artery pressure slowly and patients begin to limit their activity incrementally until they become short of breath at rest. By that time, they present to the clinic needing oxygen. Fortunately, this cause of pulmonary hypertension can be treated with pulmonary endarterectomy and/or pulmonary arterial angioplasty. At surgical resection, casts of the pulmonary arteries are removed, with an immediate improvement in vessel compliance and reduction in mean pulmonary artery pressure. This surgery dramatically reduces the disease-specific mortality for CTEPH.[59]

### *Problems with Noninvasive Imaging*

Currently, noninvasive imaging for pulmonary hypertension cannot reliably diagnose pulmonary hypertension because no pressure measurements or oxygen saturation levels can be obtained by imaging alone. Unless noninvasive imaging is able to acquire this additional data, it will not replace right heart catheterization for accurate diagnosis.

Echocardiography has a very important role in noninvasive cardiovascular imaging. It is portable, of similar price to cardiovascular MR, and can be performed in the emergent setting at the bedside.[60] In the scenario of severe massive PE, this test can show findings of severe right heart strain and McConnell's sign.[61] McConnell's sign at echocardiography has a distinct regional pattern of right ventricular dysfunction, with akinesia of the mid free wall and normal motion at the apex.[62]

### *Indirect Findings*

When CT, CTA, MR imaging, or MRA demonstrate pulmonary arterial enlargement and/or right-sided cardiac chamber enlargement, transthoracic echocardiography is recommended for estimation of mean pulmonary artery pressure. This estimate is accomplished by obtaining the velocity of the tricuspid regurgitation jet and using the modified Bernoulli equation to calculate the pressure gradient, then interpolating the end-systolic pressure of the right ventricle from that measurement.[63] The right ventricular end-systolic pressure is a proxy for the mean pulmonary arterial pressure.

Main pulmonary artery diameter greater than 3.15 cm only suggests the possibility of pulmonary hypertension (**Table 5**).[55,64,65] On chest CT examinations, Mahammedi and colleagues[64] studied 298 patients with known pulmonary hypertension from right heart catheterization and 102 controls. They found that the mean pulmonary artery diameter and mean pulmonary artery diameter/ascending aorta diameter ratio had the highest correlation with pulmonary artery pressure ($r = 0.51$ and 0.53, respectively; $P < .001$). Using a cutoff value of mean pulmonary artery diameter greater than 31.5 mm had a sensitivity of 52.0% and specificity of 90% for pulmonary hypertension (see **Table 5**). A mean pulmonary artery diameter to ascending aorta diameter ratio greater than 1 was found to be 71% sensitive and 77% specific for this disease.[64] Use of this ratio is problematic in the setting of ascending aortic ectasia and aneurysms, however.

## SUMMARY

It is interesting that the application of MRA methods in the chest has not been adopted as readily as in other body parts. For example, it is part of daily practice to use MRA for the diagnosis of acute stroke and thrombosis of the cranial venous sinuses. Renal arterial diseases and renal transplant arteries are routinely imaged with MRA. Although most institutions commonly use MRA for aortic measurements in the setting of aneurysmal dilatation, one may wonder why the MRA-PE examination is so rarely used. The results of the PIOPED III prospective study answer this question.[34] This study showed that the overall efficacy of MRA was lower than that of CTA, particularly for subsegmental PE. At Wisconsin, we were performing MRA-PE before the PIOPED III results were published and have continued to use this examination as an alternative to CTPA when appropriate, with continued excellent buy-in from our providers/reception and favorable effects on clinical management.[35,36]

Although pulmonary hypertension is difficult to diagnose and requires a right heart catheterization for accurate measurement of mean pulmonary artery pressure and diagnostic confirmation, noninvasive imaging using MR imaging and MRA can help to triage these patients once the diagnosis has been established and can be used to follow-up treatment response of patients without further exposure to ionizing radiation.

## CLINICS CARE POINTS

- Over a decade ago, PIOPED III showed that MR angiography for pulmonary embolism (MRA-PE) was less sensitive than computed tomography pulmonary angiography (CTPA) for the diagnosis of subsegmental pulmonary emboli.
- MRA-PE has similar outcomes to CTPA after 6 months of follow-up.
- Gibbs artifact may simulate a non-occlusive PE on MRA-PE examinations.
- Ferumoxytol is an alternative to gadolinium-based contrast agents for patients with contrast allergies or pregnancy needing an MRA examination.
- MRA of the pulmonary vasculature, combined with cardiovascular MR imaging, is powerful methods for the study of pulmonary hypertension and its treatment response.

## DISCLOSURES

Dr S. Reeder has no relevant conflicts. Unrelated to this work, Dr S. Reeder has ownership interests in Calimetrix, Reveal Pharmaceuticals, Cellectar Biosciences, Elucent Medical, Inc HeartVista, and RevOps. Dr M.L. Schiebler has no relevant conflicts. Unrelated to this work, Dr M.L. Schiebler has ownership interests in Healthmyne, Inc; Stemina Biomarker Discovery, Inc; X-Vax, Inc and Elucent Medical, Inc. Dr J.B. Ackman has no relevant conflicts. Unrelated to this work, Dr J.B. Ackman receives royalties from Elsevier for associate editorship of a textbook. Dr L.L. Bergmann, Dr J. Starekova, Dr A. Moeller, and Dr S.K. Nagle have nothing to disclose.

## REFERENCES

1. Bell LC, Wang K, Munoz Del Rio A, et al. Comparison of models and contrast agents for improved signal and signal linearity in dynamic contrast-enhanced pulmonary magnetic resonance imaging. Invest Radiol 2015;50(3):174–8.
2. Bell LC, Johnson KM, Fain SB, et al. Simultaneous MRI of lung structure and perfusion in a single breath-hold. J Magn Reson Imaging 2015;41(1):52–9.
3. Bauman G, Puderbach M, Deimling M, et al. Non-contrast-enhanced perfusion and ventilation assessment of the human lung by means of Fourier decomposition in proton MRI. Magn Reson Med 2009;62(3):656–64.
4. Bauman G, Scholz A, Rivoire J, et al. Lung ventilation- and perfusion-weighted Fourier decomposition magnetic resonance imaging: in vivo validation with hyperpolarized 3He and dynamic contrast-enhanced MRI. Magn Reson Med 2013;69(1):229–37.
5. Voskrebenzev A, Gutberlet M, Klimes F, et al. Feasibility of quantitative regional ventilation and perfusion mapping with phase-resolved functional lung (PREFUL) MRI in healthy volunteers and COPD, CTEPH, and CF patients. Magn Reson Med 2018;79(4):2306–14.
6. Pohler GH, Loffler F, Klimes F, et al. Validation of Phase-Resolved Functional Lung (PREFUL) Magnetic Resonance Imaging Pulse Wave Transit Time Compared to Echocardiography in Chronic Obstructive Pulmonary Disease. J Magn Reson Imaging 2022;56(2):605–15.
7. Heiss R, Tan L, Schmidt S, et al. Pulmonary Dysfunction after Pediatric COVID-19. Radiology 2022;221250. https://doi.org/10.1148/radiol.221250.
8. Prince MR, Lee HG, Lee CH, et al. Safety of gadobutrol in over 23,000 patients: the GARDIAN study, a global multicentre, prospective, non-interventional study. Eur Radiol 2017;27(1):286–95.

9. Behzadi AH, Zhao Y, Farooq Z, et al. Immediate Allergic Reactions to Gadolinium-based Contrast Agents: A Systematic Review and Meta-Analysis. Radiology 2018;286(2):731.
10. Heshmatzadeh Behzadi A, Prince MR. Preventing Allergic Reactions to Gadolinium-Based Contrast Agents. Top Magn Reson Imaging 2016;25(6): 275–9.
11. Soulez G, Bloomgarden DC, Rofsky NM, et al. Prospective Cohort Study of Nephrogenic Systemic Fibrosis in Patients With Stage 3-5 Chronic Kidney Disease Undergoing MRI With Injected Gadobenate Dimeglumine or Gadoteridol. AJR Am J Roentgenol 2015;205(3):469–78.
12. McDonald RJ, Levine D, Weinreb J, et al. Gadolinium Retention: A Research Roadmap from the 2018 NIH/ACR/RSNA Workshop on Gadolinium Chelates. Radiology 2018;289(2):517–34.
13. Lersy F, Boulouis G, Clement O, et al. Consensus Guidelines of the French Society of Neuroradiology (SFNR) on the use of Gadolinium-Based Contrast agents (GBCAs) and related MRI protocols in Neuroradiology. J Neuroradiol 2020;47(6):441–9.
14. Maki JH, Prince MR, Londy FJ, et al. The effects of time varying intravascular signal intensity and k-space acquisition order on three-dimensional MR angiography image quality. J Magn Reson Imaging 1996;6(4):642–51.
15. Nguyen KL, Yoshida T, Kathuria-Prakash N, et al. Multicenter Safety and Practice for Off-Label Diagnostic Use of Ferumoxytol in MRI. Radiology 2019; 293(3):554–64.
16. Starekova J, Nagle SK, Schiebler ML, et al. Pulmonary MRA During Pregnancy: Early Experience With Ferumoxytol. J Magn Reson Imaging 2022. https://doi.org/10.1002/jmri.28504.
17. Benson DG, Schiebler ML, Repplinger MD, et al. Contrast-enhanced pulmonary MRA for the primary diagnosis of pulmonary embolism: current state of the art and future directions. Br J Radiol 2017; 90(1074):20160901.
18. Pressacco J, Papas K, Lambert J, et al. Magnetic resonance angiography imaging of pulmonary embolism using agents with blood pool properties as an alternative to computed tomography to avoid radiation exposure. Eur J Radiol 2019;113:165–73.
19. American College of Radiology (ACR) manual on Contrast Media. Available at: https://www.acr.org/-/media/ACR/Files/Clinical-Resources/Contrast_Media.pdf.
20. Starekova J, Bruce RJ, Sadowski EA, et al. No Cases of Nephrogenic Systemic Fibrosis after Administration of Gadoxetic Acid. Radiology 2020; 297(3):556–62.
21. McDonald JS, McDonald RJ. MR Imaging Safety Considerations of Gadolinium-Based Contrast Agents: Gadolinium Retention and Nephrogenic Systemic Fibrosis. Magn Reson Imaging Clin N Am 2020;28(4):497–507.
22. Kobayashi M, Levendovszky SR, Hippe DS, et al. Comparison of Human Tissue Gadolinium Retention and Elimination between Gadoteridol and Gadobenate. Radiology 2021;300(3):559–69.
23. Tweedle MF. Gadolinium Retention in Human Brain, Bone, and Skin. Radiology 2021;300(3):570–1.
24. Winterstein AG, Thai TN, Nduaguba S, et al. Risk of fetal or neonatal death or neonatal intensive care unit admission associated with gadolinium magnetic resonance imaging exposure during pregnancy. Am J Obstet Gynecol 2022. https://doi.org/10.1016/j.ajog.2022.10.005.
25. Gerb J, Strauss W, Derman R, et al. Ferumoxytol for the treatment of iron deficiency and iron-deficiency anemia of pregnancy. Ther Adv Hematol 2021;12. https://doi.org/10.1177/20406207211018042. 20406207211018042.
26. U.S.Food & Drug Administration. FERAHEME® (ferumoxytol injection) Fpi. Available at: https://www.accessdata.fda.gov/drugsatfda_docs/label/2018/022180s009lbl.pdf.
27. Zhu A, Reeder SB, Johnson KM, et al. Quantitative ferumoxytol-enhanced MRI in pregnancy: A feasibility study in the nonhuman primate. Magn Reson Imaging 2020;65:100–8.
28. Food and Drug Administration: Drug safety and Administration. Available at: https://www.fda.gov/drugs/drug-safety-and-availability/fda-drug-safety-communication-fda-strengthens-warnings-and-changes-prescribing-instructions-decrease.
29. Fereheme: Dosing information. Available at: https://www.feraheme.com/dosing-administration/.
30. Maki JH, Neligan PC, Briller N, et al. Dark Blood Magnetic Resonance Lymphangiography Using Dual-Agent Relaxivity Contrast (DARC-MRL): A Novel Method Combining Gadolinium and Iron Contrast Agents. Curr Probl Diagn Radiol 2016; 45(3):174–9.
31. Vaikom House A, David D, Aguet J, et al. Quantification of lymphatic burden in patients with Fontan circulation by T2 MR lymphangiography and associations with adverse Fontan status. Eur Heart J Cardiovasc Imaging 2022. https://doi.org/10.1093/ehjci/jeac216.
32. Spencer FA, Emery C, Lessard D, et al. The Worcester Venous Thromboembolism study: a population-based study of the clinical epidemiology of venous thromboembolism. J Gen Intern Med 2006;21(7):722–7.
33. Prologo JD, Gilkeson RC, Diaz M, et al. CT pulmonary angiography: a comparative analysis of the utilization patterns in emergency department and hospitalized patients between 1998 and 2003. AJR Am J Roentgenol 2004;183(4):1093–6.
34. Stein PD, Chenevert TL, Fowler SE, et al. Gadolinium-enhanced magnetic resonance angiography

for pulmonary embolism: a multicenter prospective study (PIOPED III). Ann Intern Med 2010;152(7): 434–43.
35. Schiebler ML, Nagle SK, Francois CJ, et al. Effectiveness of MR angiography for the primary diagnosis of acute pulmonary embolism: clinical outcomes at 3 months and 1 year. J Magn Reson Imaging 2013; 38(4):914–25.
36. Repplinger MD, Nagle SK, Harringa JB, et al. Clinical outcomes after magnetic resonance angiography (MRA) versus computed tomographic angiography (CTA) for pulmonary embolism evaluation. Emerg Radiol 2018;25(5):469–77.
37. Schiebler ML, Benson D, Schubert T, et al. Noncontrast and contrast-enhanced pulmonary magnetic resonance angiography. In: Kauczor H, Wielpuetz MO, Eds., MRI of the lung, 2nd Ed, Springer, Cham, Switzerland; 2018: 21–52
38. Pijpe A, Andrieu N, Easton DF, et al. Exposure to diagnostic radiation and risk of breast cancer among carriers of BRCA1/2 mutations: retrospective cohort study (GENE-RAD-RISK). BMJ 2012;345: e5660.
39. Carrier M, Righini M, Wells PS, et al. Subsegmental pulmonary embolism diagnosed by computed tomography: incidence and clinical implications. A systematic review and meta-analysis of the management outcome studies. J Thromb Haemost 2010; 8(8):1716–22.
40. Tsuchiya N, Benson DG, Longhurst C, et al. Interobserver agreement for the direct and indirect signs of pulmonary embolism evaluated using contrast enhanced magnetic angiography. Eur J Radiol Open 2020;7:100256.
41. Schiebler ML, Ahuja J, Repplinger MD, et al. Incidence of actionable findings on contrast enhanced magnetic resonance angiography ordered for pulmonary embolism evaluation. Eur J Radiol 2016; 85(8):1383–9.
42. Stein PD, Matta F, Sedrick JA, et al. Ancillary findings on CT pulmonary angiograms and abnormalities on chest radiographs in patients in whom pulmonary embolism was excluded. Clin Appl Thromb Hemost 2012;18(2):201–5.
43. Schiebler ML, Listerud J. Common artifacts encountered in thoracic magnetic resonance imaging: recognition, derivation, and solutions. Top Magn Reson Imaging 1992;4(3):1–17.
44. Bannas P, Schiebler ML, Motosugi U, et al. Pulmonary MRA: differentiation of pulmonary embolism from truncation artefact. Eur Radiol 2014;24(8): 1942–9.
45. Swift AJ, Rajaram S, Marshall H, et al. Black blood MRI has diagnostic and prognostic value in the assessment of patients with pulmonary hypertension. Eur Radiol 2012;22(3):695–702.
46. Khadir MM, Chaturvedi A, Nguyen MS, et al. Looking beyond the thrombus: essentials of pulmonary artery imaging on CT. Insights Imaging 2014;5(4): 493–506.
47. Mader MT, Poulton TB, White RD. Malignant tumors of the heart and great vessels: MR imaging appearance. Radiographics 1997;17(1):145–53.
48. Kacl GM, Bruder E, Pfammatter T, et al. Primary angiosarcoma of the pulmonary arteries: dynamic contrast-enhanced MRI. J Comput Assist Tomogr 1998;22(5):687–91.
49. Leitman EM, McDermott S. Pulmonary arteries: imaging of pulmonary embolism and beyond. Cardiovasc Diagn Ther 2019;9(Suppl 1):S37–58.
50. Atasoy C, Fitoz S, Yigit H, et al. Radiographic, CT, and MRI findings in primary pulmonary angiosarcoma. Clin Imaging 2001;25(5):337–40.
51. Pugh D, Karabayas M, Basu N, et al. Large-vessel vasculitis. Nat Rev Dis Primers 2022;7(1):93.
52. Expert Panels on C, Thoracic I, Kirsch J, et al. ACR Appropriateness Criteria((R)) Acute Chest Pain-Suspected Pulmonary Embolism. J Am Coll Radiol 2017;14(5S):S2–12.
53. Nagle SK, Schiebler ML, Repplinger MD, et al. Contrast enhanced pulmonary magnetic resonance angiography for pulmonary embolism: Building a successful program. Eur J Radiol 2016;85(3): 553–63.
54. Griffin L, Swift AJ, Tsuchiya NF, et al. Multimodality imaging of pulmonary hypertension: prognostication of therapeutic outcomes, In: Ohno Y, Hatabu H, Kauczor H, Eds. Pulmonary Functional Imaging: basics and clinical applications, 2021, Springer, 225-257. Cham, Switzerland.
55. Remy-Jardin M, Ryerson CJ, Schiebler ML, et al. Imaging of Pulmonary Hypertension in Adults: A Position Paper from the Fleischner Society. Radiology 2021;298(3):531–49.
56. Humbert M, Kovacs G, Hoeper MM, et al. 2022 ESC/ERS Guidelines for the diagnosis and treatment of pulmonary hypertension. Eur Heart J 2022;43(38): 3618–731.
57. Tian L, Kellihan HB, Henningsen J, et al. Pulmonary artery relative area change is inversely related to ex vivo measured arterial elastic modulus in the canine model of acute pulmonary embolization. J Biomech 2014;47(12):2904–10.
58. Schiebler ML, Bhalla S, Runo J, et al. Magnetic resonance and computed tomography imaging of the structural and functional changes of pulmonary arterial hypertension. J Thorac Imaging 2013;28(3): 178–93.
59. Song W, Zhu J, Zhong Z, et al. Long-term outcome prediction for chronic thromboembolic pulmonary hypertension after pulmonary endarterectomy. Clin Cardiol 2022;7. https://doi.org/10.1002/clc.23900.

60. Zhang L, Wang B, Zhou J, et al. Bedside Focused Cardiac Ultrasound in COVID-19 from the Wuhan Epicenter: The Role of Cardiac Point-of-Care Ultrasound, Limited Transthoracic Echocardiography, and Critical Care Echocardiography. J Am Soc Echocardiogr 2020;33(6):676–82.
61. Ramirez-Arias E, Rosas-Peralta M, Borrayo-Sanchez G, et al. [Pulmonary thromboembolism: Recent experience of 4 years at a cardiology hospital]. Rev Med Inst Mex Seguro Soc 2017;55(1): 52–62. Tromboembolismo pulmonar: experiencia reciente de 4 anos en un hospital de cardiologia.
62. McConnell MV, Solomon SD, Rayan ME, et al. Regional right ventricular dysfunction detected by echocardiography in acute pulmonary embolism. Am J Cardiol 1996;78(4):469–73.
63. Laver RD, Wiersema UF, Bersten AD. Echocardiographic estimation of mean pulmonary artery pressure in critically ill patients. Crit Ultrasound J 2014; 6(1):9.
64. Mahammedi A, Oshmyansky A, Hassoun PM, et al. Pulmonary artery measurements in pulmonary hypertension: the role of computed tomography. J Thorac Imaging 2013;28(2):96–103.
65. Haimovici JB, Trotman-Dickenson B, Halpern EF, et al. Relationship between pulmonary artery diameter at computed tomography and pulmonary artery pressures at right-sided heart catheterization. Massachusetts General Hospital Lung Transplantation Program. Acad Radiol 1997;4(5): 327–34.

# MR Angiography

## Contrast-Enhanced Acquisition Techniques

Prashant Nagpal, MD[a,*], Thomas M. Grist, MD[b]

**KEYWORDS**

• MR angiography • Technique • Contrast-enhanced MR angiography • Bright-blood MRA • 3D MR angiography • Time-resolved MRA • Renal artery • Peripheral artery • Gadolinium

**KEY POINTS**

- Contrast-enhanced MR angiography (CE-MRA) has undergone significant technical advances that have improved the resolution, speed, and extent of its applications.
- Knowledge of the fundamental physics of fast T1-weighted spoiled gradient echo sequence and filling of k-space can help in a better understanding of the technique.
- Further, an understanding of the image acquisition and acceleration techniques will help to better understand the pitfalls, artifacts, and future development in CE-MRA.

**Video content accompanies this article at http://www.mri.theclinics.com.**

## INTRODUCTION

The use of non-invasive imaging techniques for cardiovascular imaging is now routine practice. Among the available imaging tests, contrast-enhanced MR angiography (CE-MRA) is one of the frequently used techniques for diagnosing and following up vascular diseases. Since its development in the 1990s,[1–3] technical improvements in contrast agents and better MR engineering techniques have led to improved spatial and temporal resolution with an improved signal-to-noise ratio (SNR) and decreased scan time. Similar to other advances in imaging, CE-MRA has evolved over time. However, it is considered technically challenging which reduces the routine availability of CE-MRA to patients, especially at community imaging facilities. With early detection of genetic vascular diseases, an increasing aging population, and an overall increase in atherosclerosis and other vascular diseases that need frequent follow-up, knowledge of CE-MRA principles among radiologists is critical for the appropriate use of this high-resolution non-invasive technique for appropriately selected patients. In this review, we will highlight the basic principles of CE-MRA, the timing of acquisition, sequences utilized, acceleration techniques, pitfalls, and future developments. The knowledge of these principles continues to guide the upcoming advances in CE-MRA.

## MR ANGIOGRAPHY TECHNIQUES

Conventionally, MRA techniques can be divided into black-blood imaging and bright-blood imaging. Black-blood imaging is invaluable for vessel wall assessment and cardiac imaging, while bright-blood imaging is used to evaluate course, caliber, and luminal vascular information.[4] This review is focused on CE-MRA, which is a bright-blood imaging technique. CE-MRA utilizes the administration of the intravenous contrast agent (most frequently gadolinium-based contrast agents, GBCA) that provide an increase in the signal in the

[a] Cardiovascular Imaging, Department of Radiology, University of Wisconsin-Madison, School of Medicine and Public Health, 600 Highland Avenue, Madison, WI 53705, USA; [b] Radiology, University of Wisconsin Madison, E3/366 600 Highland Avenue, Madison, WI 53792, USA
* Corresponding author. 600 Highland Avenue, Madison, WI 53705.
*E-mail address:* pnagpal@wisc.edu

Magn Reson Imaging Clin N Am 31 (2023) 493–501
https://doi.org/10.1016/j.mric.2023.04.007

T1-weighted gradient echo sequence. The time to echo (TE) and the repetition time (TR) are minimized to produce T1-weighing and shorten time scan time.

The timing of the acquisition of the 3D image volume relative to the arrival of contrast media in the vascular territory of interest is critical to the success of the CE-MRA study. The acquisition can be time-resolved (4D), or obtained after a pre-decided time delay using a test bolus, or fluoroscopically triggered in real-time when contrast reaches the specific vascular territory.[5] For the test bolus, a small volume (2 mL or less) of contrast is injected with a saline flush. Then the vessel of interest is imaged. The timing of the acquisition is decided based on the optimal time delay. The primary advantage of this technique is that it offers information regarding patient-specific physiology. However, it requires more time and more technical expertise and leads to background contamination by the presence of contrast media in the vessels from the test bolus. Fluoroscopic triggering uses a real-time fluoroscopy-like acquisition of the vascular territory of interest using a rapid 2D gradient echo technique, as the contrast is injected. The arrival of the contrast is seen as an increase in the signal intensity of the vessel and the acquisition can be triggered manually or automatically. In our experience, fluoroscopic triggering is most commonly used and is easier for technologists to learn as the method is frequently used in computed tomography angiography (CTA) as well.[6–8] An alternative acquisition method to solve this problem, time-resolved MRA, is an angiographic technique in itself and is detailed later in this review. The vendor-specific fluoroscopy triggered CE-MRA technique nomenclature is summarized in **Table 1**.

## PRINCIPLES OF CONTRAST-ENHANCED MR ANGIOGRAPHY

CE-MRA is the most used method of evaluating vessels using MR imaging outside intracranial vascular imaging. CE-MRA can be performed with a high spatial and temporal resolution, allowing multiphasic imaging with separation of the arterial and venous system and assessment of flow dynamics. Given these advantages, CE-MRA is the non-invasive imaging test of choice for dynamic compression syndromes like popliteal artery entrapment, thoracic outlet compression, or median arcuate ligament compression syndrome. Compared to non-contrast MRA, CE-MRA can generate high vascular signal intensity irrespective of vessel orientation and is significantly less sensitive to artifacts.[6] Compared to CT angiography, MRA images are more challenging to acquire, but avoid ionizing radiation and iodine contrast media. MRA is less sensitive to the detection of vascular calcification but is more accurate for luminal assessment of heavily calcified vessels like calcified lower extremity vasculature.[9,10]

## CONTRAST MEDIA

CE-MRA's image quality (IQ) primarily depends on using an intravenous (IV) contrast agent and the choice of scan parameters. *Paramagnetism* is the intrinsic property of certain materials by which they exhibit temporary magnetization when they encounter a magnetic field. Unlike CT imaging, MR imaging does not image the contrast agent directly. Instead, MR measures the shortening of T1 upon administration of GBCA or Ferumoxytol.[11–13] The characteristics and properties of contrast agents are detailed in a separate review and are beyond the scope of this review.

At 1.5 T, the T1 time of blood is approximately 1200 msec. Gadolinium (Gd) has paramagnetic properties which creates a local magnetic field and affects the H+ (proton) in the blood. When GBCA is administered, the blood T1 time can lower to less than 50 msec (on 1.5 T). The strength of the signal enhancement is proportional to the T1 shortening. And the contrast-to-noise ratio is dependent on the difference in the T1 time between the blood pool and the adjacent soft tissue (**Fig. 1**). Although the T1 shortening by GBCA is dose-dependent, a higher concentration of Gd causes T2* shortening, which can override the T1 shortening leading to loss of signal.[14]

Additionally, the degree of contrast enhancement is related to the timing of acquisition (related to the vascular territory of interest), injection rate, patient-specific hemodynamics, and sequence parameters. For CE-MRA, the GBCA is injected intravenously, usually into the antecubital vein or

**Table 1**
**Vendor-specific names for contrast-enhanced MR angiography sequences**

| MRA Technique | GE | Siemens | Philips | Canon | Hitachi |
|---|---|---|---|---|---|
| Fluoroscopy triggered CE-MRA | SmartPrep | CARE[a] Bolus | Bolus Trak | Visual Prep | FLUTE[b] |

[a] CARE, combined applications to reduce exposure.
[b] FLUTE, FLUoro Triggered Examination.

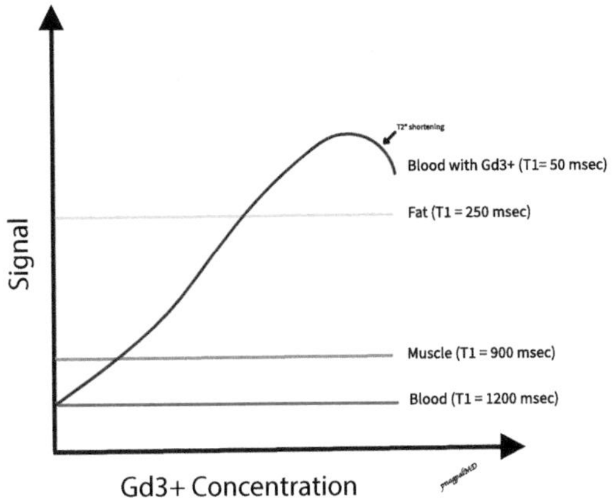


**Fig. 1.** Graphical representation of signal (y-axis) vs gadolinium concentration (x-axis) depicting T1 time of various tissues (values on 1.5 T). As shown, the native T1 time of the blood is approximately 1200 msec, hence the signal is low. However, when GBCA are injected, they lead to T1 shortening (T1 time approx. 50 msec) which is measured as a bright signal on T1-weighted images.

central catheter (if available). If possible, the right antecubital vein is preferred for contrast injection, as right-side veins have a straighter path to the right heart. This allows for a more coherent bolus. Also, if injected from the left upper extremity, the residual contrast in the left innominate vein can interfere with aortic arch vessel visualization. The contrast dose is followed by a saline chaser to ensure emptying of GBCA from the peripheral veins. The goal is to inject a compact bolus of contrast into the central circulation. An injection rate of 1 to 1.5 mL/second using power injectors is suitable for CE-MRA studies. The faster injection can lead to higher Gd3+ concentration and higher SNR but is also associated with shorter first-pass perfusion time and earlier venous contamination. The arterial Gd3+ concentration and hence enhancement is inversely related to cardiac output. Patients with lower cardiac output have a more compact contrast bolus and hence have a greater degree of arterial enhancement for the given injection rate.[15,16] MRA is timed to match image acquisition with the time of peak Gd3+ of the vascular territory of interest. **Fig. 2** shows a diagram which highlights the change in MR imaging signal with respect to contrast injection. If performed in an 'ideal' acquisition window, the MRA maximizes the signal in the arterial and venous systems. This principle is used to identify the appropriate phase of the MRA series, depending on the clinical question and the vascular territory. As GBCA recirculates from the vessels to the extracellular tissue, MRA is timed for first-pass perfusion. Early image acquisition leads to low signal intensity with poor vessel delineation. Acquisition of central k-space too early or during the rapid rise of Gd3+ concentration leads to ringing artifact with alternating bright and dark lines or peripheral hyperintensity and central hypointensity (**Fig. 3**). Other the other end, late acquisition leads to an overall low signal in the vessel of interest, more artifacts and higher venous contamination (**Fig. 4**). Additionally, some specific organ systems have unique physiologic considerations. For example, pulmonary MRA contrast bolus can get interrupted due to the patient taking a deep breath, leading to the return of non-enhanced blood from the inferior vena cava (IVC) and poor pulmonary arterial enhancement (**Fig. 5**), similar to transient interruption of the contrast described on pulmonary artery CTAs.[17]

## MR ANGIOGRAPHY SEQUENCE BASICS

A gradient sequence (GRE) is a sequence in which dephasing and rephasing gradients are used after a radiofrequency (RF) pulse to generate an echo. However, if the TR is shorter than the T1 time of the excited tissue, the protons do not fully relax before the subsequent RF pulse. The spoiled gradient echo (SGRE) sequence involves using the gradient or RF-spoiling to disrupt transverse (T2) coherences of the excited tissue. This makes SGRE sequences less sensitive to flow and motion artifacts.[18] The pulse sequence diagram of spoiled-GRE sequence is shown in **Fig. 6**. SGRE is the primary sequence that is used for CE-MRA imaging. The sequence parameters are adjusted for maximum signal (maximum T1 weighting), fastest acquisition, and high SNR and spatial resolution (depending on the size of the vascular territory being imaged). Both the spin density and T2*-weighting may be impacted by parameters on the spoiled-GRE sequence. Short TE minimizes the T2* signal loss, which tends to reduce the vascular signal. For CE-MRA, strong T1-weighting is needed; hence short TR (3–6 msec) and short TE (1–2 msec) are used. Higher T1 weighting translates to higher vascular to background contrast. A flip angle between 25° and 45° provides the maximum difference between the contrast and background tissues that translates to high SNR and contrast-to-noise ratio (CNR).[19] Vendor-specific spoiled-GRE sequences nomenclature is summarized in **Table 2**.

## 3D MR ANGIOGRAPHY

Another critical technical parameter for CE-MRA is spatial resolution and 3D acquisition. The desired voxel resolution of CE-MRA depends on the size

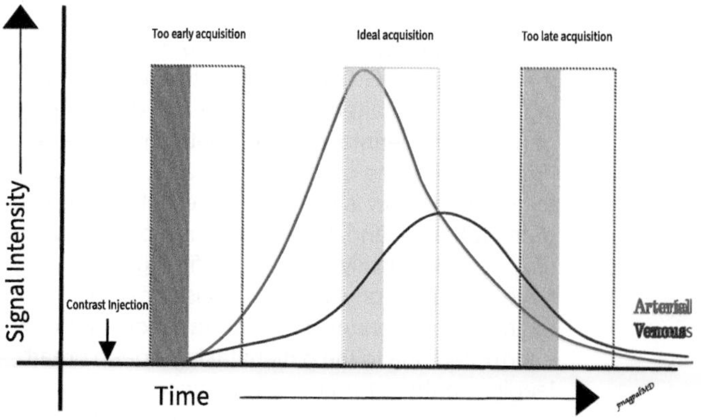


Fig. 2. Illustration showing a change in arterial and venous signal after contrast injection. Too early acquisition (brown box) leads to low signal in arterial and venous systems while too late acquisition (blue box) misses the peak signal in vessels and hence leads to low arterial and venous signals. An ideally timed acquisition is associated with peak arterial and venous signals (green box).

of the vascular system being imaged and the suspected pathology. Acquisition of CE-MRA with isovolumetric voxels is the standard practice as it allows post-processing and subsequent reconstruction in any plane. To acquire isovolumetric voxels, CE-MRA is acquired in a 3D mode.[20] 3D-MRA is typically acquired using a rectangular (Cartesian) grid with one frequency encoding and two phase-encoding directions. The second phase-encoding acts as a slice selection. To minimize the scan time, the fewest phase-encoding steps (shortest distance) are acquired along the slice selection direction (second phase-encoding). The second shortest distance is along the phase-encoding direction. And the longest distance is kept along the frequency encoding direction. The k-space ordering for the sequence can be linear or radial. Elliptical-centric ordering (a type of radial ordering) is the preferred type of k-space sampling for most CE-MRA. A modification of the elliptic-centric approach, known as recessed elliptic-centric k-space filling that involves an asymmetric collection of the central k-space data, is one of the most optimum methods for the majority of CE-MRA. Irrespective of the ordering method and modifications, the primary goal is that the central portion of the k-space (lowest spatial frequency), which contributes most to the image contrast, is sampled early in the CE-MRA acquisition. It is timed to correspond to the arrival of the contrast bolus.[21] This centric ordering maximizes the arterial enhancement and minimizes the venous enhancement as peripheral k-space data (that provides edge detail) are acquired later, at the time of venous enhancement.

## TIME-RESOLVED MR ANGIOGRAPHY

Time-resolved MRA is a technique that allows rapid multiphase scanning of an area of interest by repeated sampling of the center of the k-space. The sequence is typically started before the contrast reaches the vascular territory of interest and is repeated multiple times. Due to the lack of

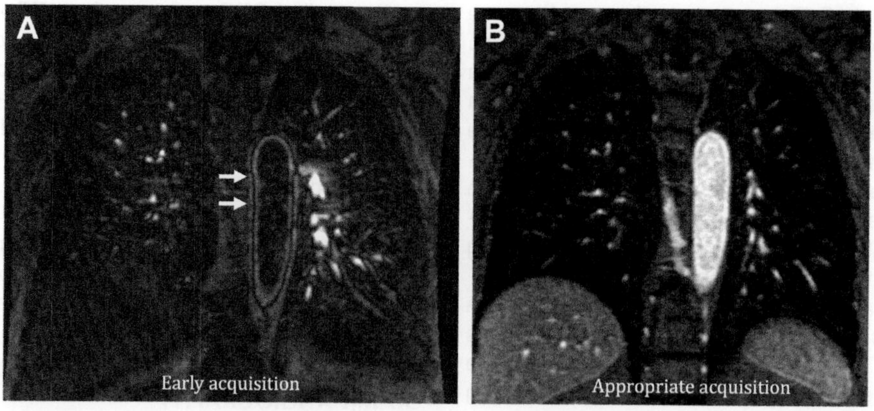


Fig. 3. MR angiography performed for aortic sizing. Panel *A* showing early acquisition (as the contrast concentration is increasing in the vessel of interest) leading to peripheral high signal and central low signal in the aorta (*white arrows*, 'ringing' artifact). Immediate repeat acquisition. Panel *B* showing the appropriate phase of acquisition for aortic MRA.

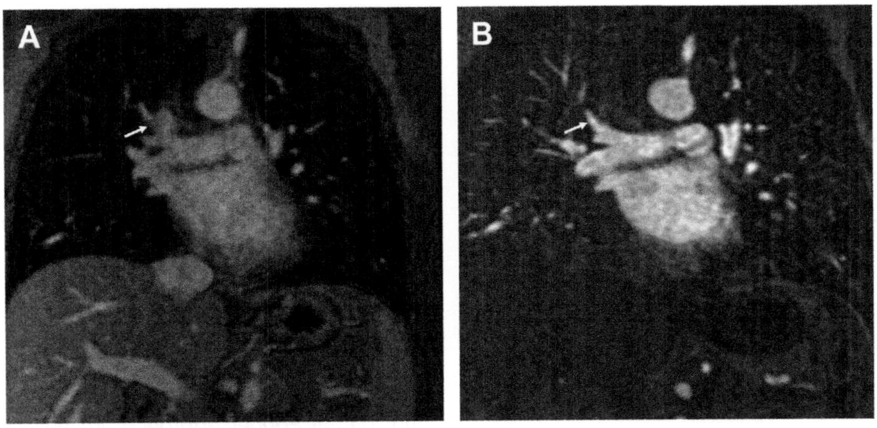


Fig. 4. Pulmonary MR angiography performed to rule out pulmonary embolism. Panel *A* showing delayed acquisition due to technical factors that led to poor pulmonary arterial enhancement with areas that may mimic embolism (*white arrows*) and extensive venous enhancement. Repeat contrast bolus performed with appropriate timing for pulmonary artery. Panel *B* showing excellent pulmonary arterial enhancement and confirming the absence of embolism and artifactual appearance on the delayed acquisition (*white arrow*).

ionizing radiation, it is possible with MR imaging to run the MRA sequence repeatedly. This allows dynamic visualization of the vascular flow (usually both arterial and early venous) as well as the directionality of the blood flow (Video 1).[22]

Typically, an inherent trade-off exists between temporal and spatial resolution. As highlighted earlier, the center of the k-space provides information on image contrast, and the periphery of the k-space provides information on fine detail. So, conventionally, improvement of spatial resolution requires more k-space sampling. However, acceleration techniques can be used to acquire multiphasic acquisition with relatively high spatial resolution.[23] It should be noted that the spatial resolution of time-resolved MRA is still typically lower than 3D MRA (**Fig. 7**).

Time-resolved MRA sequences can use multiple acceleration techniques, the most important of which is view sharing. View sharing is a process that involves filling the center of the k-space over a short period and filling the edges of the k-space less frequently. The peripheral k-space data are recorded only periodically, but frequently enough to gather data to allow image reconstruction. The images obtained before the contrast reach the vascular territory act as mask images for eventual subtraction. As there is continuous k-space filling in the sequence, one of the prerequisites is that the patient must stay still between multiphase

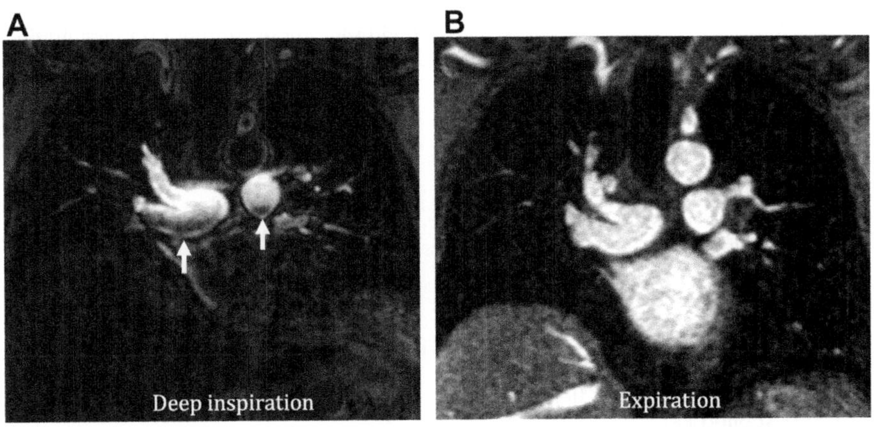


Fig. 5. Pulmonary MRA to rule out pulmonary embolism. Panel *A* showing linear low signal in the pulmonary arteries (*white arrows*) due to non-enhanced blood coming from the inferior vena cava due to patient taking a deep breath. A repeat acquisition (Panel *B*) performed in expiration showing appropriate enhancement of the pulmonary arteries.

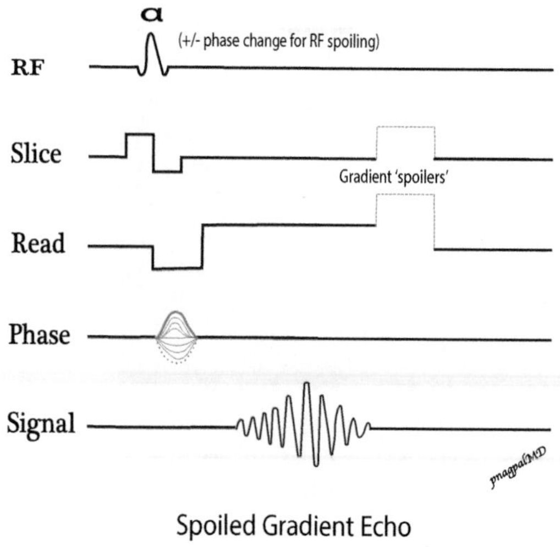


**Fig. 6.** A simplified pulse sequence diagram of an SGRE showing both gradient and RF-spoiling.

acquisitions. Time-resolved MRA images are frequently visualized as a reconstructed subtracted maximum intensity projection series of the whole volume. However, each time-point acquisition is also available for the reader to evaluate and interpret. The vendor-specific time-resolved MRA technique nomenclature is summarized in **Table 3**.

## ACCELERATION TECHNIQUES

Although one of the premises for contrast-enhanced MRA is fast acquisition with short TR, acceleration techniques are still needed. For thoracic and abdominal MRA, breath-holding is critical for optimum IQ. Additionally, in some organ systems like the brain and renal circulation, the transit of contrast through the arterial circulation is fast, due to which acceleration techniques are needed to allow appropriate arterial phase imaging. For a basic understanding, scan time on MR imaging = TR x phase-encoding steps x slices (simplified equation). The acceleration techniques focus on achieving the shortest possible acquisition time, assuming the shortest TR is limited by the performance of the magnetic field gradients or reducing the number of phase-encoding steps. Reducing the number of phase-encoding steps translates to under-sampling of the k-space and is a frequently used technique for acceleration beyond the minimum acquisition time for full sample data. Examples of such acceleration techniques include parallel imaging, partial Fourier approach, keyhole, and view-sharing approaches.[24]

**Table-2**
**Vendor-specific names for spoiled-gradient sequences**

| Vendor | Spoiled-GRE Sequence |
|---|---|
| GE | Spoiled gradient-recalled acquisition sequence (SPGR)<br>Multiplanar spoiled gradient-recalled acquisition in steady state (MPSPGR) |
| Siemens | Fast low-angle shot (FLASH) |
| Philips | T1 fast field echo (T1-FFE) |
| Canon | Radiofrequency spoiled field echo (RF-spoiled FE) |
| Hitachi | Radiofrequency spoiled steady state acquisition rewound gradient echo (RSSG) |

Parallel imaging involves decreasing the number of phase-encoding steps using a specific type of receiver coil. A phased-array coil with multiple coil elements for the body of interest is needed to use parallel imaging. A reference scan is needed to generate coil sensitivity information, and appropriate software is needed to unfold image wrap-around, or aliasing artifacts due to under-sampling of the data. Generally, parallel imaging can occur in two domains—the image domain (most frequently used) and the frequency or k-space domain. *SENSE* (*SENS*tivity *E*ncoding) is the original general acronym for image domain parallel imaging. The data are used from individual coil elements of the phased-array coil to accelerate the acquisition. A reduced number of k-space lines are acquired to decrease the scan time. The reference scan provides the coil sensitivity information or the coil sensitivity map. The sensitivity map of the individual coil is used to unfold the full image. There may be some specific differences between image domain parallel imaging and k-space domain parallel imaging. For example, image domain parallel imaging may be less effective at eliminating artifacts if there is patient motion between the calibration scan and acquisition scan, even though the patient may be perfectly still during each of these sequences separately. The k-space domain parallel imaging tends to be somewhat longer to perform as it requires extra time for the self-calibration of k-space lines. Parallel imaging results in a reduction of SNR, which is equivalent to $1/\sqrt{R}$, where R = the acceleration factor. So, if the acceleration of four times is desired (one-fourth of the time to perform a specific sequence), the SNR will be 0.5 of the original sequence. At higher acceleration factors, the artifacts also increase (**Fig. 8**). One way to decrease artifacts with high acceleration factors is to split the acceleration, wherever possible. For example, instead of applying the acceleration

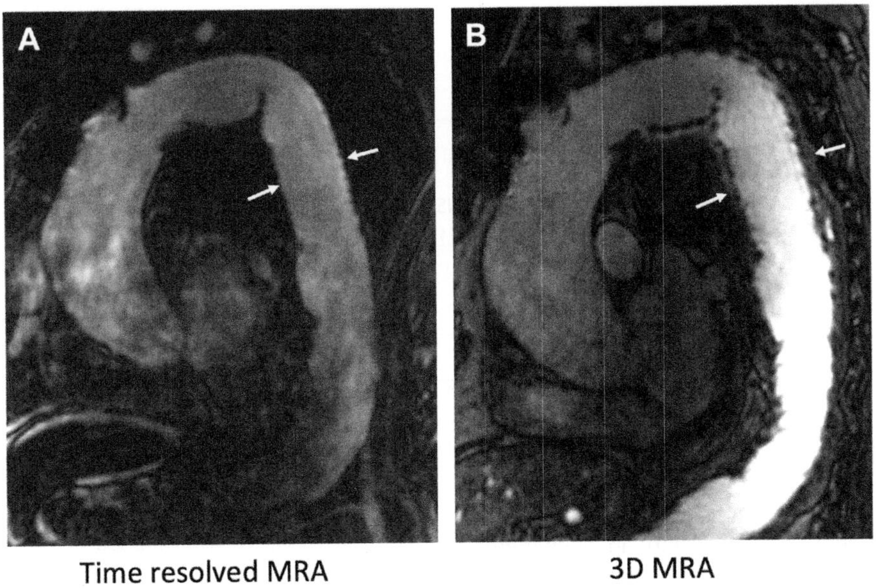


Fig. 7. Aortic MR angiogram performed in a patient with descending thoracic aortic stent. Oblique sagittal time-resolved MRA image (panel-*A*) and 3D MRA (panel-*B*) highlighting the subtle difference in enhancement and resolution of these MR angiography techniques. Notice how the stent outline (*white arrows*) and fine details are better appreciated on 3D MRA.

factor of four in one phase-encoding direction, it is better to use an acceleration factor of two in one phase-encoding direction and an acceleration factor of two in another phase-encoding direction (for a total acceleration factor of four). In practice, parallel imaging can be used to increase the spatial resolution while keeping the scan time similar or decreasing motion or breathing artifacts, keeping spatial resolution unchanged.[25] The vendor-specific parallel imaging technique nomenclature is summarized in **Table 4**.

The partial Fourier approach is another acceleration method in which the MR image is reconstructed using a fraction of k-space. This is possible because of the feature that any two points diagonally opposite in k-space are symmetric, also known as conjugate symmetry. Therefore, if half of the k-space is filled, the other half can be estimated to generate the image. A partial Fourier approach can be achieved by reduction of the phase-encoding steps, also called partial Fourier phase-encoding. Due to the decrease in phase-encoding steps, there is a reduction in the scan time. In practice, the acquisition of 60% of the k-space leads to much better IQ rather than 50% acquisition. Hence,

**Table 3**
**Vendor-specific names for time-resolved MR angiography sequences**

| Vendor | Time-resolved MRA Sequence |
|---|---|
| GE | Time-Resolved Imaging of Contrast KineticS (TRICKS) |
| Siemens | Time-resolved angiography With Stochastic Trajectories (TWIST) |
| Philips | 4D Time-Resolved Angiography using Keyhole (4D-TRAK) |
| Canon | Freeze Frame |
| Hitachi | Time-Resolved AcQuisition (TRAQ) |

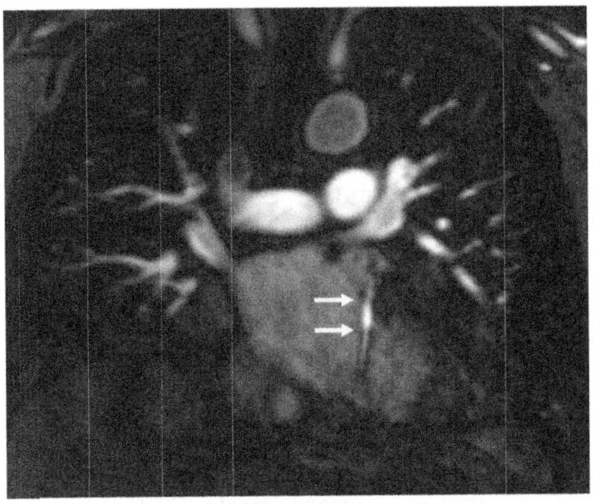

Fig. 8. Coronal pulmonary MR angiogram imaging in a patient with suspected pulmonary embolism. High parallel imaging factor (GE ASSET, R = 3) was used to decrease the breath-hold time. The use of parallel imaging factor leads to higher residual aliasing with central linear artifact (*white arrows*) and an overall decrease in image noise (was not an issue on this exam).

**Table 4**
**Vendor-specific names for parallel imaging techniques**

| Vendor | Image Domain Unfolding | k-space Unfolding |
|---|---|---|
| GE | Array Spatial Sensitivity Encoding Technique (ASSET) | Autocalibrating Reconstruction for Cartesian imaging (ARC) |
| Siemens | modified SENSitivity Encoding (SENSE) | Generalized autocalibrating partial parallel acquisition (GRAPPA) |
| Philips | SENSitivity Encoding (SENSE) | |
| Canon | SPEEDER | EXSPER |
| Hitachi | Rapid Acquisition through Parallel Imaging Design (RAPID) | |

a nearly 40% time reduction is achieved by this technique.[26]

Another method of partial Fourier acceleration may be implemented by using an asymmetric echo with the prediction of k-space data in the frequency encoding direction. This technique involves sampling only during the later part of the echo. This can be thought of as using an asymmetric echo and recording only the right half (later half) of the k-space and then using the conjugate symmetry principle to estimate the left half of the k-space.[19,26] Partial Fourier phase-encoding does not lead to a decrease in phase encoding steps but allows the shortening of the TE and the TR. It is the decrease in TR that leads to a reduction in the scan time with the use of this acceleration technique. The view-sharing acceleration technique is detailed in the time-resolved MRA section.

## SUMMARY

There are various upcoming advances in MR angiography. Some advances, like compressed sensing, allow highly accelerated acquisitions (acceleration factor up to 10–15) with inbuilt denoising to achieve an adequate SNR. Similarly, deep learning algorithms are also being developed to improve image SNR and CNR but have not been implemented on a widespread basis due to the substantial computing infrastructure requirements for 3D acquisitions. Newer techniques like in-phase proton density SGRE with radial k-space ordering can be used to visualize the vessel wall calcium,[27] one of the inherent limitations of MRA, due to which many surgeons prefer CT for vascular pre-surgical planning. Knowledge of basic MRA principles and the sequences can help better understand MRA-related artifacts, appropriately use different techniques based on their strengths and limitations, and help understand various upcoming advances in this field.

## CLINICS CARE POINTS

- Non-invasive imaging techniques, including contrast-enhanced MR angiography (CE-MRA), are commonly used for cardiovascular imaging.
- Contrast enhanced-MRA is a bright-blood imaging technique that utilizes intravenous contrast agents to enhance the signal in the T1-weighted gradient echo sequence, allowing for evaluation of course, caliber, and luminal vascular information with minimized TE and TR to shorten scan time.
- CE-MRA has improved over time due to advancements in contrast agents and MR engineering techniques, resulting in better resolution and decreased scan time.
- Knowledge of CE-MRA principles is crucial for radiologists to appropriately use this high-resolution non-invasive technique for patients with genetic vascular diseases, atherosclerosis, and other vascular conditions requiring frequent follow-up.

## SUPPLEMENTARY DATA

Supplementary data related to this article can be found online at https://doi.org/10.1016/j.mric.2023.04.007.

## REFERENCES

1. Prince MR. Gadolinium-enhanced MR aortography. Radiology 1994;191(1):155–64.
2. Korosec FR, Frayne R, Grist TM, et al. Time-resolved contrast-enhanced 3D MR angiography. Magn Reson Med 1996;36(3):345–51.
3. Willig DS, Turski PA, Frayne R, et al. Contrast-enhanced 3D MR DSA of the carotid artery bifurcation:

preliminary study of comparison with unenhanced 2D and 3D time-of-flight MR angiography. Radiology 1998;208(2):447–51.
4. Jara H, Barish MA. Black-blood MR angiography. Techniques, and clinical applications. Magn Reson Imag Clin N Am 1999;7(2):303–17.
5. Griffin M, Grist TM, Francois CJ. Dynamic four-dimensional MR angiography of the chest and abdomen. Magn Reson Imag Clin N Am 2009; 17(1):77–90.
6. Carroll TJ, Grist TM. Technical developments in MR angiography. Radiol Clin North Am 2002;40(4): 921–51.
7. Du J, Thornton FJ, Mistretta CA, et al. Dynamic MR venography: an intrinsic benefit of time-resolved MR angiography. J Magn Reson Imag 2006;24(4):922–7.
8. Swan JS, Carroll TJ, Kennell TW, et al. Time-resolved three-dimensional contrast-enhanced MR angiography of the peripheral vessels. Radiology 2002; 225(1):43–52.
9. Jens S, Koelemay MJ, Reekers JA, et al. Diagnostic performance of computed tomography angiography and contrast-enhanced magnetic resonance angiography in patients with critical limb ischaemia and intermittent claudication: systematic review and meta-analysis. Eur Radiol 2013;23(11):3104–14 [published Online First: 20130626].
10. Young PM, Mostardi PM, Glockner JF, et al. Prospective comparison of cartesian acquisition with projection-like reconstruction magnetic resonance angiography with computed tomography angiography for evaluation of below-the-knee runoff. J Vasc Intervent Radiol 2013;24(3):392–9.
11. Lehrman ED, Plotnik AN, Hope T, et al. Ferumoxytol-enhanced MRI in the peripheral vasculature. Clin Radiol 2019;74(1):37–50 [published Online First: 20180503].
12. Maki JH, Chenevert TL, Prince MR. Contrast-enhanced MR angiography. Abdom Imag 1998; 23(5):469–84.
13. Knobloch G, Colgan T, Schiebler ML, et al. Comparison of gadolinium-enhanced and ferumoxytol-enhanced conventional and UTE-MRA for the depiction of the pulmonary vasculature. Magn Reson Med 2019;82(5): 1660–70 [published Online First: 20190622].
14. Kuo AH, Nagpal P, Ghoshhajra BB, et al. Vascular magnetic resonance angiography techniques. Cardiovasc Diagn Ther 2019;9(Suppl 1):S28–36.
15. Ghouri MA, Gupta N, Bhat AP, et al. CT and MR imaging of the upper extremity vasculature: pearls, pitfalls, and challenges. Cardiovasc Diagn Ther 2019;9(Suppl 1):S152–73.
16. Bae KT. Peak contrast enhancement in CT and MR angiography: when does it occur and why? Pharmacokinetic study in a porcine model. Radiology 2003; 227(3):809–16 [published Online First: 20030417].
17. Wittram C, Yoo AJ. Transient interruption of contrast on CT pulmonary angiography: proof of mechanism. J Thorac Imag 2007;22(2):125–9.
18. Hargreaves BA. Rapid gradient-echo imaging. J Magn Reson Imag 2012;36(6):1300–13 [published Online First: 20121023].
19. Francois CJ, Hecht EM, Roditi G, et al. MR Angiography Series: Noncardiac Chest MR Angiography. Radiographics 2022;42(2):E48–9 [published Online First: 20220218].
20. Baden JG, Racy DJ, Grist TM. Contrast-enhanced three-dimensional magnetic resonance angiography of the mesenteric vasculature. J Magn Reson Imag 1999;10(3):369–75.
21. Zhang H, Maki JH, Prince MR. 3D contrast-enhanced MR angiography. J Magn Reson Imag 2007;25(1):13–25.
22. Grist TM, Mistretta CA, Strother CM, et al. Time-resolved angiography: Past, present, and future. J Magn Reson Imag 2012;36(6):1273–86 [published Online First: 20120507].
23. Mazaheri Y, Carroll TJ, Du J, et al. Combined time-resolved and high-spatial-resolution 3D MRA using an extended adaptive acquisition. J Magn Reson Imag 2002;15(3):291–301.
24. Biglands JD, Radjenovic A, Ridgway JP. Cardiovascular magnetic resonance physics for clinicians: Part II. J Cardiovasc Magn Reson 2012;14(1):66 [published Online First: 20120920].
25. Glockner JF, Hu HH, Stanley DW, et al. Parallel MR imaging: a user's guide. Radiographics 2005;25(5): 1279–97.
26. Hu HH, Madhuranthakam AJ, Kruger DG, et al. Combination of 2D sensitivity encoding and 2D partial fourier techniques for improved acceleration in 3D contrast-enhanced MR angiography. Magn Reson Med 2006;55(1):16–22.
27. Serhal A, Koktzoglou I, Aouad P, et al. Cardiovascular magnetic resonance imaging of aorto-iliac and iliofemoral vascular calcifications using proton density-weighted in-phase stack of stars. J Cardiovasc Magn Reson 2018;20(1):51 [published Online First: 20180806].

Printed and bound by CPI Group (UK) Ltd, Croydon, CR0 4YY
08/05/2025
01864715-0015